Molecular Techniques and Approaches in Developmental Biology

Molecular Techniques and Approaches in Developmental Biology

Edited by MAARTEN J. CHRISPEELS
Department of Biology, University of California
San Diego, California.

A Wiley-Interscience Publication
JOHN WILEY & SONS
New York   London   Sydney   Toronto

Copyright © 1973, by John Wiley & Sons, Inc.

All rights reserved. Published simultaneously in Canada.

No part of this book may be reproduced by any means, nor transmitted, nor translated into a machine language without the written permission of the publisher.

Library of Congress Cataloging in Publication Data

Chrispeels, Maarten, J.   1938-
   Molecular techniques and approaches in developmental biology.

   "A Wiley–Interscience publication."
   1. Molecular biology–Technique.   2. Developmental biology–Technique.   I. Title.   [DNLM: 1. Molecular biology–Congresses.   2. Research–Congresses. 3. Technology, Medical–Congresses. QH506 Llllm 1973].

QH506.C49   574.3'028   73-9939
ISBN 0-471-15618-3

Printed in the United States of America

10 9 8 7 6 5 4 3 2 1

To all the instructors who gave so
generously of their time to make the
La Jolla Summer Workshops
an interesting experience for the participants.

Foreword

The contents of this book originate in the La Jolla Summer Workshop on Molecular Techniques in Developmental Biology, an annual enterprise which is addressed to the contemporary needs of developmental biologists. Current trends in the national support of science might make the book a memorial to an exciting past, or hopefully, it might yet become a testimonial to the ways of the future. Why each of the authors should have thus exposed a little parcel of his teaching practice is a question best explained by the individual author and most usefully answered by the readers. Whether this partial reincarnation of the workshop into a book is a successful transfiguration remains to be seen. I strongly wish that the reincarnation be partial, a mitosis of the soul in which the workshop remains the stem line and the book a differentiated product.

Diplomacy dictates and sincerity compels that I single out the National Science Foundation as the primary agent in the birth of the workshop. Years ago, back in 1968, when training still fell short of being regarded as a superfluous practice, NSF not only perceived its general value but also recognized that without recurrent training, trained individuals became victims of obsolescence. Miniscule though the workshop operation has been, it has made it possible for developmental biologists from many small and some big institutions to replenish their mental furniture with the most modern items of theory and practice in studies of development. In a technological society, the human being must run to stand still and must gallop to edge ahead. When society becomes disinclined to pay the price it becomes parasitic upon the past and imposes a handicap on the future. If I could cleanly disengage my vested interests in science education from my attitudes toward the demise of training activity, I would be much more passionate in my claims. Perhaps the humanists will take up our cause when we are intellectual enough to take up theirs.

The curious reader might well peruse the Table of Contents and ask himself whether the methodologies described are the ones he would choose in setting up a workshop for the current year. If he finds the contents adequate, he should know that he is already out-of-date, and if all his colleagues agree with him, then we are all out-of-date and the crisis is with us.

As a final and personal note, I would like to single out Tom Humphreys who was the first *de facto* director and organizer of the Summer Workshop series.

La Jolla, California
June, 1973

Herbert Stern

Contributors

MAARTEN J. CHRISPEELS, Department of Biology, University of California, San Diego, California 92037.

R. B. CHURCH, Divisions of Medical Biochemistry and Biology, Faculty of Medicine, The University of Calgary, Calgary, Alberta, Canada.

I. JOHN DAVIES, Department of Obstetrics and Gynecology, School of Medicine, University of California, San Diego, California 92037.
Present address: Department of Obstetrics and Gynecology, Harvard Medical School, Boston Hospital for Women, Boston, Massachussetts.

LEON S. DURE, III. Department of Biochemistry, University of Georgia, Athens, Georgia 30601.

R. L. EASTERDAY, Pharmacia Fine Chemicals, Piscathaway, New Jersey.

STEPHEN H. HOWELL, Department of Biology, University of California, San Diego, La Jolla, California 92037.

TOM HUMPHREYS, Kewalo Marine Laboratory, Pacific Biomedical Research Center, University of Hawaii, 41 Ahui Street, Honolulu, Hawaii 96813.

W. F. LOOMIS, JR. Department of Biology, University of California, San Diego, California 92037.

D. JAMES MORRÉ, Departments of Botany and Plant Pathology and Biological Sciences, Purdue University, Lafayette, Indiana 47907.

EDWARD E. PENHOET, Department of Biochemistry, University of California, Berkeley, California 94720.

S. S. PONG, Department of Biology, University of California, San Diego, La Jolla, California 92037.

DOUGLAS W. SMITH, Department of Biology, University of California, San Diego, La Jolla, California 92037.

J. E. VARNER, Atomic Energy Commission Plant Research Laboratory, Michigan State University, East Lansing, Michigan 48823.

Contents

List of Abbreviations — xiii

Isolation and Purification of Organelles and Endomembrane Components from Rat Liver — 1
D. JAMES MORRÉ

Analysis of Specific Proteins in Differentiating Tissues of the Rat — 29
EDWARD E. PENHOET

The Measurement of Cytoplasmic Steroid "Receptor" Proteins — 39
I. JOHN DAVIES

Separation of Proteins According to Size by Gel Filtration — 55
RICHARD L. EASTERDAY

A Test for de novo Synthesis of Enzymes in Germinating Seeds: Density Labeling with D_2O — 79
MAARTEN J. CHRISPEELS and J. E. VARNER

Isolation of Multiple RNA Polymerases from Dictyostelium Discoideum — 93
S. S. PONG and W. F. LOOMIS, JR.

The Isolation and Analysis of DNA from Eukaryotic Cells — 117
STEPHEN H. HOWELL

Quantitative Measurement of RNA Synthesis — 141
TOM HUMPHREYS

DNA—RNA and DNA—DNA Hybridization, with Emphasis on
Filter Techniques   165
DOUGLAS W. SMITH

Methods to Study Isoaccepting Transfer RNA Species During
Development   199
LEON S. DURE III

Methods for the Study of Hybridization and Reassociation of
Nucleic Acids Extracted from Cells of Higher Animals   223
R. B. CHURCH

Index   303

Table of Abbreviations

ATP	adenosine 5'-triphosphate
Bis	methylene-bis-acrylamide
cpm	counts per minute
CTP	cytidine 5'-triphosphate
dpm	disintegrations per minute
DEAE	diethylaminoethyl
EDTA	ethylenediaminetetra-acetic acid
GTP	guanosine 5'-triphosphate
HA	hydroxyapatite
NAD	nicotinamide adenine dinucleotide
NADH	nicotinamide adenine dinucleotide
PB	phosphate buffer
PCA	perchloric acid
SDS	sodium dodecyl sulfate
SSC	citrate buffer
TCA	trichloroacetic acid
TES	tris(hydroxymethyl)methyl-2-amino ethane sulfonic acid
TEMED	N,N,N',N'-tetramethyl ethylene diamine
Tris	tris(hydroxymethyl)amino-methane
UTP	uridine 5'-triphosphate

Isolation and Purification of Organelles and Endomembrane Components from Rat Liver

D. JAMES MORRÉ

Procedures are described for isolation of the principal endomembrane components: endoplasmic reticulum (ER) (rough and smooth), Golgi apparatus, and plasma membrane (as well as nuclei and mitochondria) from rat liver. The methods may be useful for tissues other than rat liver but require modification as specific difficulties are encountered. The procedures fractionate decisively yet are sufficiently mild to prevent gross modification or loss of structural and functional properties.

The isolation media are minimal media. Buffering and osmotic concentration are not critical, and both sucrose and buffer concentrations may be varied by at least a factor of two without serious consequences. The pH may be varied over the range 6.2–7.5. Various ions, sulfhydryl protectants etc., may be added to aid in enzymatic studies. Fixatives are not required.

The method of homogenization is critical and it is essential that all steps following tissue homogenization be carried out as rapidly as possible. Considerable losses of Golgi apparatus through unstacking and of rough ER through vesiculation and/or loss of ribosomes may occur if homogenates are not processed immediately.

Choice of centrifuge and rotor is not critical. Swinging bucket rotors are preferred to minimize wall effects and to sediment particles perpendicular to the axis of centrifugation. Centrifuges must be refrigerated (0–4°C). For individual livers, the Sorvall HS rotor may be used for differential centrifugation steps and the Spinco 39SW for gradient steps. To process larger volumes of liver, a combination of the Sorvall HB-4 and the Spinco 27SW rotor may be used. Zonal rotors are impractical because of excessive time required for loading and unloading the rotors. Isolations are carried out more efficiently, in less time and in higher yields with large-volume, swinging bucket rotors.

Sucrose gradients are simple step gradients where each layer serves a specific function and unnecessary layers have been eliminated. They are based on studies with continuous gradients and multistep gradients; however, once the sedimentation characteristics of a cell component have been determined, continuous gradients offer no particular advantage over step gradients. Step gradients are fast and efficient with greater capacity than linear gradients (less subject to overloading). Step gradients can be poured using ordinary pipets. Slight mixing at the interfaces may be advantageous and extreme care in preparation of step gradients is not required. Gradients are usually prepared immediately before use or during preliminary centrifugation steps.

Unless indicated otherwise, all operations are at 0–4°C, but temperature control is not critical. It is not necessary to work in a cold room. An ice bath to hold tubes, solutions, homogenizers, etc., is sufficient.

Centrifugal forces are calculated for the middle of the tube. All solutions are prepared in deionized water.

At least two different homogenates are required. One is for Golgi apparatus and ER (and/or mitochondria). The other is for plasma membrane, nuclei, and mitochondria. Crude fractions of lysosomes, microbodies, glycogen, and cytoplasmic polysomes are also obtained from these homogenates.

A. TOTAL HOMOGENATE

Rats are provided with standard diet and drinking water ad libitum, weighed to the nearest 1 g, killed by decapitation, and drained of blood. The livers are then removed and weighed to the learest 0.1 g. These operations are at ambient temperature.

Fed male rats of the Holtzman strain (The Holtzman Company, Madison, Wisconsin) are used at Purdue, but both male and female rats of a variety of ages and strains (Wistar, Sprague-Dawley, Long-Evans), fed or fasted, have given good preparations. Pathological and postmortem tissue changes are a frequent source of difficulty with many tissues, but with liver the manner in which the animal is sacrificed is largely a matter of convenience.

Preparation of the total homogenate is one of the most critical steps of cell fractionation. Overhomogenization yields membrane fragments of uniform size and limited functional capacity. Small uniform fragments cannot be resolved by differential centrifugation and tend to sediment with the microsome fraction. Underhomogenization leaves large numbers of unbroken cells and

ISOLATION OF ORGANELLES

tissue fragments so that yields of isolated cell components are low. Also, for each method of homogenization, it is necessary to establish the appropriate centrifugal forces and times necessary to sediment components during the initial differential centrifugation steps. Thus, with any procedure that involves a differential centrifugation step, the conditions of homogenization must be carefully regulated and reproducible.

A mechanical homogenizer, the Polytron 20ST or Polytron 10ST (Kinematica, Lucerne, Switzerland), is definitely superior to other types of homogenizers commonly used for cell fractionation. It disrupts cells efficiently with a minimum of shear and is fast. A single liver is homogenized in a minute or less. Each Polytron must be calibrated. Thereafter, speed settings and times can be reported with precision so that homogenization conditions may be reproduced exactly in laboratories other than the one where the homogenization procedure was developed. Preparations of useful quantity and purity have been obtained using loose-fitting, all-glass or glass-Teflon homogenizers, but these devices tend to be slow and variable. The Polytron may be calibrated by converting flashing light reflected from the rotating, half-blackened shaft into an electric signal by means of a photocell and an audiosignal generator matching the frequency of this signal with an oscilloscope.

Method A (for Golgi apparatus, ER, etc.): The livers are minced rapidly with razor blades (a cork board or petri plate cover serves as a convenient chopping surface). The minced tissue (~5 mm cubes), in lots of approximately 10 g each, is mixed with 12–25 ml of chilled homogenization medium A contained in a 50 ml lusterloid centrifuge tube. Homogenization is for 30–50 sec at 10,000 rpm using the Polytron homogenizer. The homogenization process should be watched carefully so that the tube can be moved up and down slowly to guide unhomogenized bits of liver through the blades of the Polytron. Homogenization is complete when all liver bits have been homogenized and the Polytron motor begins to run free. With minimum practice, homogenization can be completed in exactly 40 sec.

Method B (for plasma membrane, nuclei, etc.): 40 g of liver are minced coarsely into 1 cm cubes and mixed in lots of 5–6 g each with 15 ml of chilled homogenization medium B contained in a 50 ml lusterloid centrifuge tube. Homogenization is for 90 sec at 6000 rpm (speed may be adjusted using a rheostat at approximately half line voltage and a Polytron setting of 2.5). The tube should be moved up and down slowly to guide unhomogenized bits of liver through the blades of the Polytron. Immediately after homogenization, the homogenate is poured into 700 ml of bicarbonate and the mixture is swirled. The homogenization step is repeated until all the liver is homogenized. The total homogenate is made to a final volume of 1000 ml and stirred slowly for 5 min to complete cell breakage and facilitate removal of cytoplasm from ruptured cell membranes.

Note: Either homogenization method A or method B can be scaled up or down to process larger or smaller amounts of liver but the ratio of tissue to medium should not be varied beyond the limits indicated. With the Polytron 20ST, the minimum volume for homogenization is about 10 ml. The maximum volume is about 25 ml. For method A, the minimum quantity is 1/2 liver (~5–6 g) in 10–12 ml of medium. For method A, the maximum quantity is 2 livers (20–25 g) in 25 ml of medium. In method B, the ratio is critical and should not be varied so that ~1/2 liver is homogenized at a time. To process larger quantities of tissue, the homogenization step is repeated.

In method A, a concentrated homogenate is obtained. In method B, emphasis is on a diluted homogenate. The lower homogenization speed of method B favors preservation of large fragments of plasma membrane but less than complete tissue disruption. Method A gives more complete tissue disruption but most of the plasma membrane fragments enter the microsome fraction.

Medium A: Stock Solutions.
   (a) Buffer: Mix 50 ml of a 0.2 M solution of tris(hydroxymethyl) aminomethane (Tris) maleate (24.2 g of Tris + 23.2 g of maleic acid or 19.6 g of maleic anhydride in 1000 ml) and 37 ml of 0.2 N NaOH, dilute to a total of 200 ml, and adjust to pH 6.4 with NaOH.
   (b) Sucrose, 2 M, prepared in buffer (a).
   (c) Dextran (average molecular weight 225,000, Sigma Chemical Company), 10%.
   (d) Magnesium chloride, 50 mM (required for isolation of ER fragments).
   (e) Sulfhydryl protectants (mercaptoethanol or dithiothreitol) must be added if sugar transferase activity is to be measured.

The homogenization medium is prepared by combining 50 ml of buffer (a), 25 ml of 2 M sucrose (b), 10 ml of dextran (c), 10 ml of 10 mM $MgCl_2$ (d) or water, and 5 ml of sulfhydryl protectant solution (e) or water.

Medium B: 1 mM sodium bicarbonate, pH 7.4 (168 mg of sodium bicarbonate makes 2 liters of medium which is enough to process 40 g of liver).

Yield: The volume of the total homogenate should be determined and recorded and a portion (~1 ml) retained for determination of relative specific activities of marker enzymes (ratio of specific activity of cell fraction to that of the total

ISOLATION OF ORGANELLES

homogenate). Relative specific activity gives an indication of recovery and degree of purification and corrects for differences in assay procedures, protein determinations, animals, etc., to permit more meaningful comparisons among different experiments and among experiments from different laboratories. The absolute activity of a 1 ml portion of the homogenate multiplied by total homogenate volume gives the total activity of the tissue homogenized.

Note: Once the total homogenate has been prepared, proceed as quickly as possible through the differential centrifugation step to the sucrose gradient. Delays are costly in terms of yield and fraction purity. To avoid delays:

(1) Reserve centrifuges in advance.
(2) Make sure centrifuges are turned on, cooled down, and operational.
(3) Make sure appropriate rotors, adaptors, solutions, etc., are available and precooled.
(4) Prepare all solutions and locate necessary tubes and glassware in advance.

B. GOLGI APPARATUS

Cells are first disrupted by low shear homogenization and the Golgi apparatus are concentrated by differential centrifugation. Final purification is achieved by sucrose gradient centrifugation. Degradation by lysosomal enzymes is minimized by the presence of dextran in the medium and the rapidity with which homogenization and centrifugation are carried out. Structural preservation is favored by use of concentrated homogenates and a sucrose gradient where the Golgi apparatus collect at the gradient/homogenate interface without actually entering the sucrose layer. The development of the method and references are given by Morré [1971].

Homogenization Medium: Medium A (see p. 4 for preparation of stock solutions).

37.5 mM Tris maleate, pH 6.5
0.5 M Sucrose
1% Dextran
(5 mM $MgCl_2$ and sulfhydryl protectants optional)

Homogenization Procedure: Method A (1/2 to 1 liver in the ratio of 1 g tissue/2 ml of medium) for 40 sec at 10,000 rpm with the Polytron 20ST.

Low-speed Differential Centrifugation: The homogenate is transferred to 50 ml lusterloid tubes for the Sorvall HB-4 rotor (or 5.4 ml lusterloid tubes for the Spinco 39SW rotor for small volumes) and centrifuge for 15 min at 5000 × g

(5500 rpm, HB-4) to concentrate the Golgi apparatus. Most of the supernatant fluid is removed into another tube and saved while care is taken not to remove any of the loosely packed pellet. The supernatant from this step is used as a source of ER fragments in procedure D and also to resuspend the crude Golgi apparatus.

The yellow-brown phase of the pellet (upper 1/2 to 2/3) which lies above the red to pink (containing whole cells) and dark brown (containing nuclei and large mitochondrial fragments) layers is resuspended in a portion of the supernatant (final volume of about 6 ml per 10 g liver) by squeezing in and out of a large-bore pasteur pipet. Do not hand-homogenize. Once the yellow-brown phase has been removed and mixed with the appropriate amount of supernatant, 15–20 additional "slurps" with the pasteur pipet are sufficient to achieve adequate resuspension of the Golgi apparatus. The remainder of the crude Golgi apparatus pellet ("debris" fraction) may be retained for the recovery of either the mitochondria or the ER fragments under procedures C or E.

Sucrose Gradient Centrifugation. The suspension of the crude Golgi apparatus in supernatant is then layered on 1.5–2 vol of 1.2 M sucrose and centrifuged for 30 min at 90,000–150,000 × g (39SW rotor at 30,000 rpm is sufficient). Gradients are prepared by filling the tube approximately 2/3 full with 1.2 M sucrose and layering the crude Golgi apparatus fraction on top of the sucrose to fill the tube. After centrifugation, Golgi apparatus are collected as a "rug" from the 1.2 M sucrose/homogenate interface using a pasteur pipet fitted with a rubber bulb. The best procedure is to come in from the top of the tube with the tip of the pipet next to the portion of the tube wall directly in front of you at eye level. Remember to squeeze the bulb to dispel air before going into the tube and not after. Holding the tube up in front of a diffuse light source, the rug can be lifted off the 1.2 M sucrose layer without removing any of the 1.2 M sucrose layer. Remove as much of the overlying particle-free supernatant as is convenient. The 1.2 M sucrose layer and the pellet from the gradient step may be combined with the debris fraction from the differential centrifugation step for the recovery of the mitochondrial and the ER fragments under procedures C or E.

Note: The 1.2 M sucrose layer should be clear at the end of the centrifugation. Occasionally it is cloudy with microsomal fragments. Under these conditions, special care must be taken to avoid removing any of the 1.2 M sucrose layer with the Golgi apparatus rug. A concentration of 1.2 M sucrose is used so that the contaminating cell components enter the sucrose layer while the Golgi apparatus

ISOLATION OF ORGANELLES

collect at the 1.2 M sucrose/homogenate interface. The equilibrium density of Golgi apparatus varies from animal to animal and according to definite diurnal and seasonal patterns due in part to the numbers of secretory vesicles or peripheral tubules and to the nature of the secretory products contained within

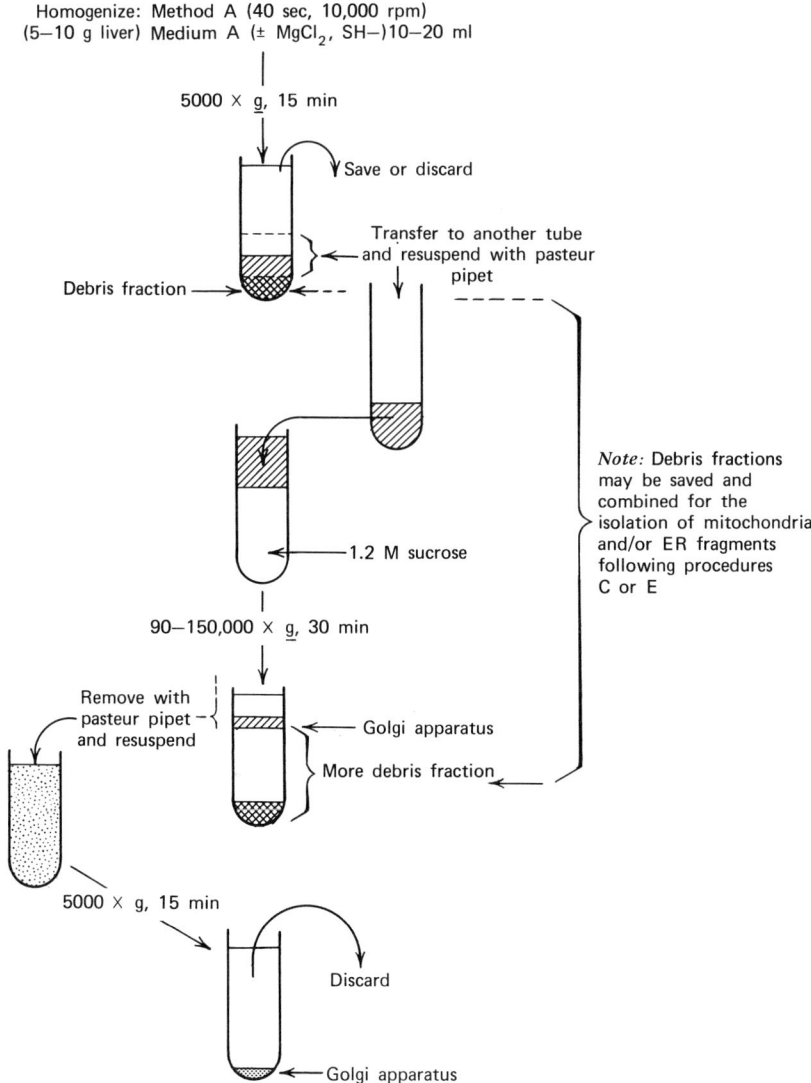

Flow Diagram   Procedure B: Golgi Apparatus

these elements. Cell structure, enzyme activities, etc., all follow definite daily and seasonal patterns associated with the animal's metabolism. This is a fact of life to be recognized and lived with. Occasionally, lipoprotein-rich preparations of Golgi apparatus will float on a layer of 1.0 M sucrose. However, 1.2 M sucrose is necessary to ensure that the Golgi apparatus membranes are recovered over a range of physiological conditions. Fraction purity is not greatly affected over the range 1.0–1.25 M in the sucrose layer. At Purdue University, yield and fraction purity of the Golgi apparatus is greatest between 8 and 10 A.M. during the months of March–mid-June and September–November.

The purified Golgi apparatus are resuspended in ~5 ml of one of the following:

(a) Clear supernatant from the sucrose gradient for the optimum preservation of morphology
(b) Distilled water for the highest fraction purity (to vesiculate ER fragments)
(c) Homogenization medium or enzyme assay "cocktail" for the preservation of enzymatic activities

The Golgi apparatus are then collected by centrifugation at 5000 × g for 15–20 min.

Yield: 4–8 mg Golgi apparatus protein from 10 g liver.

Recovery: Based on estimates of galactosyl transferase activity [Morré, 1972; Morré, Merlin and Keenan, 1969] the recovery of Golgi apparatus ranges from 25 to 70%, with 40% being an acceptable recovery.

Purity: When properly carried out, intact portions of the Golgi apparatus (dictyosomes) which sediment at low centrifugal force are obtained in high yield. The identification of the isolated Golgi apparatus can be based on their morphology which is characteristic and serves as a reliable marker (Plate I). Morphological assays of Golgi apparatus fractions are carried out most rapidly and accurately by the technique of negative staining (Plate I, 3). Details of morphological analysis are provided by Morré [1971] and Cunningham, Morré, and Mollenhauer [1966].

Based on analysis of marker enzymes (Table I), fraction purity is at least 80%. Contamination by ER, mitochondrial inner membrane, mitochondrial outer membrane, and plasma membranes is estimated by assaying glucose-6-phosphatase, succinate-INT-reductase [Morré, 1971], monoamine oxidase [Stahn, Maier, and Hannig, 1970] and 5′-nucleotidase [Morré, 1971], respectively. Purified fractions give specific activities of approximately 34 (glucose-6-phosphatase: ER), 25 (succinate -2-[p-indophenyl]-3-[p-nitrophenyl]-5-phenyl tetrazolium (INT)-reductase: mitochondrial inner membrane), 33 (monoamine oxidase: mito-

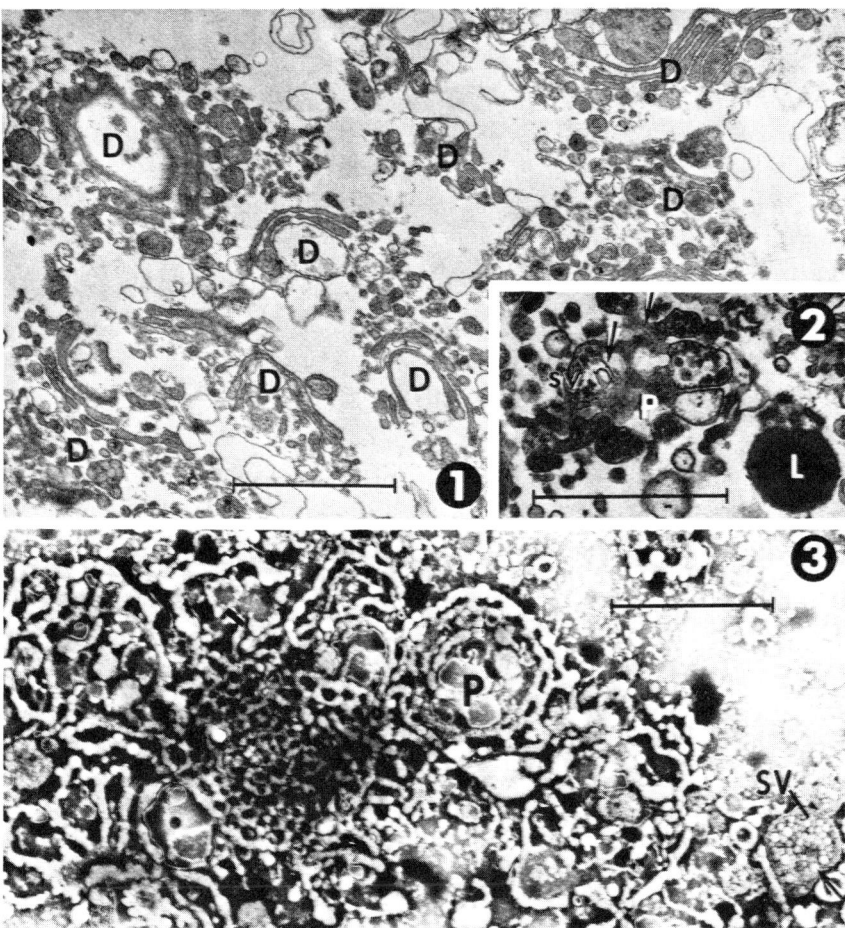

PLATE I. Golgi Apparatus. (1) Electron micrograph showing the appearance of the intact dictyosomes (D) of Golgi apparatus isolated from rat liver. A portion of the final pellet was fixed in glutaraldehyde (2.5% in 0.1 M sodium phosphate buffer, pH 7.2) for 2 hr at 4°C (fixation time may be extended to 18 hr or longer if more convenient) followed by osmium tetroxide (1% in 0.1 M sodium phosphate, pH 7.2) at 4°C for 1/2-16 hr; dehydrated through an acetone series and embedded in Epon-Araldite [Mollenhauer, 1964]. Thin sections were positively stained with alkaline lead citrate [Reynolds, 1963]. Bar = 1 μ. (2) A dictyosome in face view. Arrows show tubular connections between secretory vesicles (SV) and the central plate-like portion (P) of a cisterna. L = lysosome. Bar = 1 μ. (3) Portion of a Golgi apparatus from rat liver after negative staining with 1% phosphotungstic acid neutralized to pH 6.5 with potassium hydroxide. The dictyosome is partially unstacked to show both the system of peripheral tubules and the central plate-like portions (P) of cisternae. The form of cisternae varies from typically plate-like with few peripheral tubules to almost entirely tubular. Secretory vesicles (SV) contain the very low density lipoprotein particles (arrow) of the secretory product. Details of negative staining are given by Morré [1971]. Bar = 1 μ.

chondrial outer membrane), and 80 (5' nucleotidase: plasma membrane) μmole product/hr/mg protein. The estimates of contamination of the Golgi apparatus by ER and plasma membranes represent maximum upper limits, since both 5'-nucleotidase and glucose-6-phosphatase may be enzymes endogenous to the Golgi apparatus. A high level of acid phosphatase is expected since lysosomes are derived, at least in part, as vesicles from the Golgi apparatus.

Uridine-5'-diphosphate galactose: N-Acetylglucosamine galactosyl transferase (galactosyl transferase) is a convenient marker enzyme for rat liver Golgi apparatus. This activity is enriched 90- to 100-fold in purified Golgi apparatus relative to the total homogenate (Table I).

TABLE I. Enzymatic Activities of Golgi Apparatus-Rich Fractions from Rat Liver

Enzyme[a]	Specific activity Homogenate	Specific activity Golgi apparatus	Relative specific activity
5'-Nucleotidase	7.1	11.4	1.6
Glucose-6-phosphatase	6.7	4.0	0.6
Succinate-INT-reductase	2.6	0.2	0.08
Monoamine oxidase	0.8	0.5	0.6
Acid phosphatase	1.0	3.4	3.4
Galactosyl transferase	2.4	220.0	91.5

[a]Units of specific activity are micromoles of inorganic phosphorus formed per hour per milligram of protein for glucose-6-phosphatase, 5'-nucleotidase, and acid phosphatase; micromoles of INT reduced per hour per milligram of protein for succinate-INT-reductase; micromoles of benzaldehyde formed per hour per milligram of protein for monoamine oxidase and millimicromoles of glucosamine-dependent hydrolysis of UDP-galactose for galactosyl transferase. From Huang and Morré [unpublished]; Merritt and Morré [in press] and Cheetham, Morré, and Yunghans [1970].

C. ENDOPLASMIC RETICULUM AND MICROSOMES

Endoplasmic reticulum can be isolated from liver as large sheets only when conditions are very carefully regulated (Plate II, 1). Under more general conditions of homogenization, especially with media of low tonicity, the cisternae fragment and vesiculate. Smooth vesicles (vesicles lacking ribosomes) are called smooth microsomes. Rough vesicles (vesicles with attached ribosomes) are called rough microsomes. Rough microsomes are derived exclusively from rough ER. In addition to smooth ER, Golgi apparatus, plasma membranes, mitochondria, and any other membranes lacking ribosomes may contribute to the smooth microsome fraction.

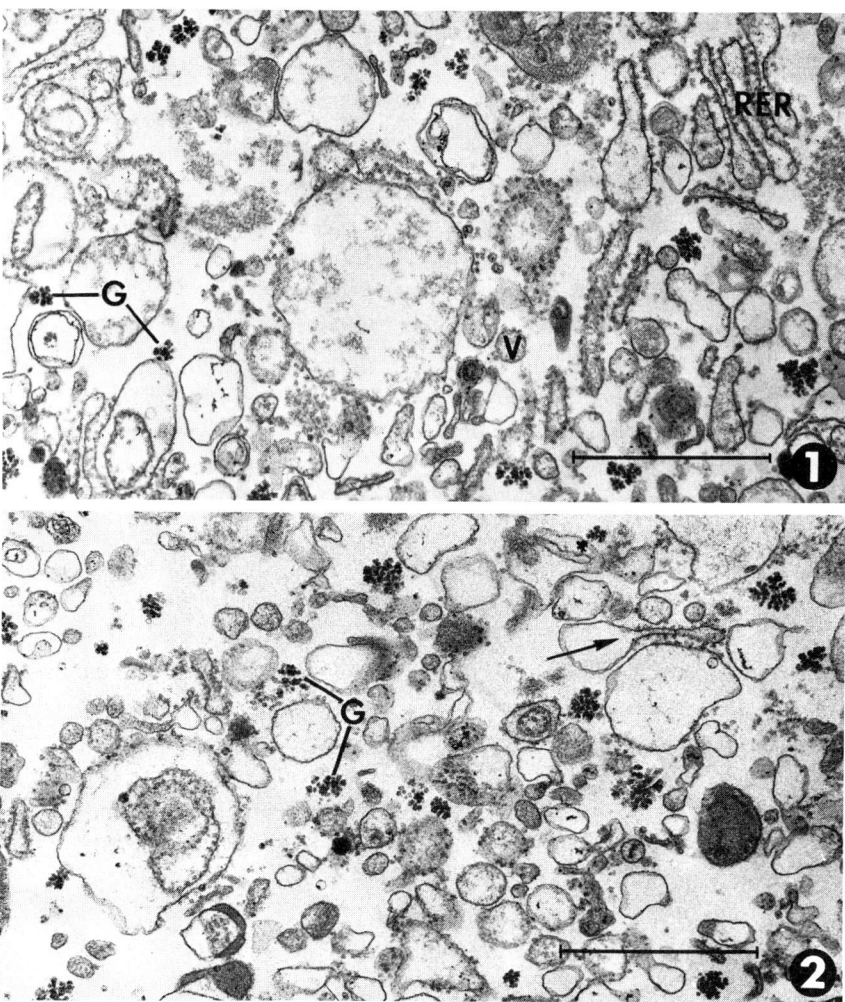

PLATE II. Endoplasmic reticulum. (1) Predominantly rough ER (with ribosomes attached; ER-I) collected from 1.5 M sucrose/2.0 M sucrose interface of a preparative sucrose gradient (Figure 1). The composition of the fraction varies from sheets, sometimes partially stacked (RER), to what appear as small vesicular profiles (V). Prepared for electron microscopy as in Plate I-1 and embedded in Epon [Spurr, 1969]. Glycogen rosettes (G) contaminate the fraction. The vesicle interiors contain electron dense material, presumably protein such as albumin, which may contribute to their density and help account for their occurrence in a density fraction distinct from ER-II vesicles (below) which generally lack electron dense contents. From rat liver. Bar = 1 μ. (2) A fraction containing both rough ER and smooth ER (lacking ribosomes) referred to as ER-II. This fraction is collected from the 1.3 M sucrose/1.5 M sucrose interface of the preparative sucrose gradient of Figure 1. Transition elements consisting of part rough and part smooth ER (arrow) are a predominant characteristic of the fraction. G = glycogen. (1) and (2) are from the same experiment. Bar = 1 μ.

Total Microsomes

Total microsome fractions consist of bits and pieces of ER and associated ribosomes plus other membrane fragments of similar sedimentation characteristics. Generally, any particles sedimenting between 15,000 and 250,000 × g are referred to as microsomes (the pellet when the supernatant fluid from the mitochondrial fraction is centrifuged at 100,000–250,000 × g for 60–120 min.). With liver cells, where ER is abundant, rough and smooth ER constitute the bulk of the microsome fraction. With other cell types, other types of membrane may predominate. Golgi apparatus, plasma membranes, lysosomes, nuclear envelope, mitochondria, membrane-enclosed bags of cytoplasm, microbodies, cytoplasmic polysomes, glycogen, and even chromatin may all contribute to the microsome fraction. The composition of the microsome fraction varies most from tissue to tissue, but with a specific tissue such as liver, the physiological state of the animal and the conditions of homogenization are also important. As a result, data from total microsome fractions frequently accomplishes little in defining the intracellular localization of the constituents analyzed.

There is no standard procedure for preparing microsome fractions. The procedure varies with the investigator, the tissue under investigation, the age and type of organism, and the purpose of the study. It is a common practice to starve animals for about 24 hr, especially for preparations from liver, to reduce contamination of the fractions with glycogen. However, starvation is not recommended for physiological or functional studies since changes other than reduction of glycogen occur. Homogenization is carried out in a medium containing 0.25–0.5 M sucrose (0.35 M sucrose), 5–10 mM $MgCl_2$, buffer (50 mM Tris HCl, pH 6.5–7.5) and other additives (25 mM KCl, 1% dextran) in a ratio of 2.5–10 ml of homogenization medium/g liver. The procedure for homogenization is to disrupt the tissue in either all-glass or glass-Teflon homogenizers or mechanized homogenizers such as the Polytron 20ST.

Once a homogenate has been prepared, it is necessary to remove whole cells, nuclei, mitochondria, and other large particles. This is usually accomplished by differential centrifugation according to the basic procedure of Palade and Siekevitz [1956]. Using a 10% homogenate [weight/volume (w/v)] in 0.25 M sucrose, 10,000 × g for 10 min is required for complete removal of intact mitochondria. This centrifugation step may sediment ER as well (up to 50% with some homogenates), but so far cell biologists have regarded this loss of microsomal vesicles as an undesirable but necessary aspect of the procedure. Sometimes, centrifugal forces of under 8000 × g are used to reduce the loss of microsomal vesicles and yet remove most of the mitochondria.

ISOLATION OF ORGANELLES

To obtain total microsomes, the mitochondria-free supernatant is centrifuged at 100,000–250,000 × g for 60–120 min. There are several alternate methods, based on different principles, which may be used to obtain microsomal subfractions once the large particles have been removed. Two such methods follow.

Endoplasmic Reticulum Subfractions from Golgi Apparatus Supernatant

This procedure was developed to permit isolation of Golgi apparatus and ER subfractions from the same homogenates. It is a modification of the method of Bloemendahl et al. [1967] in which mitochondria- and Golgi apparatus-free supernatants are centrifuged on a discontinuous sucrose gradient. It yields a highly purified fraction of rough ER vesicles [Cheetham et al., 1970] referred to here as ER-I and a fraction enriched in smooth ER vesicles (ER-II) that is not heavily contaminated by the Golgi apparatus.

Homogenization Medium: Same as for the isolation of the Golgi apparatus except that 5 mM $MgCl_2$ must be included to retard loss of ribosomes from rough membranes. (See p. 4 for details.)

37.5 mM Tris maleate, pH 6.5
0.5 M Sucrose
1% Dextran
5 mM $MgCl_2$

Homogenization Procedure: Method A

Low-Speed Differential Centrifugation: 20 min at 5000 × g (or 10 min at 10,000 × g) to remove Golgi apparatus, mitochondria, and other large particles or use Golgi apparatus supernatant (15 min at 5000 × g). The supernatant is then diluted 1:3–1:5 with homogenization medium (or diluted 1:5 with a medium containing 37.5 mM Tris maleate, pH 6.5, 0.35 M sucrose, 1% dextran, and 5 mM $MgCl_2$ to give a final sucrose concentration of ~0.35 M). At this point, the Golgi apparatus supernatant may be centrifuged at 10,000 × g for 10 min to remove residual mitochondria.

Sucrose Gradient Centrifugation: The diluted supernatant from the differential centrifugation is then top-loaded onto a discontinuous sucrose gradient consisting of 2.0 M sucrose, 1.5 M sucrose, and 1.3 M sucrose in a volume/volume (v/v) ratio of 3:4:4 (for a 40 ml centrifuge tube, 6 ml: 8 ml: 8 ml). The remainder of the tube is filled with diluted Golgi apparatus supernatant. The gradient is then centrifuged for 8–9 × 10⁶ g·min (for example, 90,000 × g for 90 min). Rough ER fragments (ER-I) are recovered from the 1.5/2.0 M sucrose interface. Free ribosomes and glycogen enter the 2.0 M sucrose layer and with longer centrifugation times will form a pellet at the bottom of the tube. Smooth microsomes collect at the other interfaces, the 1.3 M sucrose/homogenate interface being especially rich in plasma membrane and other contaminants while smooth ER is concentrated at the 1.3/1.5 M sucrose interface (ER-II). The fractions are collected from the gradient using a pasteur pipet, diluted 1:1 with buffer or distilled water and pelleted by centrifugation at 90,000 × g [26,000 rpm, Spinco SW 27 Rotor] for 30 min. The gradient centrifugation step and the presumed origins of the ER-I and ER-II fractions are summarized in Figures 1 and 2.

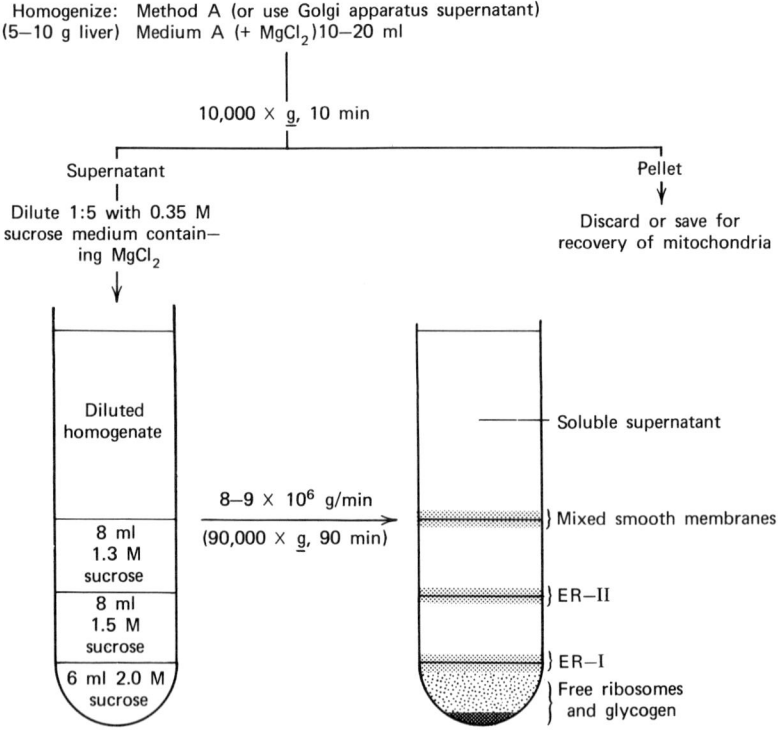

FIGURE 1. Sucrose gradient procedure for preparing ER from the Golgi apparatus supernatant.

ISOLATION OF ORGANELLES

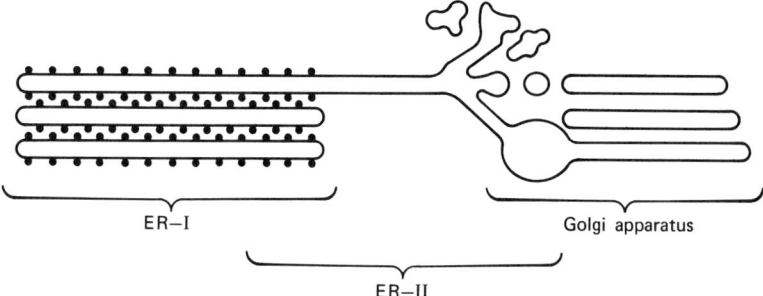

FIGURE 2. Diagrammatic interpretation of the origin of ER-I, ER-II, and Golgi apparatus fractions. The composition of each of the fractions was verified from electron microscope examination of fixed and embedded pellets.

Yield: 10–15 mg of protein/10 g fresh weight of liver. The ratio of ER-I to ER-II is about 1.

Recovery: The total recovery of ER fragments based on recovery of glucose-6-phosphatase is approximately 50%. The bulk of the remainder is found in the low-speed pellet especially in the "under Golgi apparatus" fraction. To recover some of this activity, the material remaining after removal of the crude Golgi apparatus fraction may be combined with the material passing through 1.2 M sucrose on the Golgi apparatus gradient, rehomogenized in the 0.35 M sucrose medium (see Low-Speed Differential Centrifugation, p. 5) using an all-glass or glass-Teflon homogenizer, centrifuged for 20 min at 5000 × g to remove mitochondria and purified by the sucrose gradient procedure described above (Figure 1).

Purity: The appearance of the ER-I and ER-II fractions in the electron microscope are illustrated in Plate II, 1 and 2. ER-I is predominantly vesicles derived from rough ER uncontaminated by plasma membrane (5′-nucleotidase), mitochondria (succinate-INT-reductase), or Golgi apparatus (galactosyl transferase) activities (Table II). Glycogen is the principal contaminant with smaller amounts of nuclear envelope fragments and collagen fibers also present. ER-II is a mixture of rough and smooth ER vesicles and contains the membranes which respond to phenobarbital injections by increased drug detoxification activities (a characteristic of smooth ER). Studies with an O-demethylase system of drug detoxification suggest that cross contamination between ER-I and ER-II is normally less than 10% [Morré and Hocker, unpublished].

TABLE II. Enzyme Activities of Rough ER-Rich Fractions (ER-I)

Enzyme	Specific activity[a]	Relative specific activity[b]
Glucose-6-phosphatase	34	12
5′-Nucleotidase	0.1	0.1
Succinate-INT-reductase	0.2	0.2
Galactosyl transferase	3.0	1.2

[a]Units of specific activity are given in Table I.
[b]Ratio of specific activity of ER fraction to that of total homogenate. From Cheetham et al. [1970], Morré et al. [1969] and Huang and Morré [unpublished].

Dallner Procedure for Microsomal Subfractionation

The procedure developed by Dallner and Ernster (Figure 3) utilizes monovalent cations to cause selective aggregation of the rough microsomes. In the presence of cesium ions, the mean radius of the sedimentating rough vesicles is doubled or trebled, causing a 4- to 9-fold increase in sedimentation velocity. Thus, the addition of CsCl to the mitochondrial supernatant followed by centrifugation in a discontinuous sucrose gradient of 0.25 M and 1.3 M sucrose results in an almost complete separation of smooth and rough microsomes. The smooth vesicles appear at the interface and the rough vesicles sediment through the 1.3 M sucrose layer to form a pellet. The method of preparation is not time-consuming and the yield is high.

The smooth microsome fraction prepared by the Dallner procedure contains less rough membrane than ER-II of the Golgi apparatus supernatant but tends to be more heterogeneous in that the plasma membrane and the Golgi apparatus

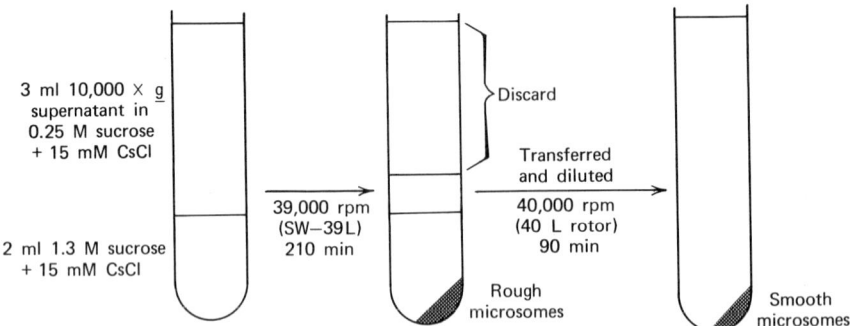

FIGURE 3. Procedure for preparation of rough and smooth microsomal subfractions by density gradient centrifugation in the presence of CsCl [Dallner, Siekevitz, and Palade, 1966; Ernster, Siekevitz, and Palade, 1962].

ISOLATION OF ORGANELLES

fragments are not removed. Except for the presence of cesium, rough microsomes by the Dallner method and ER-I appear to be approximately equivalent fractions.

D. PLASMA MEMBRANE (NUCLEI AND MITOCHONDRIA)

Procedures developed for isolation of plasma membranes from rat liver employ all-glass or glass-Teflon homogenizers to disrupt the tissues. Tissue homogenization is frequently the most difficult, critical and time-consuming step. The procedure presented here [Yunghans and Morré, unpublished results] provides for homogenization using the Polytron and eliminates a major source of variability and uncertainty in the preparation of plasma membrane fractions. Except for the homogenization step, the procedure follows closely that described by Neville [1960] and Emmelot et al. [1964].

Homogenization Medium: 1 mM sodium bicarbonate, pH 7.4.

Homogenization Procedure: Method B (1/2 liver in the ratio of 5–6 g tissue/15 ml of medium) for 90 sec at 6000 rpm with the Polytron 20ST. The homogenate is diluted immediately to a final volume of 125 ml of cold 1 mM bicarbonate; or alternatively, if 40 g of liver is processed, the homogenate is poured into 700 ml of cold 1 mM bicarbonate and swirled. The procedure is repeated until all of the liver is homogenized. The homogenate from 40 g liver is made to a total of 1000 ml and stirred. For the rest of the procedure, volumes are for 40 g of liver. If more or less liver is processed, volumes must be adjusted accordingly. The dilution and mixing are necessary to increase cell breakage and to help disperse the contents of ruptured cells.

Low-Speed Differential Centrifugation: The diluted homogenate is filtered through cheesecloth premoistened with bicarbonate, transferred to four 250 ml centrifuge bottles (Sorvall GSA rotor) and centrifuged 10 min at 3500 rpm accelerating slowly (1 min 1000 rpm; 1 min 2000 rpm, 1 min 3000 rpm). With smaller amounts of homogenate, 50 ml tubes and the SS-34 rotor may be used for this step. The supernatant is removed by aspiration leaving about 50 ml of liquid and the pellet undisturbed. This is primarily a concentration step and the supernatant is left to avoid losing any of the pellet. The portion of the pellet enriched in plasma membrane is loose and friable and overlies a reddish-brown, packed layer of nuclei and unbroken cells. The supernatant solution remaining in the bottle is gently swirled over the pellet to resuspend the friable layer without disturbing the pellet of nuclei and debris. A rubber policeman or glass "hockey stick" may be used to loosen the friable layer. The supernatant containing the resuspended plasma membrane is poured through a double layer of cheesecloth premoistened with bicarbonate (to trap fragments of the nuclear pellet) while the main mass of nuclei and debris is held back with a rubber policeman. The nuclear mass should be transferred to a small beaker and held on ice until the sucrose gradient step. Resuspension of the plasma membrane is completed using a glass-Teflon homogenizer (avoid ground glass; a test tube fitting loosely around a Teflon pestle works quite well), and the homogenate is made to a final volume of 300 ml (again for 40 g liver). The resuspended crude plasma membrane is distributed among eight 50 ml tubes and centrifuged for 10 min at 3000 rpm (Sorvall SS-34 rotor, RC2B centrifuge). After centrifugation, the supernatant is aspirated and discarded leaving a loosely packed pellet which is resuspended by swirling the tube. The combined resuspended pellets are made to a final volume of 300 ml bicarbonate. This step is repeated two additional times, followed by resuspension in 150 ml bicarbonate. The material resuspended in 150 ml bicarbonate is distributed among four 50 ml tubes, centrifuged for 10 min at 3000 rpm and resuspended in 150 ml, etc. The pellet from this step is resuspended in 80 ml, transferred to two tubes, etc. This step is also repeated. The final pellets from the differential centrifugation steps are resuspended in a final volume of 3.6 ml and homogenized briefly (2–3 strokes with a 5 ml, loose-fitting glass-Teflon homogenizer; a 5 ml test tube works well). The differential centrifugation steps are summarized as follows:*

Step number	Initial volume	Final volume	Number and size of tubes	Number times
1	1,000 ml	300 ml	4 X 250 ml bottles	1
2–4	300 ml	150 ml	8 X 50 ml tubes	3
5–6	150 ml	80 ml	4 X 50 ml tubes	2
7–8	80 ml	2 X 3.6 ml	2 X 50 ml tubes	2

*Volumes are for 40 g liver. All centrifugations are at 3000 rpm (SS-34 rotor) for 10 min except for the initial centrifugation with the GSA rotor which is at 3500 rpm.

Note: There is always a great temptation to cut short the procedure and eliminate some of the differential centrifugation steps. These steps remove mitochondria and are necessary. If eliminated, the final gradient step will be overloaded with mitochondria and a fraction heavily contaminated with mitochondria will result. The big loss of plasma membrane occurs in step 1 where small plasma membrane fragments are lost to the low-speed supernatant and large fragments of plasma membrane become trapped among the nuclei.

Sucrose Gradient Centrifugation (Figure 4): To the 3.6 ml of resuspended plasma membrane are added 10 ml of sucrose of density (d) = 1.3 (81 g sucrose

ISOLATION OF ORGANELLES

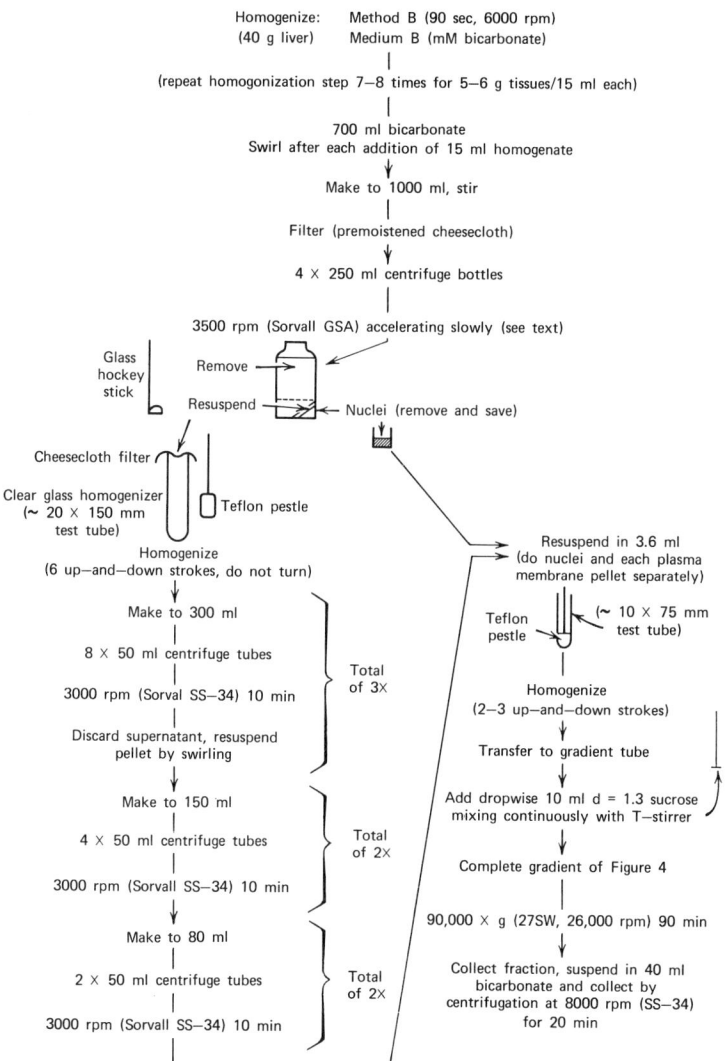

Flow Diagram   Procedure D: Plasma Membrane

in a final volume of 100 ml) dropwise with constant mixing. This mixture forms the bottom layer of the gradient (final d = 1.22). Successive sucrose solutions are then added; for a 40 ml cellulose nitrate tube, 8 ml sucrose d = 1.2 (53.4 g sucrose in 100 ml), 8 ml sucrose d = 1.18 (48 g sucrose in 100 ml), 3 ml sucrose d = 1.173 (46 g in 100 ml), 3 ml d = 1.166 (44 g in 100 ml), and enough sucrose d = 1.16 (42.6 g in 100 ml) to fill the tube. Two gradients are

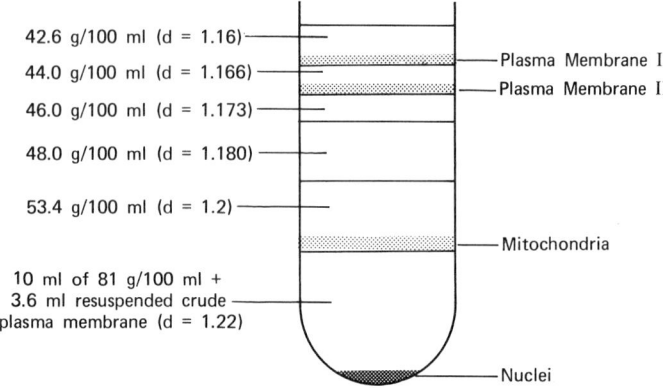

FIGURE 4. Sucrose gradient for preparing plasma membranes, mitochondria, and nuclei.

prepared for 40 g liver. For 20 g of liver or less one gradient is prepared. In contrast to other steps, gradient volumes are not adjusted for liver weight. The fraction containing nuclei from step 1 of the differential centrifugation is homogenized in a final volume of 3.6 ml and applied to a third (or second) gradient tube in the same fashion as crude plasma membrane. The gradients are then centrifuged for 90 min (Spinco 27SW rotor, 26,000 rpm, ~90,000 × g). Purified plasma membranes (PM-I of Figure 4) are collected as a thick rug from the 1.16/1.166 interface of all three gradient tubes using a pasteur pipet. The membranes are resuspended in 40 ml of 1 mM bicarbonate and collected by centrifugation for 20 min at 8000 rpm (Sorvall SS-34 rotor, RC2B centrifuge). Purified mitochondria are recovered from the 1.2/1.22 interface of tubes 1 and 2. Purified nuclei form a pellet in gradient tube 3. The 1.166/1.173 interface contains plasma membrane mixed with mitochondria (PM-II of Figure 4). If a quick check shows mitochondrial contamination not to be excessive (10% or less by succinate-INT-reductase or negative staining electron microscopy), this layer can be combined with the plasma membrane fraction from the 1.16/1.166 interface. The purity of the second plasma membrane layer depends on the efficiency of the differential centrifugation steps in removing mitochondria.

Yield: 1–3 mg plasma membrane protein/10 g fresh weight of liver.

Recovery: Based on electron microscope morphometry, a 100% yield of about 20 mg/10 g fresh weight of liver would be expected so that the actual yield is on the order of 10–15%. The recovery of 5′-nucleotidase is much less; only 1–2% of the total liver 5′-nucleotidase is recovered in the plasma membrane fraction.

ISOLATION OF ORGANELLES

One problem is that 5'-nucleotidase activity is exhibited by membrane fractions other than plasma membrane, for example, Golgi apparatus, ER, and mitochondria.

Purity: The purified plasma membrane fractions are at least 90% plasma membrane-derived material with mitochondria being the principal source of contamination (Table III). Small ER-derived vesicles (attached to or closely associated with the plasma membrane) constitute a second serious source of contamination. For enzymes associated exclusively with the plasma membrane, a 100-fold purification would constitute an acceptable value [Lauter, Solyom, and Trams, 1972]. That 5'-nucleotidase is concentrated less than 25-fold in the plasma membrane fraction merely provides additional argument for the non-localization of this enzyme in the plasma membrane. A 20- to 25-fold purification of 5'-nucleotidase relative to total homogenate is indicative of 90%+ purity of the isolated membrane fraction.

TABLE III. Enzymatic Activities of Plasma Membrane-Rich Fractions

Enzyme	Specific activity[a]	Relative specific activity[b]
Glucose-6-phosphatase	1.3	0.2
Succinate-INT-reductase	1.3	0.7
Galactosyl transferase	Not detected	-
5'-Nucleotidase	77.5	23.2

[a]Units of specific activity are given in Table I.
[b]Ratio of specific activity of plasma membrane fraction to that of total homogenate.
From Yunghans and Morré [unpublished results].

In thin sections, junctional complexes identify long undulating profiles of membranes as being derived from plasma membrane (Plate III, 1). When negatively stained with phosphotungstic acid, collapsed vesicles with a smooth to fibrous-mottled appearance characterize the fraction (Plate III, 2). Contaminating mitochondria are easily recognized from the presence of internal cristae with the attached 90 A adenosinetriphosphatase particles or knobs. Plasma membrane margins sometimes exhibit globular knobs (quite distinct from mitochondrial knobs) or the hexagonal array of subunits as reported by Benedetti and Emmelot [1968]. These structures are associated with microvilli and junctional complexes, and most plasma membrane fragments lack them.

E. MITOCHONDRIA (MICROBODIES AND LYSOSOMES)

Perhaps more investigators have isolated mitochondrial fractions from rat liver than any other cell component from any other tissue. Lysosomes, peroxisomes,

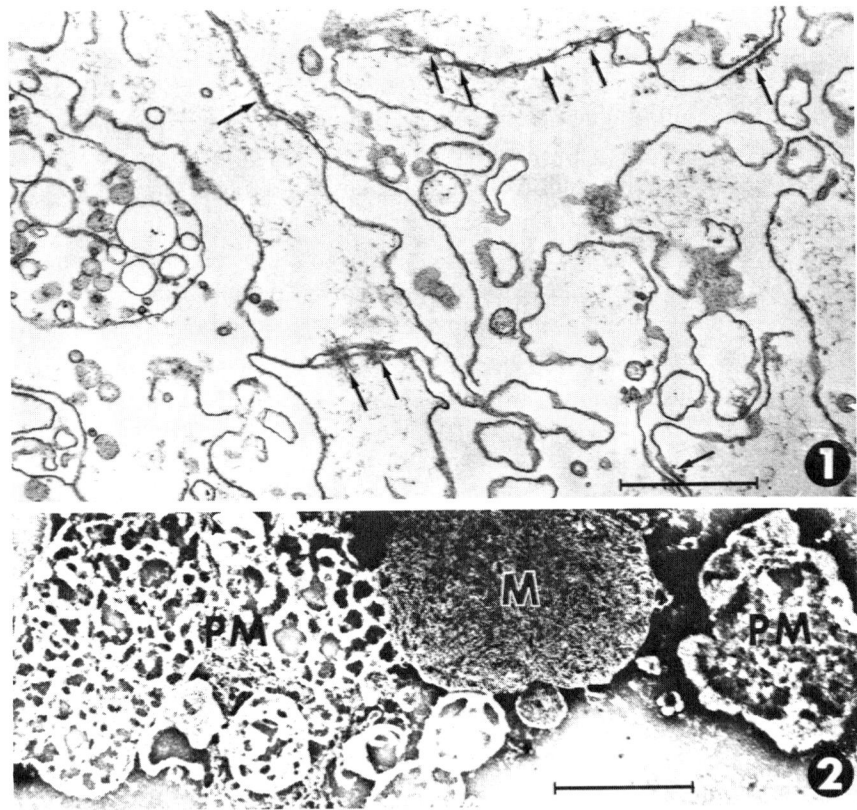

PLATE III. Plasma membrane. (1) Plasma membrane-rich fraction from rat liver in thin section. Junctional complexes (arrows) identify the long undulating membrane profiles as plasma membrane. Prepared for electron microscopy as in Plate II-1. Bar = 1 μ. (2) A plasma membrane fraction negatively stained with potassium phosphotungstate (see Plate I-3 for details of procedure). Collapsed vesicles are embedded in a thin amorphous film of stain and show a fibrous texture with smooth peripheries (PM). A contaminating mitochondrial fragment (M) is included for comparison. Swollen mitochondria are frequently difficult to distinguish from plasma membrane fragments in thin sections but can be readily identified in negatively stained preparations from the characteristic knob structure of the inner membranes of the mitochondria. Bar = 1 μ.

and ER are common contaminants of such mitochondrial preparations. Most mitochondrial isolations from liver involve homogenization in buffered 0.25 M sucrose, centrifugation at 1000–4000 × $\underline{g}$ to remove debris, whole cells, and nuclei, and centrifugation at 10,000–15,000 × $\underline{g}$ to obtain the crude mitochondrial pellet. In my experience, little additional purification is achieved by placing such fractions on sucrose gradients. Endoplasmic reticulum and mito-

ISOLATION OF ORGANELLES

chondria, as well as ER and microbodies, are so firmly associated that all one obtains is a smear of large ER fragments with small mitochondria and large mitochondria with small ER fragments. Lysosomes, being normally heterogeneous, and microbodies tend to distribute among the mitochondria. One approach, in addition to recovery of mitochondria from the plasma membrane gradient (procedure D), is repeated resuspension cycles until the fractions "look right," that is, all fluffy material is removed and the fraction has a uniform dark brownish color. The mitochondria remain largely intact through this process.

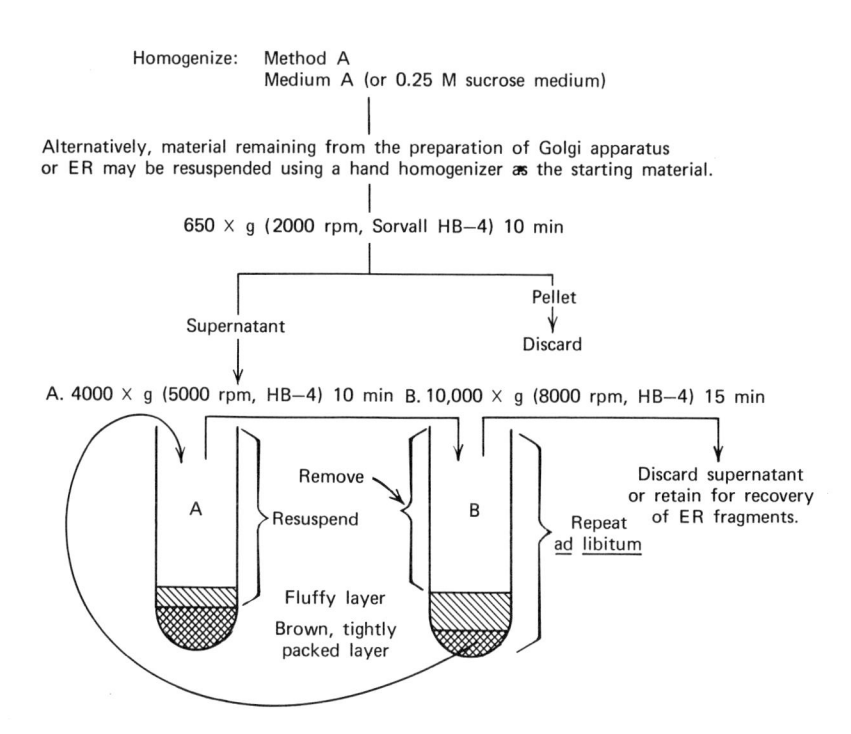

```
              Homogenize:   Method A
                            Medium A (or 0.25 M sucrose medium)
                                   |
Alternatively, material remaining from the preparation of Golgi apparatus
or ER may be resuspended using a hand homogenizer as the starting material.
                                   |
              650 X g (2000 rpm, Sorvall HB-4) 10 min
                                   |
                    ┌──────────────┴──────────────┐
                                                Pellet
              Supernatant                          ↓
                    │                           Discard
                    ↓
A. 4000 X g (5000 rpm, HB-4) 10 min   B. 10,000 X g (8000 rpm, HB-4) 15 min
```

Tube A should eventually contain a homogeneous pellet of brown tightly packed material = mitochondria. The fluffy layer concentrated in tube B may be used as a source of crude lysosomes or microbodies or discarded.

Flow Diagram   Procedure E: Mitochondria

Homogenization Medium:

0.25 M sucrose
0.01 M Tris HCl, pH 7.4
0.1 mM ethylenediaminetetraacetic acid (EDTA)

Homogenization Procedure: Method A. Alternatively, the combined residues from the Golgi apparatus isolation step or any material removed in the microsomal precentrifugation can be combined, resuspended in the above medium using a hand homogenizer, and diluted to about 40 ml with medium. Distilled water or 0.25 M sucrose alone can be used for resuspension with about equal success.

Low-Speed Differential Centrifugation: The homogenate is centrifuged for 10 min at 650 × g (2000 rpm, SB-4 rotor, Sorvall RC2B) to remove residual nuclei and debris. The supernatant is decanted carefully and the pellet discarded. The supernatant is centrifuged at 5000 rpm (4000 × g) for 10 min to collect the crude mitochondrial pellet. The supernatant is placed in another tube and recentrifuged for 15 min at 8000 rpm. The pellet is retained and the supernatant is either discarded or retained for isolation of microsomes. If the supernatant is to be used for recovery of ER fragments or microsomal subfractionation, the 0.1 mM EDTA should be replaced by 5 mM $MgCl_2$. The centrifugation steps are then repeated beginning with the 6000 rpm centrifugation of the resuspended 5000 rpm pellet. The supernatant from this centrifugation is combined with the 8000 rpm pellet and the 8000 rpm centrifugation is repeated. At this point, both pellets should contain two layers. The top layer will be fluffy and gray. The bottom layer will be tightly packed and brown. The objective is to end up with a tightly packed and brown mitochondrial fraction free of the fluffy gray material. This can be hastened by resuspending the fluffy layer with the supernatant from the 5000 rpm centrifugation and combining this with the fluffy layer from the 8000 rpm centrifugation. The brown mitochondrial layer from the 8000 rpm centrifugation can be resuspended with the brown mitochondrial layer from the 5000 rpm centrifugation, etc. The resuspension-recentrifugation is repeated until the 5000 rpm tube contains only homogeneous brown material (usually a minimum of 4–5 times); this fraction contains purified mitochondria (Plate IV, 1). The fluffy layer is either discarded or used for the preparation of crude lysosome or microbody fractions (Figure 5). The organelles present in the fluffy layer are shown in Plate IV, 2.

F. SOLUBLE SUPERNATANT AND FLOATING LIPID

Nonparticulate activities or constituents are frequently assayed on samples of a "soluble supernatant" from which membranes, ribosomes, glycogen, etc., have been removed. The supernatant obtained after preparation of total microsomes or preparation of ER subfractions from the Golgi apparatus supernatant will

ISOLATION OF ORGANELLES 25

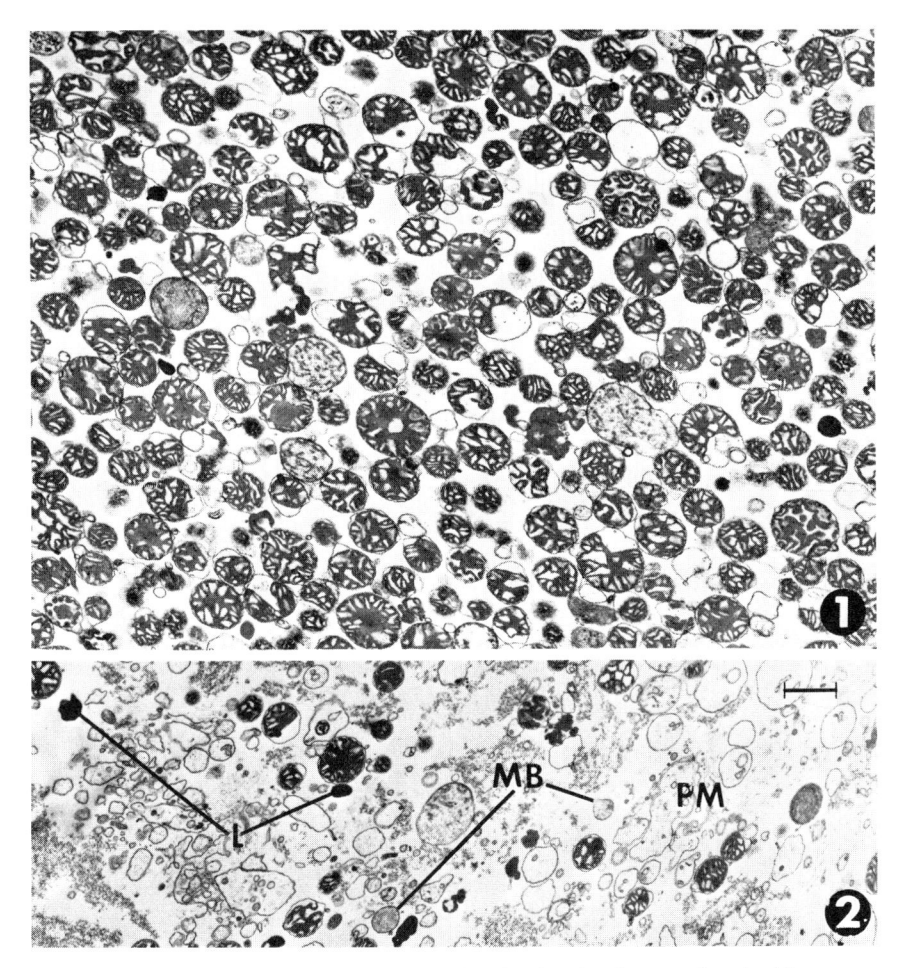

PLATE IV. Mitochondria. (1) Mitochondrion-rich fraction from rat liver in thin section after four resuspension cycles according to procedure D. Prepared for electron microscopy as in Plate II-1. Bar = 1 μ. (2) Fluffy layer remaining after removal of mitochondria illustrated in 1. L = lysosome. MB = microbody. PM = plasma membrane. Bar = 1 μ.

suffice. To determine total supernatant activity it is usually necessary to centrifuge a known volume of total homogenate as if preparing microsomes and then determine accurately the volume of supernatant recovered.

The floating lipid contains primarily the reserve triglycerides of the liver (in the form of lipid bodies) and liposomes plus smaller amounts of secretory

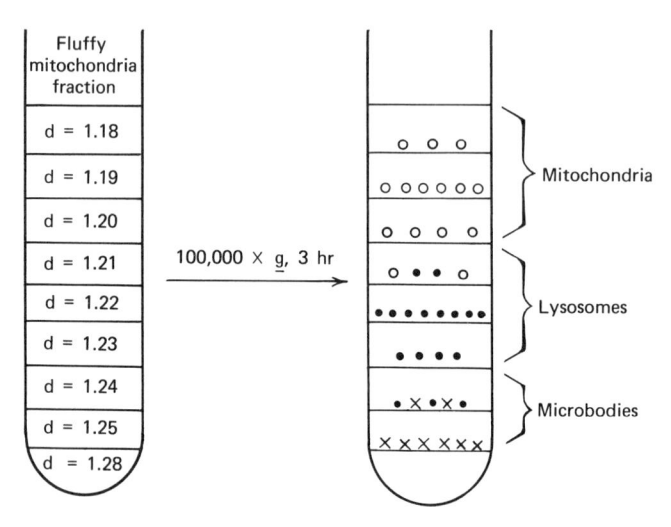

FIGURE 5. Simple linear sucrose gradient for separation of mitochondria, lysosomes, and microbodies. Separation of mitochondria, lysosomes, and microbodies must be verified in any given experiment, for example, by determinations of succinate-INT-reductase, acid phosphatase, and uric acid oxidase (uricase), respectively. Lysosomes especially exhibit variable sedimentation characteristics.

lipoproteins and released membrane lipids. This fraction is usually discarded but may be separated from the microsomal supernatant by adding a layer of deionized water over the homogenate prior to the microsomal centrifugation. In this manner, the floating lipid layer may be removed from the top of the water layer without contamination from other supernatant constituents.

REFERENCES

Benedetti, E. L., and P. Emmelot. 1968. Structure and function of plasma membranes isolated from liver. In A. J. Dalton and F. Haguenau, (ed.), Ultrastructure in biological systems. The membranes. Academic Press, New York. 4:33–120.

Bloemandal, H., W. S. Bont, M. De Vries, and E. L. Benedetti. 1967. Isolation and properties of polyribosomes and fragments of the endoplasmic reticulum from rat liver. Biochem. J. 103:177–182.

Cheetham, R. D., D. J. Morré, and W. N. Yunghans. 1970. Isolation of a Golgi apparatus-rich fraction from rat liver. II. Enzymatic characterization and comparison with other cell fractions. J. Cell Biol. 44:492–500.

Cunningham, W. P., D. J. Morré, and H. H. Mollenhauer. 1966. Structure of isolated plant Golgi apparatus revealed by negative staining. J. Cell Biol. 28:169–179.

Dallner, G., P. Siekevitz, and G. E. Palade. 1966. Biogenesis of endoplasmic reticulum membranes. I. Structural and chemical differentiation in developing rat hepatocytes. J. Cell Biol. 30:73–96.

de Duve, C. 1963. The lysosome. Sci. Am. 208:64–72.

Emmelot, P., C. J. Box, E. L. Benedetti, and P. Ruemke. 1964. Studies on plasma membranes. I. Chemical composition and enzyme content of plasma membranes isolated from rat liver. Biochim. Biophys. Acta 90:126–145.

Ernster, L., P. Siekevitz, and G. E. Palade. 1962. Enzyme-structure relationships in the endoplasmic reticulum of rat liver. A morphological and biochemical study. J. Cell Biol. 15:541–562.

Huang, C. M. and D. J. Morré. 1972. Unpublished observation. Purdue University Lafayette, Indiana.

Lauter, C. J., A. Solyom, and E. G. Trams. 1972. Comparative studies on enzyme markers of liver plasma membranes. Biochim. Biophys. Acta 266:511–523.

Merritt, W. and D. J. Morré. 1973. Biochem. Biophys. Acta. In press.

Mollenhauer, H. J. 1964. Stain Technol. 39:111–115.

Morré, D. J. 1971. Isolation of Golgi apparatus. Meth. Enzymol. 22:130–148.

Morré, D. J., R. D. Cheetham, S. E. Nyquist, and L. Ovtracht. 1972. A simplified procedure for isolation of Golgi apparatus from rat liver. Prep. Biochem. 2:61–69.

Morré, D. J. and S. Hocker. 1972. Unpublished. Purdue University, Lafayette, Ind.

Morré, D. J., L. M. Merlin, and T. W. Keenan. 1969. Localization of glycosyl transferase activities in a Golgi apparatus-rich fraction isolated from rat liver. Biochem. Biophys. Res. Comm. 37:813–819.

Nevelle, D. M. 1960. The isolation of a cell membrane fraction from rat liver. J. Biophys. Biochem. Cytol. 8:413–422.

Palade, G. E., and P. Siekevitz. 1956. Pancreatic microsomes. An integrated morphological and biochemical study. J. Biophys. Biochem. Cytol. 2:671–690.

Reynolds, E. S. 1963. The use of lead citrate at high pH as an electron opaque stain in electron microscopy. J. Cell. Biol. 17:208–212.

Spurr, A. R. 1969. A low-viscosity epoxy resin embedding medium for electron microscopy. J. Ultrastr. Res. 26:31–43.

Stahn, R., K. Maier, and K. Hannig. 1970. A new method for the preparation of rat liver lysosomes. Separation of cell organelles of rat liver by carrier-free continuous electrophoresis. J. Cell Biol. 46:576–591.

Yunghans, W. and D. J. Morré. 1973. A rapid and reproducible procedure for isolation of plasma membranes from rat liver. Prep. Biochem. In press.

Analysis of Specific Proteins in Differentiating Tissues of the Rat

EDWARD E. PENHOET

ANALYSIS OF SPECIFIC PROTEINS IN DIFFERENTIATING TISSUES

The process of cytodifferentiation may be viewed as the acquisition of a specific pattern of macromolecular synthesis which results in the expression of a characteristic morphology and physiology in a given tissue. These differentiated characteristics, although undoubtedly genetically controlled, are expressed primarily as the result of the synthesis and accumulation of specific sets of enzymes and other protein species. Therefore the analysis of the proteins which exist in a given tissue and the way in which these proteins change during a developmental transition is an important part of the science of developmental biology. In order to determine the nature of the regulation of protein complement taking place during development in a tissue, one must be able to distinguish the protein whose regulation he is studying from all other proteins present in the cells from which it was derived. This may be accomplished by analyzing properties which are unique to the protein in question, such as its catalytic activity, electrophoretic mobility, molecular weight, and/or immunochemical properties. In the experiments described here, measurement of catalytic and electrophoretic properties of mammalian fructose-1, 6-diphosphate aldolases will be described. The methodologies can be adapted to other enzymes with slight modifications of the protocol.

Biochemical pathways such as glycolysis are present in virtually all vertebrate cells. However, the metabolic functions of these pathways are often different in different tissues of a higher organism. Glycolysis in vertebrate muscle, for example, is directed almost exclusively toward the generation of energy through the catabolic utilization of glucose. Thus, the major flow of small molecules through this pathway occurs in the direction of glucose breakdown. In the cells of tissues such as liver and kidney, on the other hand, the flow of metabolites through glycolysis takes place in both directions, that is, for the degradation and synthesis of glucose molecules. This type of metabolic diversity among the organs of a single animal is made possible partially by the existence of multiple enzyme forms which catalyze the same basic reactions, but which have different molecular and catalytic properties. Enzymes of this sort which are structurally and catalytically distinct, but which catalyze the same basic reaction, are known as "isoenzymes" or "isozymes." Fructose diphosphate (FDP) aldolase is an example of such an enzyme in the glycolytic pathway. The levels of the enzymatic activity are different in different tissues and there are three distinct aldolase isoenzyme forms distributed in specific ways among the various tissues of an organism. The reaction catalyzed by this enzyme is fructose 1,6-diphosphate $\rightleftharpoons$ glyceraldehyde-3-phosphate + dihydroxyacetone phosphate. The basic catalytic, physical, and immunochemical properties of the three mammalian aldolase forms isolated from adult rabbit tissues are presented in Table I along with their tissue distribution in the major organ systems of adult mammals. Aldolase A is a protein molecule which appears well equipped for a role in catabolic glycolysis, cleaving FDP at a high rate and having little activity with other substrates. Aldolase B, which exists in liver and kidney, is more effec-

TABLE I. Properties of Homologous FDP Aldolases (Rabbit)

	A (muscle)	B (liver)	C (brain)
Maximal rate of FDP cleavage	2,900	250	1,000
Maximal rate of F-1-P cleavage	58	250	100
FDP/F-1-P activity ratio	50	1	10
Molecular weight (native enzyme)	160,000	160,000	160,000
Subunit molecular weight	40,000	40,000	40,000
Immunological reaction with anti-A	+	−	−
Immunological reaction with anti-B	−	+	−
Immunological reaction with anti-C	−	−	+
Electrophoretic mobility in pH 8.6 veronal buffer	slightly cathodic	moderately cathodic	very anodic
Number of polypeptide chains	4	4	4
Tissue distribution (adult rabbit)	muscle, spleen, brain, kidney, etc.	liver, kidney, intestine	brain, adrenal

tive in synthesis of FDP from the triose phosphates and has a broader substrate specificity which confers upon it more metabolic flexibility. It quite effectively cleaves fructose-1-phosphate, for example, which is an intermediate in the metabolism of fructose in liver tissue, while aldolase A is a poor catalyst for the cleavage of this substrate. Aldolase C is found primarily in nervous tissue in mammals and has catalytic properties intermediate between those of A and B. Recent data indicate that it may be specifically associated with subcellular particles in this type of tissue.

Aldolases A, B, and C, purified from rabbit muscle, liver, and brain, respectively, have different electrophoretic mobilities and can be conveniently separated from each other by electrophoresis on cellulose acetate strips or polyacrylamide gels. Following electrophoretic separation, the aldolases may be located on the strips or gels by use of an activity stain which works according to the following reactions:

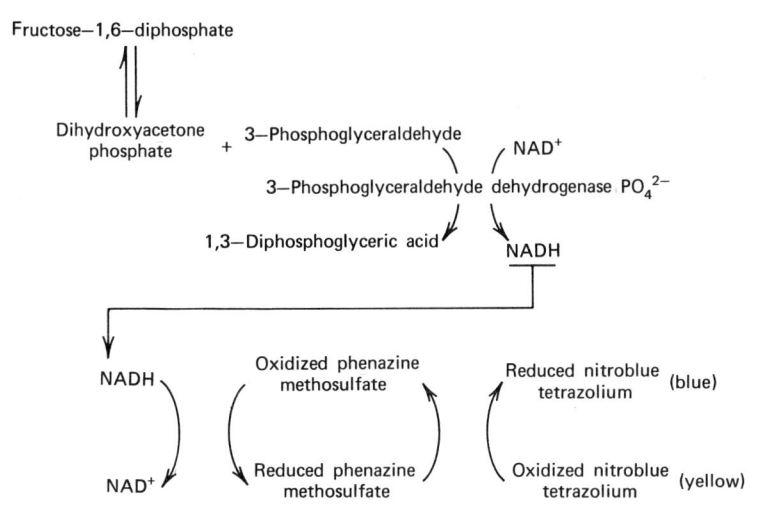

Fructose–1,6–diphosphate

↓

Dihydroxyacetone phosphate + 3–Phosphoglyceraldehyde

3–Phosphoglyceraldehyde dehydrogenase, NAD$^+$, PO$_4^{2-}$

1,3–Diphosphoglyceric acid, NADH

NADH / NAD$^+$ ⇌ Oxidized phenazine methosulfate / Reduced phenazine methosulfate ⇌ Reduced nitroblue tetrazolium (blue) / Oxidized nitroblue tetrazolium (yellow)

The various assay components are mixed in a soft agar solution to which a cellulose acetate strip containing an aldolase solution or tissue extract is applied. The aldolase on the strip comes in contact with the FDP in the agar and cleaves it to dihydroxyacetone phosphate and 3-phosphoglyceraldehyde. The 3-phosphoglyceraldehyde is then oxidized to 1,3-diphosphoglyceric acid by the enzyme 3-phosphoglyceraldehyde dehydrogenase (present in the agar) with the concomitant reduction of NAD$^+$ to NADH (nicotinamide adenine dinucleotide). The NADH thus produced in turn reduces oxidized phenazine methosulfate which then reduces oxidized nitroblue tetrazolium to the reduced form which is a highly colored blue compound. Thus, wherever aldolase activity is present on a cellulose acetate strip, a blue band appears in the adjacent agar. Any enzyme which is an oxido reductase using NAD^+ as a cofactor or an enzyme (such as aldolase) which can be linked to such an oxidoreductase can be assayed in this way using appropriate substrates.

Each of these aldolase enzymes is composed of four polypeptide chains (subunits). In a tissue that synthesizes only one type of aldolase subunit, the active enzymatic form is a homogeneous tetramer containing only one type of subunit. In muscle, for example, only A subunits are synthesized and the enzyme is present as A_4. In tissues synthesizing only B subunits, the active species would be B_4, and in a similar way those tissues which synthesize only C subunits have their aldolase in the form of C_4. In tissues in which two types of aldolase subunits are synthesized simultaneously, the subunit types can combine with each other to form hybrid tetramers which are composed of mixtures of the parental subunits. Thus, in a tissue like brain where both A and C subunits are synthesized, five aldolase species are present which have the subunit composition A_4, A_3C, A_2C_2, AC_3, and C_4. This ability to form hybrid molecules is shared by other multimeric enzymes such as lactate dehydrogenase, for example, and can be duplicated in the laboratory by subjecting mixtures of two homogeneous tetramers (A_4 and C_4, for example) to reversible dissociation by a variety of techniques. Electrophoresis of rabbit tissue extracts on cellulose acetate followed by activity staining as described above results in the patterns of aldolase activity depicted in Figure 1.

```
brain
heart
liver
etc.
```

The equipment and methodology used to perform such analyses is presented below.

Preparation of Tissue Extracts

Dissect out the organ or tissue to be analyzed and drop into a beaker containing 10 mM Tris Cl pH 8.0, 1 mM ethylenediaminetetra-acetic acid (EDTA) at 0°C. Remove the tissue and weigh it. Mince into small pieces with dissecting scissors and suspend in 2 vol of the above buffer. Pour into a glass homogenizing vessel and homogenize for 10 strokes. Pour the resulting homogenate into appropriate-

PROTEINS IN DIFFERENTIATING TISSUES

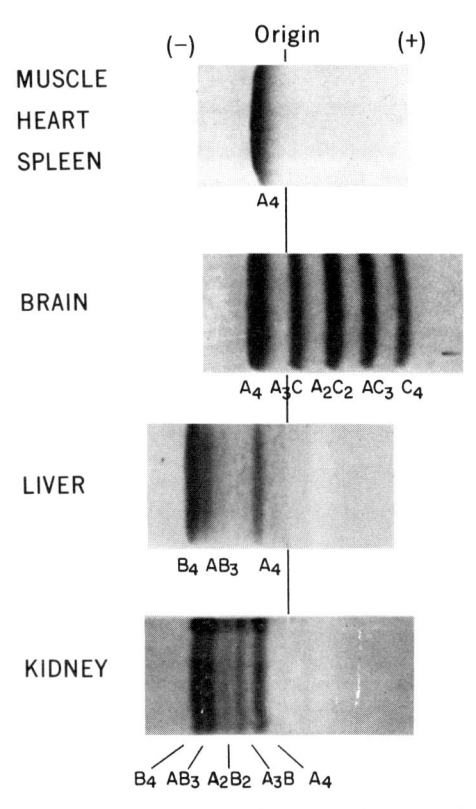

FIGURE 1. Patterns of aldolase activity of adult rabbit tissues after cellulose acetate electrophoresis. Electrophoresis and activity staining for aldolase was performed as indicated in the text.

sized ultracentrifuge tubes and spin in an ultracentrifuge for 60 min at 100,000 X g and 0°C to remove subcellular particles and debris. For embryonic tissues, small homogenizers are necessary as are small centrifuge tubes with appropriate adapters. After the centrifugation is complete, remove the supernatant for electrophoretic analysis.

Cellulose Acetate Electrophoresis

Equipment Required:

Regulated dc power supply
Cellulose acetate electrophoresis chamber

Supplies:

Cellulose acetate strips (1 × 6 1/2 in.)
Blotter paper cut to 2 × 9 in. strips
Sample applicator (Gelman #51220 or equivalent)
Lang–Levy type of micropipets

Conduct all operations in a cold room at 0–4°C.

Fill the electrophoresis chamber with 50 mM Na Barbital, 10 mM 2-mercaptoethanol pH 8.6 as indicated in the chamber instructions. Soak cellulose acetate strips for approximately 20 min before use by floating on top of the buffer and allowing to sink into the buffer as wetting progresses. Load the sample applicator with 1–2 μliter of solution from a capillary tube or micropipet. Transfer a soaked strip from the buffer to a piece of blotter paper and remove excess buffer with a second blotter paper laid over the top of the strip. Apply the sample to the center of the strip by holding the applicator perpendicular to the plane of the strip and pressing firmly onto the strip. Place the strip in the electrophoresis chamber with the sample equidistant from the cathode and the anode. Cover the chamber to protect yourself and others from the possibility of electrocution and to minimize evaporation of buffer from the strip. Turn on the power supply and adjust to a level of 200–250 v constant voltage. Continue electrophoresis for a period of 1–2 hr. Turn off the power supply and carefully remove the strips without allowing buffer to run onto the center portion. The strips may now be stained with a protein stain or assayed for enzymatic activity as indicated in the following sections.

Polyacrylamide Gel Electrophoresis

The most widely used polyacrylamide gel system for the resolution of proteins in their "native" states is the high pH (8.3) system described by Davis [1964]. The equipment and chemicals utilized for the system are as follows.

Equipment Required:

Regulated dc power supply
Polyacrylamide gel electrophoresis chamber (readily available commercially or may be constructed according to the designs published by Davis [1964] or Maizel [1969]
Rack for holding gel tubes

Supplies:

0.6 cm (ID) × 15 cm glass tubes

Stock Solutions for Preparing Polyacrylamide Gels:

Solution A		Solution B	
Tris	36.6 g	Tris	5.98 g
1 N HCl	48 ml	1 N HCl	48 ml
N,N,N',N'-tetramethyl-ethylenediamine (TEMED)	0.23 ml	TEMED	0.46 ml
H_2O	to 100 ml, pH to 8.9	H_2O	to 100 ml, pH to 6.7

Solution C		Solution D	
Acrylamide	28 g	Acrylamide	10 g
Methylene-bis-acrylamide (Bis)	0.735 g	Bis	2.5 g
H_2O	to 100 ml	H_2O	to 100 ml

Solution E	Solution F
4 mg Riboflavine to 100 ml c̄ H_2O	40% Sucrose

Solution G	Reservoir buffer	
28% Ammonium persulfate	Tris	6.0 g
	Glycine	28.8 g
	H_2O	to 1000 ml

Dilute 1:10 for use, adjust pH to 8.3

Preparing the Gels: Place a rubber serum cap over one end of the gel tube and place in the tube holder with the capped end down. Prepare the resolving gel by mixing the following components in a small beaker allowing approximately 4 ml for each gel:

1 part A   1 part H_2O
2 part C   4 part G

Pour the mixture into the gel tubes to a height of approximately 10 cm and carefully overlay the gel solution with distilled water so that the top of the gel does not solidify in the shape of a meniscus. After the gel has solidified (30 min or so at room temperature) pour off the H_2O from the top of the gel and prepare the stacking gel which will be layered on the top of the running gel or resolving gel. To prepare the stacking gel, mix the following components: 1 part B, 2 parts D, 1 part E, and 4 parts F. Pour approximately 1.5 cm of the stacking gel mixture onto the resolving gel and overlay the mixture with water as done previously. Polymerize the stacking gel by photoxidation of the riboflavin in the stacking gel with an ordinary fluorescent lamp placed 6 in. or so from the gel. After 30 min or so of the photoxidation, the gels are ready to be used. At this time, carefully pour off the water from the tops of the gels and insert the gels into the electrophoresis chamber after carefully removing the serum caps from the bottom of the tubes. Fill the reservoirs of the electrophoresis chamber with the diluted reservoir buffer. Mix the sample containing approximately 100 μg of protein in a volume of 0.1 ml of 10 mM Tris·Cl, 5 mM 2-mercaptoacetic acid pH 8.0 with 25 μliter of 50% w/v sucrose and 5 μliter of 0.1% bromphenol blue, which is used as a marker. Using a Lang–Levy type of micropipet with a suction tube and mouthpiece, apply the sample to the top of the stacking gel by inserting the micropipet through the reservoir buffer to the top of the gel and carefully expressing the dense solution so as not to mix it with the overlying reservoir buffer. The mercaptoacetic acid is added to the sample to prevent oxidation of the enzymes by unreacted persulfates remaining in the gel. When all the samples have been applied, begin the electrophoresis by applying a voltage of approximately 300 v dc or a constant current of approximately 3.5 mamp per gel with the anode at the bottom of the gels and the cathode at the top. Terminate the electrophoresis when the bromphenol blue marker comes within 1/2–1 cm of the bottom of the gels. At this time, turn off the power and remove the gels for analysis of proteins by staining with Coomassie Blue or analysis of enzymatic activity using an appropriate activity stain.

Activity Stain for Fructose Diphosphate Aldolase on Cellulose Acetate Strips

Prepare 20 ml of a solution containing 0.6% noble agar, 10 mM sodium arsenate, 50 mM Tris·Cl pH 8.0. Dissolve the agar by boiling and cool to 42°C in a water bath set to that temperature. Add the following ingredients in this order while maintaining the solution at 42°C:

2 ml 100 mM Sodium fructose-1, 6-diphosphate
2 ml 10 mg/ml Nitroblue tetrazolium chloride
2 ml 15 mg/ml NAD$^+$
0.6 ml 1 mg/ml Phenazine methosulfate
0.1 ml 10 mg/ml Glyceraldehyde-3-phosphate dehydrogenase

The phenazine methosulfate is light-sensitve, so make it up fresh and keep it in the dark until used. After adding the last ingredient, pour the mixture into five or six 100 mm plastic petri plates and place in a refrigerator to solidify. The plates may be stored in the dark for up to 24 hr before use.

Remove the cellulose acetate strips from the electrophoresis chamber. Lay the strips with the upper surface down on top of the solidified agar and place in a 37°C incubator in the dark for 10-15 min. Remove the plates and examine the pattern produced. Record the results by photography of the inverted plates.

Activity Stain of Polyacrylamide Gels

Carefully remove the gels from the gel tubes and place in empty 100 mm petri dishes. Prepare the agar assay solution as indicated above, pour it over the gel in the petri plate, and solidify by floating the plate in ice water. After the agar has solidified incubate at 37°C for 10-15 min to develop the color reaction.

A very thorough review of other polyacrylamide gel electrophoresis systems has been published recently by Maizel [1969]. This review should be consulted for methodologies of protein staining and fractionation and analysis of gels of radioactive proteins.

REFERENCES

Multiple Enzyme Forms

Kaplan, N. O. 1968. Nature of multiple molecular forms of enzymes. Proc. N.Y. Acad. Sci. 151(1):382.

Lebherz, H. G., and W. J. Rutter, 1969. Distribution of fructose diphosphate aldolase variants in biological systems. Biochemistry 8:109.

Electrophoresis

Davis, B. J. 1964. Disc electrophoresis II: method and application to human serum proteins. Ann. N.Y. Acad. Sci. 121:404.

Maizel, J. 1969. Acrylamide gel electrophoresis of proteins and nucleic acids. In K. Habel and N. P. Salzman (ed.), Fundamental techniques in virology. Academic Press, New York. p. 334.

The Measurement of Cytoplasmic Steroid "Receptor" Proteins

I. JOHN DAVIES

INTRODUCTION

For the purposes of this discussion, cytoplasmic high-affinity, low-capacity steroid-binding proteins will be referred to as "receptor" proteins without regard to whether such a functional role has been established for a particular example. Steroid-binding proteins are measured, not directly, but in terms of binding activity. For some purposes, semiquantitative methodology is used to compare different samples and relative binding activity may be expressed in terms of a binding index [1]. For quantitative purposes, the total number of binding sites in a given sample can be measured. As cytoplasmic receptor proteins have not been purified, and the number of binding sites per molecule is not known, binding site concentration is expressed in terms of some tissue parameter, such as milligrams of total cytoplasmic protein, tissue weight, or cell number. The number of binding sites is measured by determining the number of molecules of radiolabeled steroid required to "saturate" the receptor protein. A variety of methods have been used for such measurements. The appropriate application of these methods requires an appreciation of the theoretical principles of steroid-protein interaction and also the very significant methodological problems which have been encountered. The present discussion will focus on the principles and application of multiple equilibrium dialysis. This method remains the standard by which other techniques must be assessed. The theoretical basis of the method is firm, no assumptions are involved other than the applicability of the laws of mass action, and potential artifacts can be readily observed and controlled. An understanding of multiple equilibrium dialysis will provide a framework for the evaluation and appropriate application of other methods.

The protein-steroid complexes which are under consideration here are held together by noncovalent bonds. These bonds are relatively weak, their energy being of the order of hydrogen bonds [1]. The complexes readily associate and dissociate at ordinary temperatures, and a state of thermodynamic equilibrium is attained. The laws of mass action can be applied and the equilibrium can be described by the general equation:

$$K_a = \frac{[S \sim P]}{[S][P]}$$

Definitions of abbreviations:
[B]   = Bound steroid concentration
K_a = Association constant (equilibrium)
n[M]   = Binding site concentration (number of binding sites per protein molecule × concentration of binding protein)
[P]   = Steroid-binding protein concentration
[S]   = Steroid concentration
[S ∼ P] = Steroid-protein complex concentration
[U]   = Unbound steroid concentration

In steroid-binding studies, K_a is applied to describe the relative concentration of reactants at equilibrium; it therefore reflects the affinity of the steroid and protein for each other. The constant K_a is sometimes referred to as an intrinsic association constant, an equilibrium constant, or an affinity constant. Insofar as the laws of mass action are applicable, K_a is constant for a given steroid-protein pair with varying concentrations of steroid or protein. Experimental factors which alter K_a are ionic strength, pH, and temperature. The affinity of steroid-protein binding is generally inversely related to temperature. For all cytoplasmic receptor proteins which have been described, the affinity is much greater, and the dissociation rate is much slower, at 0–5°C as compared to ambient or physiological temperatures. This fact is applied to advantage in binding measurements, but it is important to recognize that the limitation of dissociation by cooling is relative, and it is variable in degree with different steroid-protein combinations.

Steroid-binding proteins tend to fall into two observationally defined groups: (1) specific, high-affinity, low-capacity, and (2) nonspecific, low-affinity, high-capacity. The term, specific, indicates that the protein binds only a specific steroid and biologically active analogs or inhibitors. This specificity is not always complete. Specific is also used to indicate that the protein is tissue-specific, being found only in biologically responsive tissues, and it therefore carries the connotation that the protein has biological significance in hormone action.

The term, high-affinity, implies a K_a on the order of 10^8 M^{-1} or greater, while low-affinity implies a K_a on the order of 10^4 M^{-1} or less [1]. Low-capacity means that the binding sites can be saturated at the limited concentrations of steroids which occur physiologically, or, in the laboratory, within the limited concentrations of steroids which are soluble in aqueous media. Cytoplasmic receptor proteins are high-affinity low-capacity proteins, and their measurement resolves itself to the determination of the quantity of steroid which saturates the protein. While it is thermodynamically impossible to truly saturate the protein, the saturation point is obtained by extrapolation from lower concentrations of steroid or by adding steroid in great excess so that saturation is closely approached. Nonspecific binding is important as background "noise" which must be experimentally or analytically excluded from the specific binding. Nonspecific binding generally follows the polarity rule, that is, it is greater with less polar steroids such as progesterone [1]. It is an important methodological consideration in the measurement of cytoplasmic receptor proteins.

THE METHOD IN GENERAL

To determine the concentration of progesterone receptor sites in rat myometrial cytosol, you will prepare a number of dialysis experiments which are identical except for varying concentrations of progesterone The cytosol will comprise the inside solution, and the steroid in buffer will be the outside solution. For operational convenience, the same quantity of radiolabeled progesterone will be added to each vial and the different steroid concentrations will be obtained by adding varying amounts of unlabeled steroid. Following equilibration, the relative concentrations of radioactivity will be analyzed to compute the concentration of high-affinity binding sites.

THE METHOD IN DETAIL

Progesterone-1,2-^{3}H (Specific activity(S.A.) 40–60 Ci(Curies)/mmole) **or Progesterone 1,2,6,7-^{3}H** (S.A. 80–100 Ci/mmole). Check the purity. Impurities will be measured as unbound steroid. At low concentrations of steroid, where the proportion of progesterone which remains unbound is relatively small, a total impurity of a few percent will cause a much larger error in the apparent ratio of bound to unbound steroid. We routinely purify all ^{3}H-progesterone by paper chromatography (Ligroin/95% methanol). Prepare the ^{3}H-progesterone in 95%

ethanol at 100 pmole/ml. Store at −20°C in 10 ml aliquots in tightly capped vials. You will need 250 pmole (2.5 ml) for one experiment.

Unlabeled Progesterone. A series of dilutions are prepared such that addition of 0.1 ml, in addition to the 10 pmole of ^{3}H-progesterone, will provide a range of total steroid added from 10 to 3000 pmole. See Table I.

TABLE I. Preparation of Unlabeled Progesterone Dilutions

		pmole/ml	pmole/0.1 ml	Total steroid with 10 pmoles ^{3}H-progesterone added to 0.1 ml
31.4 mg —— 100 ml		10^6	−	−
→ 0.30	→ 10 ml	30,000	3,000	3,000
→ 0.20	→ 10 ml	20,000	2,000	2,000
→ 0.15	→ 10 ml	15,000	1,500	1,500
→ 0.10	→ 10 ml	10,000	1,000	1,000
→ 0.20	→ 20 ml	10,000	−	
→ 7.4	→ 10 ml	7,400	740	750
→ 4.9	→ 10 ml	4,900	490	500
→ 2.9	→ 10 ml	2,900	290	300
→ 1.4	→ 10 ml	1,400	140	150
→ 0.9	→ 10 ml	900	90	100
→ 0.4	→ 10 ml	400	40	50

Notes:
(1) Serial dilutions are avoided to prevent cumulative undetectable error.
(2) Dilutions are stored in 10 ml aliquots in rubber-stoppered tubes and discarded after repeated opening of the tube.

Dialysis Tubing. The dialysis tubing is seamless regenerated cellulose, 24 Å average pore size, 0.25 in. in diameter. To prepare the tubing, boil it for 5 min in 5% $NaHCO_3$ and rinse with distilled water. Wash it in 0.01 M Tris HCl. 0.002 M ethylenediaminetetra-acetic acid (EDTA) buffer, pH 7.4, for 24 hr, and rinse for 24 hr in four changes of distilled water. Tubing not used within one week is discarded. You will need 350 cm for one experiment.

Buffer. The buffer used for homogenization of tissue, dilution of cytosol, and the dialysis solution is Tris HCl 0.01 M, $CaCl_2$ 0.003 M, pH 7.4.

Cytosol. A rat in midpregnancy is a good model animal. Anesthetize the rat with ether, open the abdomen, and exsanguinate it by aortic puncture. Excise the uterus, separating it from the cervix, mesentary, and fallopian tubes. Slit it open with scissors, peel off the implantation sites and endometrium with a scal-

STEROID "RECEPTOR" PROTEINS

pel, blot gently, and weigh. Subsequent procedures are done at 0–5°C. Rinse for 30 min in two changes of normal saline. Cut up the tissue (3–4 g is sufficient) with scissors and homogenize it in 3 vol of buffer in a motor-driven, all-glass conical homogenizer (Kontes) surrounded by ice. Rinse the homogenizer with 1 vol of buffer. Centrifuge at 10,000 × $\underline{g}$ × 10 min and recentrifuge the supernatant at 105,000 × $\underline{g}$ × 60 min. Measure the volume of cytosol obtained. On a 0.1 ml aliquot, diluted 100-fold, determine the protein concentration [2]. Take a portion of cytosol sufficient to give a protein concentration of 1 mg/ml when diluted to 25 ml. Dilute this quantity of cytosol to 25 ml with buffer.

Multiple Equilibrium Dialysis. Each dialysis is done in a 20 ml screw cap liquid scintillation counting vial. Add 10 pmole (0.1 ml) of ^{3}H-progesterone to each of 24 vials. Add unlabeled progesterone, 0.1 ml of each of the 10 dilutions to 10 duplicate pairs of the vials. With 2 vials which contain only ^{3}H-progesterone, you will have 11 different steroid concentrations, each in duplicate. To the remaining 2 vials, add scintillation solution for accurate determination of ^{3}H-progesterone added. With the 22 dialysis vials, blow off the ethanol under nitrogen, add 15 ml of buffer, cap, and agitate for 30 min at 37°C (Dubnoff shaking incubator) to redissolve the steroid. Remove the vials from the incubator onto ice. Cut a segment of dialysis tubing 10–15 cm, knot one end tightly, pipet 1 ml of cold cytosol into the bag and knot the top end. Leave some air in the top of the bag (0.5–1.0 cm). Cut excess tails from the bag, place it in a dialysis vial, and cap it. Agitate the vials gently at 0–5°C (a second Dubnoff in the cold room) for about 40 hr. (See Figures 4 and 5.) After dialysis, remove the vials from the cold room $\underline{\text{on ice}}$. Remove each bag, cut off the top, and empty it into a small tube. Allow tubes and vials to come to room temperature (10 min for tubes, 60 min for vials). Pipet 0.5 ml aliquots from each of the tubes and vials into counting vials. The protein determination having been done at room temperature, the proper temperature-volume relationships have been maintained. Count for sufficient time to reduce the counting error to less than 2%, usually 1 min. Efficiency can be monitored by including 3 vials containing 10 μliter ^{3}H$_2$O and 0.5 ml of distilled water. In our system, quenching does not occur with either 0.5 ml of water or cytosol, and counter stability is monitored with a sealed standard. With a protein concentration of 1 mg/ml, the inside volume does not change during dialysis. At a higher protein concentration the final inside volume must be measured by protein determination.

Data Analysis. The derivation of the total number of high-affinity binding sites from the multiple dialyses is based on linearization of the data as described by Scatchard [3]. The parameters to be plotted are calculated as follows:

$$\frac{[B]}{[U]} = \frac{[\text{cpm inside}] - [\text{cpm outside}]}{[\text{cpm outside}]}$$

$$[B] = ([\text{cpm inside}] - [\text{cpm outside}]) \times \frac{\text{total steroid added}}{\text{total cpm added}}$$

The ratio of [B]/[U] is plotted against [B] (Figure 1). With a single binding system, to which the laws of mass action are applicable, this plot produces a straight line with a slope of $-K_a$ (the negative of the association constant), an intercept on the abscissa of n[M] (the molar concentration of binding sites), and an intercept on the ordinate of $K_a \cdot n[M]$.

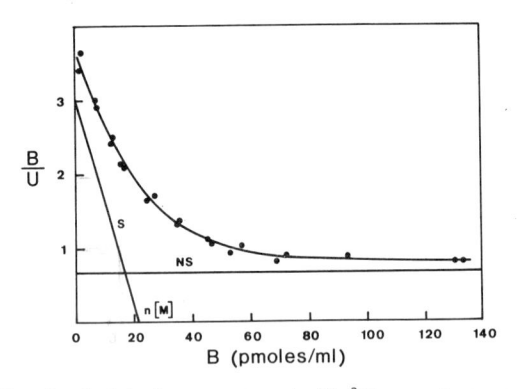

FIGURE 1. Scatchard plot of an experiment with ^{3}H-progesterone and uterine cytosol from a 9 day pregnant rat. The dots are the experimental points. The horizontal straight line is the low-affinity binding and the steeply sloping straight line is the high-affinity binding, as calculated from the experimental curve. n[M] = 21.4 × 10^{-12}/mg protein. K_a = 1.41 × 10^8 M^{-1}. S = specific. NS = Nonspecific.

The derivation of these parameters from the general equation for the association constant is simple and readily conceptualized.

$$K_a = \frac{[\text{Steroid} \sim \text{Protein}]}{[\text{Steroid}][\text{Protein}]}$$

$$K_a = \frac{[B]}{[U][\text{free binding sites}]}$$

$$\frac{[B]}{[U]} = K_a [\text{free binding sites}]$$

STEROID "RECEPTOR" PROTEINS

$$\frac{[B]}{[U]} = K_a([\text{total sites}] - [\text{occupied sites}])$$

$$\frac{[B]}{[U]} = K_a(n[M] - [B])$$

The latter equation is a straight line with a slope of $-K_a$. At the intercept on the ordinate, B has become 0 and:

$$\frac{[B]}{[U]} = K_a \cdot n[M]$$

At the intercept on the abscissa, B/U has become 0, and:

$$0 = K_a(n[M] - [B])$$

$$[B] = n[M]$$

As is evident in the example shown in Figures 1 and 2, our experimental points are not linear. High-affinity binding, which rapidly becomes saturated, is seen in the initial steep descent of the curve. As the slope levels out, non-specific, lower-affinity binding of unlimited capacity becomes apparent. The curve is the sum of the two classes of binding. The contribution of the non-specific binding to the experimental curve is appreciable, even at low steroid concentrations, and cannot be ignored.

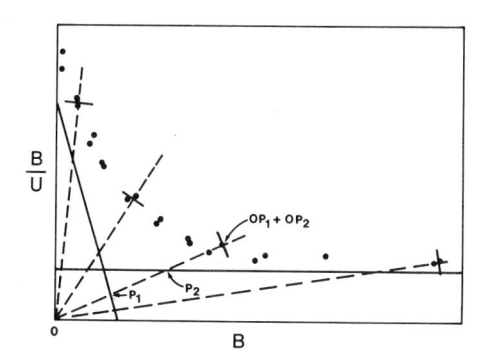

FIGURE 2. Evaluation of the fit of the calculated two-line model to the experimental data. The dotted lines drawn from the origin (O) to the experimental points intercept the two solid straight lines at P_1 and P_2. The sum of the distances, OP_1 and OP_2 is marked on each dotted line by the short bar ($OP_1 + OP_2$), confirming the fit of the two-line model to the experimental curve.

The experimental curve must be defined by a full range of points so that both the steep slope at low steroid concentrations and the almost 0 slope at high concentrations are defined. In Figures 1 and 2 the first four pairs of points at low steroid concentrations appear to be linear. If this were accepted as evidence of a single binding system, extrapolation to the baseline would overestimate the receptor concentration by about 70%. The leveling out of the curve must be observed to define the nonspecific binding.

The steeply sloping portion of the curve must include an adequate number of points to define the high-affinity binding. At low receptor concentrations this will require the use of smaller steroid concentrations. In the example shown in Figure 3, dialysis with 1 pmole of steroid was required to get below the saturation concentration, and additional points in this range would be desirable to confirm the apparent curve.

The relationship of the binding parameters for two binding systems is described by the formula [4]:

$$\frac{[B]}{[U]} = \frac{K_1 n_1 [M_1]}{K_1 [U] + 1} + \frac{K_2 n_2 [M_2]}{K_2 [U] + 1}$$

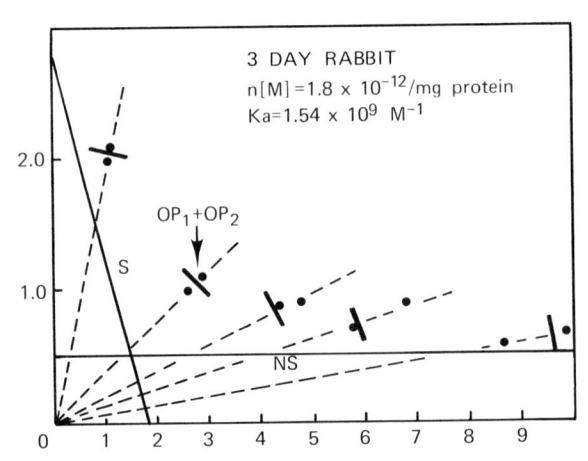

FIGURE 3. An example of application of the methodology to cytosol of a 3 day pregnant rabbit with a very low concentration of high-affinity binding sites, 1.8 pmole/mg of protein. The usual lowermost quantity of total steroid added, 10 pmole, has been supplemented by two additional dialyses, each containing 1 pmole of progesterone. Dialyses at seven higher concentrations of progesterone are off the graph to the right, but were included in the computer derivation of the two straight lines. The fit of the two-line model to the experimental curve is indicated by the short bars ($OP_1 + OP_2$). S = Specific. NS = Nonspecific.

The algebraic procedure to resolve this equation has been described [5] and computer programs have been used to perform the calculations [1,6]. The formula defines the parameters of the Scatchard plot and is the mathematical basis for our computer data analysis. The program is written in FORTRAN for the Burroughs B6700 computer. The computer first derives the Scatchard parameters, [B]/[U] and [B], from the counting data as described above. On the assumption that the observed curve represents the sum of two straight lines, the program derives these two lines by iterated trial and convergence. The printed output includes the following information: (1) the observed values of B and B/U, (2) the coordinate intercepts and slopes of the two straight lines, (3) the theoretical values of B/U for each value of B, calculated back from the proposed two straight lines, and (4) the residuals, that is, the difference between each theoretical value of B/U and the original observed value. The residuals provide a check on the fit of the observed data to the derived two line model.

To assess overall experimental precision, including both the technique of dialysis and the computer-derived analysis, the experimental points, and the calculated lines are graphed. While the theoretical B/U values from the computer could be graphed to assess the conformity of the observed curve with the theoretical curve, it is more convenient to apply graphical summation [7] of the two straight lines (Figure 2). The summation of the two binding systems is not upward from the abscissa but radially from the point of 0 binding, the origin. The distance from the origin to the first straight line, added to the distance from the origin to the second straight line, is equal to the distance from the origin to the theoretical curve and should coincide with the experimental points.

DISCUSSION OF THE METHOD

Reliability. The technical precision of the 21 dialyses shown in Figures 1 and 2 is indicated by the agreement of each point with its duplicate and with the overall curve. The graphical summation confirms the good fit of the data to the calculated to line model. In the example shown, the difference between duplicates and the means of duplicate pairs is 2.4% ± 0.5 standard error (SE). The experimental data fed to the computer 10 times gave identical results each time. The K_a of the high-affinity binding system determined individually on the cytosol fraction of 8 different 9 day pregnant animals was 1.5 ± 0.1 SE $\times 10^8$ M^{-1}. The potential precision of the method appears to be limited only by the care with which it is executed.

The accuracy of our measurement of receptor proteins cannot be directly assessed without purified preparations. However, the firm theoretical basis of multiple equilibrium dialysis justifies confidence in its accuracy [1]. A potential source of error which requires consideration is the effect of endogenous ligand. Endogenous progesterone in the cytosol in equilibrium with the added progesterone in the dialyses could artifactually decrease the apparent association constant. Considering the maximum concentration of myometrial progesterone in the pregnant rat, 22.5 µg/100 g on day 11 [8], and assuming that this progesterone were entirely in the cytosol, in the experiment shown in Figure 1 we would be adding 16 pmoles of endogenous progesterone to each dialysis. If this were true, the association constant would be underestimated by 9.7%. However, intracellular steroid hormones appear to be largely associated with the nuclei [10–14]. One hour after injection of radiolabeled progesterone into the pregnant rat, 26% of the intracellular hormone was present in the cytosol [11]. Allowing for the more likely estimate of 4 pmole of endogenous ligand, recalculation of the results of the experiment indicates that the apparent association constant would be underestimated by 2%, an insignificant error. Of greater importance in the present context is the accuracy of the determination of the concentration of binding sites, n[M]. With endogenous ligand in equilibrium with the added steroid, the value of n[M] should theoretically be unaffected. The recalculations described above, allowing for 16 and 4 pmole of endogenous ligand, indicated an error in the determination of n[M] of 0.9% and 0.2%, an artifact arising in the data analysis.

A more significant potential error exists if the endogenous ligand is bound to the receptors and does not dissociate and reach equilibrium with the added steroid. With the estimated 4 pmole of endogenous progesterone initially entirely bound to the receptor, n[M] reflected in Figure 1 would be too low by a maximum of 15%, and would gradually increase toward the true value as a function of time. As is shown in Figure 4, the dialysis equilibrium which is attained at 20 hr remains stable for 120 hr. Three explanations for this stability can be considered: (1) appreciable dissociation of endogenous complexes does not occur in 120 hr, or (2) true equilibrium of endogenous ligand with exogenous ligand has already been attained at 20 hr, or (3) bound endogenous ligand is too small to be appreciable beyond 20 hr.

The first two possibilities can be tested experimentally, and the results are shown in Figure 5. This experiment is designed to permit observation of the dissociation of ^{3}H-progesterone binding with reassociation of freed ^{3}H-progesterone largely prevented by excess unlabeled steroid. The residual binding of a small amount of radiolabeled steroid reflects reassociation with unsaturable nonspecific binders. It can be concluded that the equilibrium which is attained

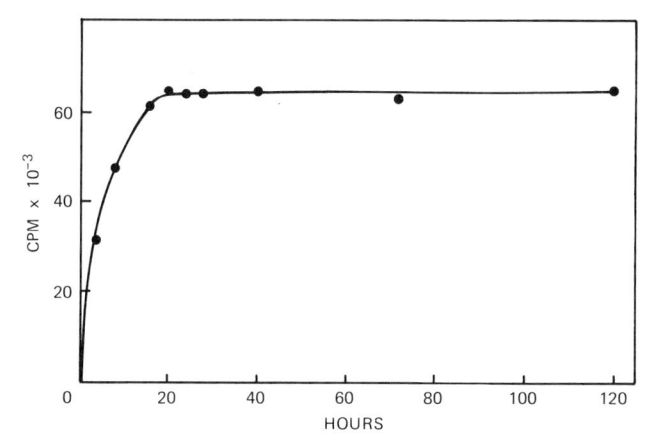

FIGURE 4. Equilibration of the dialysis in 20 hr, and stability of the equilibrium for 120 hr, is shown. A series of identical dialyses which were initiated simultaneously, were terminated sequentially at the times indicated. Ten pmole of ^{3}H-progesterone were in each outside solution and 1 ml of cytoplasm (protein 1 mg/ml) was inside the bag. The cpm inside the bags are plotted.

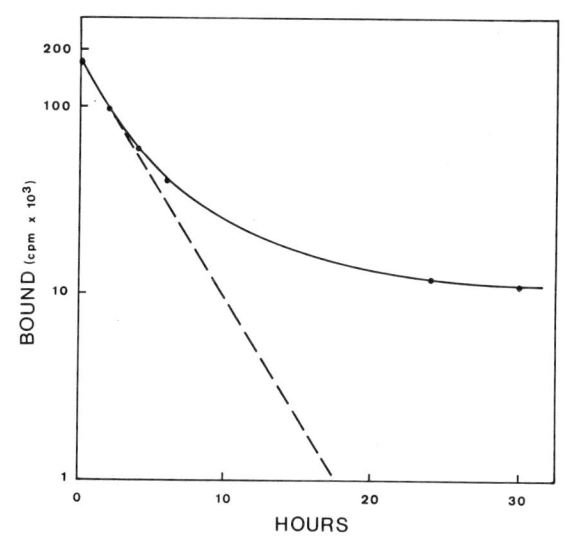

FIGURE 5. Dissociation of ^{3}H-progesterone bound by rat uterine cytosol at 5°C. Twenty ml of cytosol (protein 1 mg/ml) and 200 pmole of ^{3}H-progesterone were incubated overnight at 5°C. Unbound steroid was removed by exposure to dextran-coated charcoal for 10 min followed by centrifugation. Excess unlabeled progesterone (10^{-6} M) was added, and aliquots were dialyzed against 15 ml quantities of buffer. The dialyses were terminated sequentially at the times indicated. The solid line is the experimental curve. The dashed line is an extrapolation of the initial slope of the dissociation curve and represents an estimate of the dissociation rate of the receptor-steroid complexes and/or the diffusion rate.

in 20 hr includes equilibration of any endogenous steroid which may be present.

The specificity of the methodology relates to the question of whether a single high-affinity protein, that is the receptor, is being measured. The first consideration is the fit of the two line model to the experimental data. If the high-affinity binding is attributable to two components, which differ appreciably in their affinity for the steroid, true linearization of the data would not be possible, and a three-line model would be required to provide a fit to the data. It can be seen by comparison of Figures 2 and 3 that greater confidence in the correctness of the two-line model is warranted in Figure 2 where the high-affinity binding is defined by a full range of points. These considerations of linearity cannot exclude the presence of different components which have similar binding affinities for the steroid, and the final assessment of specificity rests on the total physiochemical evidence that a single high-affinity binding component is present in the cytosol.

The sensitivity of the method is limited only by the specific activity of the radiolabeled progesterone and the associated counting time required. This currently places the practical lower limit below 1 pmole/mg of protein.

The only assumption which we have made in the determination of n[M] is that mass action theory is applicable, that is, that the binding sites are homogeneous and noninteracting. It is recognized on the basis of theoretical considerations that this is not strictly correct, and that determination of whether the deviation from mass action theory in a given system is negligible or appreciable requires experimental assessment [14]. With the binding of cortisol to serum albumin, the binding parameters are dependent to a significant degree on steroid concentration and even more on protein concentration [15]. An influence of protein concentration in the opposite direction was found with serum α_1-acid glycoprotein (AAG), however, this is thought to be due to contaminating inhibitors [1]. With neither of these proteins are the binding sites homogeneous [1,15]. Rat corticosteroid-binding globulin (CBG) has been shown to depolymerize at low corticosterone concentrations with a decrease of binding affinity [16].

At present, while there is no evidence that receptor-steroid binding is dependent on protein concentration, comparison of observations made at significantly different total protein concentrations requires experimental justification, and it is not precluded that the concentration of high-affinity binding protein could influence the determination of K_a and n[M]. Concerning the possible influence of steroid concentration on binding, the fit of the data to the linear two-phase model, over a wide range of steroid concentration makes this possibility unlikely.

OTHER METHODS

Graphical Presentation. No single method of graphing steroid-protein binding data is ideal for all situations. The Lineweaver–Burke reciprocal plot has been used [1], but the crowding of points near the ordinate at higher steroid concentrations makes it generally unsatisfactory for steroid-protein binding studies. The Scatchard plot gives a better distribution of the full range of points, including higher steroid concentrations. This is more satisfactory for the recognition of both primary and secondary binding systems as are found in cytoplasm. However, the Scatchard plot tends to crowd the points close to the ordinate at low steroid concentrations. The relatively even distribution of points shown in Figure 1 is achieved by increasing the steroid concentration by larger increments, 5-fold, at the lowest concentrations. In Figure 5 most of the experimental points are off the graph to the right. Nonlinear logarithmic graphing permits a more even distribution of points over a wide range of steroid concentration. The procedure is more complicated and more time consuming but in complex situations, such as two or more high-affinity binding systems, it may be worthwhile [17,18]. The Scatchard plot is satisfactory for most cytoplasmic steroid-binding data and is the most widely utilized plot.

Other Analytical Methods. A variety of methods have been applied to the measurement of high-affinity steroid-binding proteins. They may be classified, generally, as either equilibrium or nonequilibrium methods, the latter differing from each other primarily in the manner by which specifically bound steroid is separated from nonspecifically bound and unbound steroid.

Ultrafiltration retains most of the theoretical advantage of equilibrium dialysis while reducing the time factor, and it has been applied to the study of plasma proteins in a manner similar to that described here [6,19,20]. The deviation from equilibrium may be minimized if the volume of the filtrate is small ($<10\%$) and if the rate of dissociation of the complexes is slow relative to filtration time. Both bound and unbound steroid can be measured. Ultrafiltration is potentially advantageous when a shortened time interval is desired, as with an unstable protein or for determinations at physiological temperatures. The problem of volume changes encountered in dialysis with higher protein concentrations is circumvented in ultrafiltration. However, departure from the experimental simplicity of dialysis increases the potential for artifact. Inattention to details such as the water content of the filtration membrane [6], temperature variation in thermo-regulated centrifuges [19], or binding of steroid to the filtration membrane [20], may introduce significant systematic error. The question of endogenous ligand must be considered as discussed above. The most serious disadvantage of ultrafiltration is the requirement for relatively large volumes of cytosol (about 10 ml per tube). This requirement, coupled with the fact that ultrafiltration is somewhat more laborious than dialysis, limits its use in the measurement of cytoplasmic receptors to situations in which the particular characteristics of the method are advantageous.

The desire for methodology which is rapid has resulted in the introduction of numerous methods for measuring steroid-binding proteins. The saving in technical time is usually achieved by using a single experiment, rather than a multipoint, approach. If a multipoint technique is used, there is no saving of technical time but the waiting time required for dialysis is substantially reduced to provide quicker availability of results. The rapid methods which have been applied to receptor protein measurement are largely nonequilibrium methods, and this is the major theoretical and practical limitation of these techniques.

The essential requirement in the nonequilibrium measurement of binding protein is to separate the protein-bound steroid from unbound steroid so that one or the other can be measured. In practice, the protein is usually incubated with an excess of radiolabeled steroid to saturate the protein, and the bound and unbound fractions are separated by physiochemical means. The receptor-steroid complexes can be precipitated with ammonium sulfate [21-23] or protamine chloride [23,24], or adsorbed onto glass beads [23,25] or a hydroxyapatite column [26]. Density gradients of sucrose [1,27] or glycerol [28] and electrophoresis [1,23,29] have been used. Two of the most rapid and widely used methods rely on removal of unbound steroid by Sephadex gel filtration [1,30-32] or adsorption onto dextran-coated charcoal [18,33,34].

By departure from equilibrium conditions, and by failure to measure both bound and unbound steroid, these methods introduce a number of potential difficulties: (1) The intended saturation of the protein is not actually complete. Excess steroid on the order of 100-fold will be required to exceed 95% saturation of the high-affinity binding in rat uterine cytosol. (2) The measurement of the macromolecule-steroid complex is made, not at equilibrium, but during the process of dissociation. (3) Rapid separation of bound and unbound steroid may not allow sufficient time for removal of free steroid by an adsorbant [18,35,36] or for dissociation of nonspecific binding [1,18,32]. A variety of technical problems arise such as binding of steroid to filtration gel [37] and centrifuge tubes [1] and binding of both steroid and steroid-receptor to charcoal [23] or laboratory equipment [12]. Usually only bound steroid is measured directly. Any estimate of unbound steroid based on what was added must be evaluated critically. As discussed above, differences in apparent binding due to variation in endogenous ligand must be considered. Jungblut [23] assayed the cytoplasmic estrogen receptors in calf uterus and mammary tumor by six different nonequilibrium methods. The highest results were obtained with agar gel electrophoresis and Sephadex gel filtration. If the results by these two methods are arbitrarily taken as 100%, the results with other methods were: charcoal 62 and 49%, glass bead adsorbtion 17 and 41%, sucrose density gradient 16 and 30%, and protamine chloride precipitation 10 and 23%. These results neither validate nor discredit any of the methods, but do serve to emphasize the importance of the problems which have been discussed and the necessity of validating any quantitative application of these methods.

These important theoretical and technical problems notwithstanding, rapid nonequilibrium methods have been applied to advantage under well defined circumstances in which the above difficulties could be circumvented or accounted for, and, generally, when only data of relative magnitude was desired. In the measurement of tissue steroid-binding proteins, circumstances are usually not well defined and, more importantly, not uniform among different samples. Variable nonspecific binding, the possibility of multiple binding systems, differences in endogenous steroid concentration, differences between tissues, and other unknown variables introduce uncertainty into any determination of binding activity in which the potential difficulties enumerated above are not adequately considered for the specific circumstances under study. When these methods are appropriately applied and interpreted within their limitations they are very useful in steroid-binding studies. Multiple equilibrium dialysis serves as a model to elucidate the principles of receptor-protein measurement and provides a standard against which other methods can be evaluated.

REFERENCES

[1] Westphal, U. 1971. Steroid-protein interactions. Springer-Verlag, New York.
[2] Lowry, O. H., N. J. Rosebrough, A. L. Farr, and R. J. Randall. 1951. J. Biol. Chem. 193:265.
[3] Scatchard, G. 1949. Ann. N. Y. Acad. Sci. 51:660.
[4] Edsall, J. T., and J. Wyman. 1958. Biophysical chemistry, vol. 1. Academic Press, New York.
[5] Hart, H. E. 1965. Bull. Math. Biophys. 27:87.
[6] Keller, N., L. R. Sendelbeck, U. I. Richardson, C. Moore, and F. E. Yates. 1966. Endocrinology 79:884.
[7] Rosenthal, H. E. 1967. Anal. Biochem. 20:525.
[8] Wiest, W. G. 1970. Endocrinology 87:43.

[9] Noteboom, W. D., and J. Gorski. 1965. Arch. Biochem. Biophys. 111:559.
[10] Fanestil, D. D., and I. S. Edelman. 1966. Proc. Nat. Acad. Sci. 56:872.
[11] Wichmann, K. 1967. Acta Endocr. Suppl. 116:1.
[12] Spelsberg, T. C., A. W. Steggles, and B. W. O'Malley. 1971. J. Biol. Chem. 246:4188.
[13] O'Malley, B. W., M. R. Sherman, and D. O. Toft. 1970. Proc. Nat. Acad. Sci. 67:501.
[14] Weber, G. 1972. Biochemistry 11:864.
[15] Brunkhorst, W. K., and E. L. Hess. 1965. Arch. Biochem. Biophys. 111:54.
[16] Chader, G. J., and U. Westphal. 1968. Biochemistry 7:4272.
[17] Baulieu, E. E., and J. P. Raynaud. 1970. Eur. J. Biochem. 13:293.
[18] Bauleiu, E. E., J. P. Raynaud and E. Milgrom. 1970. Acta Endocr. Suppl. 147:104.
[19] Doe, R. P., P. Dickinson, H. H. Zinneman, and U. S. Seal. 1969. J. Clin. Endocr. Metab. 29:757.
[20] Rosenthal, H. E., E. Pietrzak, W. R. Slaunwhite, Jr., and A. A. Sandberg. 1972. J. Clin. Endocr. Metab. 34:805.
[21] Mayes, D., and C. A. Nugent. 1968. J. Clin. Endocr. Metab. 28:1169.
[22] Heyns, W., and P. DeMoor. 1971. Steroids 18:709.
[23] Jungblut, P. W., S. Hughes, A. Hughes, and R. K. Wagner. 1972. Acta Endocr. 70:185.
[24] Steggles, A. W., and R. J. King. 1970. Biochem. J. 118:695.
[25] Clark, J. H., and J. Gorski. 1969. Biochim. Biophys. Acta 192:508.
[26] Erdos, T., M. Best-Belpomme, and R. Bessada. 1970. Anal. Biochem. 37:244.
[27] Davies, I. J., and K. J. Ryan. 1972. Endocrinology 90:507.
[28] McEwan, B. S., C. Magnus and G. Wallach. 1972. Endocrinology 90:217.
[29] Sherman, M. R., P. L. Corvol, and B. W. O'Malley. 1970. J. Biol. Chem. 245:6085.
[30] Doe, R. P., R. Fernandez, and U. S. Seal. 1964. J. Clin. Endocr. 24:1024.
[31] Gorski, J., D. Toft, G. Shyamala, D. Smith, and A. Notides. 1968. Prog. Horm. Res. 24:45.
[32] Milgrom, E., M. Perrot, M. Atger, and E. E. Baulieu. 1972. Endocrinology 90:1064.
[33] Korenman, S. G. 1970. J. Clin. Endocr. Metab. 87:1119.
[34] Schrader, W. T. and B. W. O'Malley. 1972. J. Biol. Chem. 247:51.
[35] Korenman, S. G. 1970. In discussion of Corker, C. S., D. Exley, and F. Naftolin, Acta Endocr. Suppl. 147:305.
[36] Korenman, S. G. 1970. Acta Endocr. Suppl. 147:291.
[37] Pearlman, W. H. 1970. Acta Endocr. Suppl. 147:225.

Separation of Proteins According to Size by Gel Filtration

RICHARD L. EASTERDAY

GENERAL CONSIDERATIONS

Gel filtration is a powerful technique for the fractionation and separation of molecules and other biological materials according to their size and shape. Although other techniques are available (rate zonal sedimentation, for example) gel filtration has been the preferred technique for biological molecules since the introduction of Sephadex® in 1959.

Prior to 1959, a number of workers [1-5] had observed that certain porous media, including some used for electrophoresis and ion exchange chromatography, had varying abilities to discriminate between molecules on the basis of their size. Porath and Flodin working with Tiselius at the Institute of Biochemistry in Uppsala, Sweden, realized the potential usefulness of cross-linked dextran gels for separating molecules on the basis of size while attempting to perfect an anticonvective medium for electrophoresis [6].

Gel Properties and Structure

Sephadex gels are synthesized by the cross-linking of dextrans. Dextran is a water-soluble polyglucose which is produced by the bacterium Leuconostoc mesenteroides as a protective coat. The high molecular weight native dextran is partially hydrolyzed with acid, and purified by fractional precipitation with alcohol. By reacting purified dextran fractions with epichlorohydrin in the presence of base and a reducing agent, a cross-linked, three-dimensional porous network which swells in polar solvents is produced. Figure 1 shows portions of two dextran chains which have been cross-linked with epichlorohydrin. Note that the dextran chains are made up of glucose units linked through alpha, 1,6-

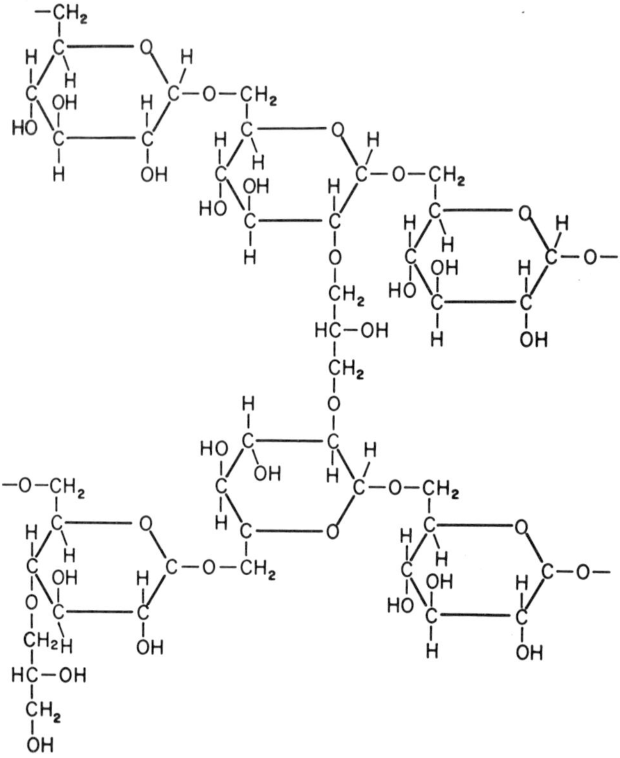

FIGURE 1. Chemical structure of cross-linked dextran chains.

glycosidic linkages. The cross-linking reaction produces very stable ether linkages between the dextran chain and the glycerol residues. The Sephadex gels can therefore be used in the wide pH range of 2–10, are insoluble in all solvents, and are stable to high salt concentrations. Sephadex can be sterilized in the wet state at neutral pH or in the dry state by autoclaving for 30 min at 120°C. Prolonged exposure of the gels to oxidizing agents will affect the gel and should be avoided. Their excellent chemical properties make the Sephadex gels well suited for a chromatographic medium. All Sephadex gels are synthesized as beads since such particles have better hydrodynamic properties than granular- or irregular-shaped materials.

A number of Sephadex gels with different average pore sizes and different abilities to swell are produced by controlling the degree of cross-linking. Table I shows that eight Sephadex gels are available for gel filtration of molecules with

TABLE I. Physical Data Sephadex Gels

Sephadex type	Particle diameter, μ	Water regain, ml H_2O/g dry Sephadex	Bed volume, ml/g dry Sephadex	Fractionation range Peptides and globular proteins	Fractionation range Dextrans
Sephadex G-10	40–120	1.0±0.1	2 – 3	700	700
Sephadex G-15	40–120	1.5±0.2	2.5– 3.5	1,500	1,500
Sephadex G-25 Coarse	100–300	2.5±0.2	4 – 6	1,000– 5,000	100– 5,000
Sephadex G-25 Medium	50–150				
Sephadex G-25 Fine	20– 80				
Sephadex G-25 Superfine	10– 40				
Sephadex G-50 Coarse	100–300	5.0±0.3	9 –11	1,500– 30,000	500– 10,000
Sephadex G-50 Medium	50–150				
Sephadex G-50 Fine	20– 80				
Sephadex G-50 Superfine	10– 40				
Sephadex G-75	40–120	7.5±0.5	12 –15	3,000– 70,000	1,000– 50,000
Sephadex G-75 Superfine	10– 40				
Sephadex G-100	40–120	10.0±1.0	15 –20	4,000–150,000	1,000–100,000
Sephadex G-100 Superfine	10– 40				
Sephadex G-150	40–120	15.0±1.5	20 –30	5,000–400,000	1,000–150,000
Sephadex G-150 Superfine	10– 40				
Sephadex G-200	40–120	20.0±2.0	30 –40	5,000–800,000	1,000–200,000
Sephadex G-200 Superfine	10– 40				

molecular weights from essentially 0 to 800,000 dalton. The superfine gels with a 10–40 μ dry particle size are used for thin layer gel filtration and high-resolution column chromatography. The coarse and medium grades are used for large-scale preparative separations, industrial applications, or where ultrahigh flow rates are required in laboratory experiments. The standard grade 40–120 μ is used for routine laboratory work. The Sephadex G number designation (that is, G-25, G-200, etc.) reflects the ability of the gel to swell in water and the relative degree of cross-linking. The amount of water taken up per gram of dry Sephadex is defined as the water regain value. Sephadex G-25 and G-200 take up 2.5 ml and 20 ml of water/g of dry gel, respectively. Doubling of the water regain value gives an approximation of the bed volume which can be expected from 1 g of dry gel. The fractionation ranges for the various gels are listed in Table I. Note that two ranges are given for the more porous gels. Since all compounds of equal molecular weight do not necessarily have the same molecular size, the fractionation range for different types of molecules such as proteins and polysaccharides may be slightly different.

For example, a 200,000 molecular weight dextran molecule, which is a randomly coiled and rather extended molecule, is so large that it cannot penetrate into the Sephadex G-200 beads. A globular protein molecule, which is more dense and tightly coiled, must have a molecular weight of almost 800,000 before it is large enough to be excluded from the inner volume of the Sephadex G-200 beads. In the low molecular weight range, only one value is listed because the tertiary structure is limited for such molecules and is less important in determining their size.

The fractionation range for gel filtration media has been extended to approximately 3×10^7 dalton with the advent of the Sepharose® gels. These gels are produced from agarose, the neutral portion of agar. Agar consists primarily of two polysaccharides [7]. The agaropectin portion contains 6% sulfate groups, pyruvic acid and gluconic acid. These charged materials make it undesirable for gel filtration or electrophoresis. The neutral portion, called agarose, is a galactose polymer consisting of alternate residues of D-galactose and 3,6-anhydro-L-galactose. By varying the concentration of hot aqueous solutions of agarose which are stirred and cooled in a mixture of toluene, carbon tetrachloride, and surfactant, spherical beads of Sepharose gels with varying fractionation ranges are produced. Unlike the Sephadex gels, Sepharose polysaccharide chains are not covalently cross-linked. Their porous structure is apparently due to molecular bonding such as hydrogen bonding formed during gel preparation.

Three Sepharose gels, 2B, 4B, and 6B, are available as aqueous suspension in 0.02% sodium azide as a preservative. The number designation refers to the fact

GEL FILTRATION

that they are beaded gels made from 2, 4, and 6% agarose. Dehydration of the gels will cause destruction of their structure. Sepharose gels can be used in the pH range of 4–9 and are stable in 1 M salt, 2 M urea, detergents such as Triton X-100, guanidine HCl, sodium dodecyl sulfate (SDS), and sodium deoxychloate. The gels should be used at temperatures between 0 and 40°C. If they are heated above 50°C, they will begin to melt.

Gel Filtration Principle

Gel chromatography with Sephadex can be considered as a kind of partition chromatography in which the gel beads are the stationary phase and the solvent used for swelling is the moving phase. The partition of solute between the very similar mobile and stationary phases is governed by several factors. The predominant factor is that of molecular size.

The porous three-dimensional dextran network of the Sephadex bead acts as a steric barrier to solute molecules as they attempt to equilibrate with the liquid inside and outside of the bead. The ability of a solute molecule to penetrate the gel network is a function of its molecular size and shape. Certain molecules are too large to penetrate the gel matrix and exist only in the liquid in the space outside of the beads called the void volume (V_0). Some molecules are so small that they can penetrate almost all of the liquid volume inside of the bead called the inner volume (V_i). All other molecules are capable of penetrating a fraction of the internal volume.

Figure 2 shows a schematic drawing of a chromatographic column which has been filled with swollen Sephadex beads. The large open circles represent the Sephadex beads. The space between the beads is also occupied with the swelling solvent. The total volume of the bed (V_t) is equal to the sum of the internal liquid volume of the beads (V_i), the void volume between the gel beads (V_0) and the volume of the gel matrix itself (V_g).

$$V_t = V_0 + V_i + V_g \tag{1}$$

In Figure 2 a mixture of two solute molecules have been added to the top of the Sephadex gel bed. The large dark circles represent molecules which are so large that it is assumed that they are restricted from penetrating the inner volume of the gel matrix. They are therefore excluded from the liquid inside the gel beads and must exist only in the void volume between the gel beads. The small dark circles represent small molecules which are so small that it is assumed they can penetrate any part of the inner liquid volume of the gel. These small molecules must spend part of their time outside of the beads and part of it inside of the

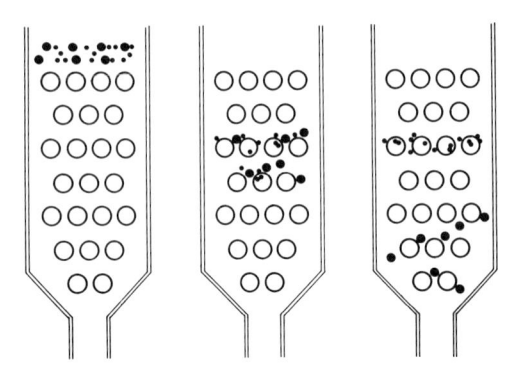

FIGURE 2. Schematic representation of gel filtration [8].

beads. They therefore take a longer path through the column bed than the larger molecules. As a result, it will take them a longer period of time to move through the gel bed than the large molecules which move only in the void volume.

Those molecules which are completely excluded from a Sephadex gel will appear after a volume equal to the void volume has been eluted. The elution volume for a compound (V_e) is equal to the amount of effluent collected from the time the sample was placed on the bed until the compound appears in the effluent. In this case V_e equals V_0. The void volume for all Sephadex gels can be determined experimentally with a solution of Blue Dextran 2000, a colored dextran with an average molecular weight of 2,000,000. Small molecules which can occupy all of the liquid volume inside of the gel will be eluted after a volume equal to $V_0 + V_i$ has been collected, that is, $V_e = V_0 + V_i$. The total volume of the gel bed is defined by (1). The total bed volume, V_t, can be calculated from the equation $V_t = \pi r^2 \cdot h$ where r and h equal the radius and height of the bed, respectively. It can also be determined experimentally by calibrating the column with eluant. The V_0 can be determined experimentally with compounds such as Blue Dextran 2000 which are excluded from the inner volume of the gel, that is, they exist only in the void volume. The Blue Dextran is not only useful for determining the column void volume but also allows one to check the quality of the column packing. The V_i can be calculated from (2) where W_r and d equal the water regain value and wet density, respectively.

$$V_i = \frac{d \cdot W_r}{1 + W_r} \cdot (V_t - V_0) \tag{2}$$

$$d = \frac{W_r + 1}{W_r + 0.61} \tag{3}$$

GEL FILTRATION

The elution of solute molecules in gel filtration experiments can be characterized in several ways. The fraction of the gel phase which is accessible to a solute molecule can be described by constants similar to the distribution coefficient in ordinary partition chromatography. The parameter K_{av} [9] is used when the whole gel ($V_g + V_i$) is considered as the stationary phase, while K_d [10] is used when only the liquid inside of the gel (V_i) is considered as the stationary phase. The constants for a given molecule may be calculated from experimentally determined elution volumes.

$$K_{av} = \frac{V_e - V_o}{V_t - V_o} \tag{4}$$

$$K_d = \frac{V_e - V_o}{V_i} \tag{5}$$

From (5) we can see that when V_e equals V_o, as for large molecules, such as Blue Dextran 2000, then K_d equals 0. If V_e equals V_o plus V_i, as for very small molecules, the K_d equals 1. All molecules which fall within the fractionation range of a given gel should have K_d values between 0 and 1. The K_d values greater than one have been observed on highly cross-linked gels for certain types of compounds such as those containing aromatic and heterocyclic ring structures. Under these circumstances, molecular sieving and/or adsorption chromatography are considered responsible for the K_d values greater than one. Advantage can often be taken of such selective interactions with the dense gels for the separation of molecules of similar size and molecular weight.

EXPERIMENTAL TECHNIQUE
—Gel and Eluant Selection

Let us now consider just how one would design and perform a gel filtration experiment. One must, of course, first select the proper gel. If the K_d or K_{av} values for the compounds of interest are known, then the gel on which we obtain the greatest numerical difference between the K_d values is the gel on which we will obtain the best separation. If the K_d values are unknown, but the approximate molecular weights are known, we can select the gel on the basis of the fractionation ranges listed in Table I. If nothing is known regarding the molecular weights of the compounds with which we are working, our first experiment should be performed with a somewhat porous Sephadex gel such as G-100 so that we can conveniently get an idea as to the range of the molecular weights of the compounds.

The amount of gel required for an experiment is easily calculated by dividing the amount of desired bed volume by twice the water regain value for the particular gel. A 10% excess of gel is recommended due to losses of gel during preparation.

The selection of eluant is usually made on the basis of the stability of the sample since the Sephadex gels are not affected by a wide range of conditions of pH, temperature, and salt concentration.

Gel Preparation

Next one must consider preparation of the gel for packing. Complete swelling of the gel under the proper conditions is important. Sephadex gels require from 3 hr to days at room temperature for complete swelling. The porous gels, such as G-200, with higher water regain values, require the longest swelling time. The swelling period may be accelerated by the use of a boiling water bath, that is, only 5 hr for G-100, G-150, and G-200. See Table II for exact recommendations.

TABLE II. Swelling Time for Sephadex Gels

Type of Sephadex	Minimum swelling time, hr	
	At room temperature	On boiling water bath
G-10, G-15, G-25, G-50	3	1
G-75	24	3
G-100, G-150, G-200	72	5
LH-20	3	

Although degassing of the buffer and Sephadex is not essential, it is advantageous in most cases. The gel should be added slowly to an excess of eluant with mixing to facilitate dispersion. The gel should be stirred, allowed to settle, and decanted intermittently. Stirring with a magnetic stirrer should be avoided since it may degrade the gel particles. The supernatant above the settled gel should always be clear before the gel is slurried for packing. Although Sepharose gels do not require swelling, they should be washed to remove the NaN_3 used as a preservative.

Antimicrobial Agents

Bacterial and fungal growth may interfere with the chromatographic properties of gel filtration media. The eluant in columns which are not in use should therefore generally contain a small amount of some bacteriostatic agent. Some of the more commonly used agents are described here.

GEL FILTRATION

Sodium azide (NaN$_3$), 0.02%, is widely used. It does not interact notably with proteins or carbohydrates or change their chromatographic behavior. Sodium azide interferes with fluorescent marking of proteins, the anthrone reaction, and inhibits certain enzymes.

Chloretone (trichlorobutanol), 0.05%, is effective only in weakly acidic solutions.

Merthiolate (thimerosal, ethyl mercuric thiosalicylate), 0.005%, is most effective in weakly acidic solutions. It is bound to and inactivated by substances containing thiol groups.

Hibitane (chlorhexidine), 0.002%, is a very effective antimicrobial agent. It is incompatible with only a few substances.

Phenyl mercuric salts (acetate, borate, nitrate), 0.001–0.01%, are effective only in weakly alkaline solutions.

Chloroform, butanol, and toluene are not recommended as antimicrobial agents for Sephadex G-100, G-150, or G-200 as they cause the gel particles to shrink slightly. In addition they are effective only in concentrated solutions. They penetrate plastic parts of chromatographic equipment, softening the plastic and leaving the liquid without antimicrobial activity. Oxidizing substances should not be used as antimicrobial agents.

Column Selection

The selection of a chromatographic column for gel filtration experiments is a vital point because, unlike most types of chromatography, during gel filtration all compounds are always moving through the bed and are usually eluted within one column volume. This means that column conditions and design must be such that they minimize uneven sample application and movement of bands. They must also minimize the dilution of compounds eluted from the bed.

The following points should be considered in the selection of a proper column for gel filtration. First, porous glass, plastic, or metal bed supports cannot be recommended because they may rupture or cut the beads and therefore can easily become clogged. This is particularly true with the more porous Sephadex gels. A 10–40 μ nylon or Teflon net or similar fabric type of material has been found to be the most ideal material for a bed support. The net is usually supported by a coarse screen. The column should be designed so that compounds eluted from all areas of the surface of the bed are collected at the same time with a minimum of dilution. In order to prevent nonuniform flow near the bottom of the column, the bed support must not be in a constricted part of the column. Large dead volumes at the bottom of the column which provide mixing or gradient chambers for the sample should be avoided. The column should also provide for (1) easy sample application, (2) connection of the reservoir and outlet tubing, and (3) venting of air from the column and connecting tubing. Jacketed columns may also be required for temperature control. Mechanical devices such as a sample applicator or flow adaptor are also extremely valuable.

On a laboratory scale the column should have a width to height ratio of 1:5 or 1:10 for most separations. Fractionation of compounds with similar molecular weights might require ratios of 1:100. Columns with lengths greater than 100 cm are usually not recommended because of the inconvenience of packing and column availability. The connection of columns in series is a more satisfactory solution to the need for increased bed length.

Column Packing

Since the Sephadex and Sepharose gels are self-regenerating and can be used for long periods of time, the time spent on careful and proper column packing procedures is well worth the effort.

The use of upward flow elution with flow adaptors has found widespread use, especially with the porous Sephadex and Sepharose gels. The column packing procedure used for this technique is as follows. Install the bottom flow adaptor and connect a valve and capillary tubing as shown in Figure 3(a). The use of a gel reservoir connected to the top of the column is recommended since it allows the addition of all the gel slurry in one step. Check the vertical alignment of the column with a spirit level. Fill the column with eluant to the desired bed height and measure this volume (V_t) for later calculation of K_{av} values. Fill the column with freshly degassed buffer to a height of 5–10 cm. Check for leaks and remove any air bubbles trapped under the net of the flow adaptor by suction from above the net. Suspend the gel in approximately twice the expected gel bed volume of buffer. The slurry should be just thin enough so that air bubbles can escape. Carefully pour all the slurry into the gel reservoir. Establish the proper hydrostatic pressure head (Table III) and open the valve. Stabilize the bed by passing at least 1 column vol of buffer through the bed. Remove or add gel to produce the desired bed height. Empty and remove the gel reservoir having approximately 2 cm of buffer above the bed surface. Carefully insert the top flow adaptor and connect a buffer reservoir as shown in Figure 3(b). Adjust the reservoir to give a hydrostatic pressure or flow rate approximately 75% of that used during stabilization. The use of pressure or flow rates greater than that used during packing can result in lifting of the gel from the bottom flow adaptor or compression of the bed with a concomitant decrease in flow rate. For complete

GEL FILTRATION

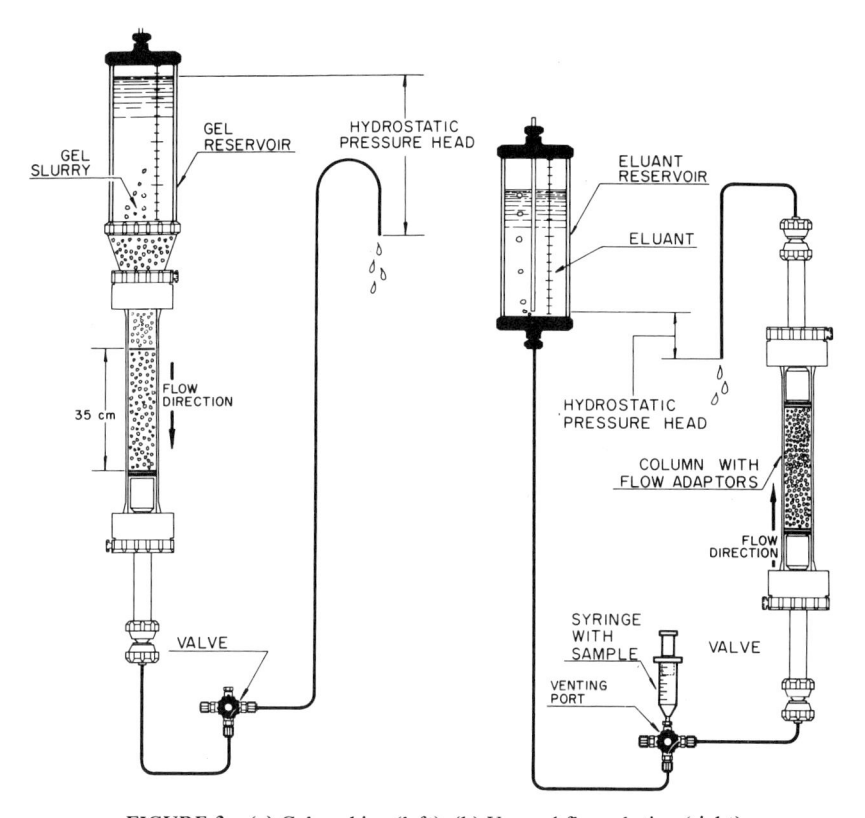

FIGURE 3. (a) Gel packing (left) (b) Upward flow elution (right)

stabilization the bed should be washed with an additional 1–2 bed vol of buffer in the upward direction.

The column void volume and homogeneity of packing should be determined by percolating a sample of 0.2% Blue Dextran 2000 (vol 1–4% of V_t) through the bed. Column irregularities such as channeling, zone packing, or trapped air bubbles are usually quite visible as the colored zone passes through the bed. Continuous ultraviolet (UV) radiation or visible monitoring of the column effluent should show the Blue Dextran 2000 zone as an almost symmetrical peak. In addition, the elution volume of the Blue Dextran should be approximately 30% of the total bed volume.

The procedure for packing the dense Sephadex gels G-10 and G-50 is the same as that described above except that it is not necessary to use a raised outlet tubing or to limit the hydrostatic pressure in laboratory scale experiments.

TABLE III. Maximum Flow Rates for G-75, G-100, G-150, and G-200 at Optimal Operating Pressures

Gel type	Column diameter 1.5 cm			Column diameter 2.5 cm			Column diameter 5.0 cm		
	Operating pressure, cm H_2O	Flow rate ml/cm².hr	ml/min	Operating pressure, cm H_2O	Flow rate ml/cm².hr	ml/min	Operating pressure, cm H_2O	Flow rate ml/cm².hr	ml/min
G-75	50–200	25	0.74	40–160	23	1.9	38–150	18	5.9
G-75 Superfine	50–200	6	0.18	40–160	5.5	0.45	38–150	4.5	1.5
G-100	25–100	16	0.47	24– 96	15	1.2	19– 76	12	3.9
G-100 Superfine	25–100	4	0.12	24– 96	3.7	0.3	19– 76	3	1
G-150	10– 40	7.4	0.22	9– 36	7	0.57	8– 32	5.5	1.8
G-150 Superfine	10– 40	1.8	0.05	9– 36	1.7	0.14	8– 32	1.4	0.45
G-200	5– 20	4	0.12	4– 16	3.6	0.3	3– 12	3	1
G-200 Superfine	5– 20	1	0.03	4– 16	0.9	0.07	3– 12	0.8	0.26

GEL FILTRATION

Sample Application

After stabilizing the bed with at least 2–3 column vol of eluant and checking the quality of the packing with Blue Dextran, we are ready to apply our sample. There are three commonly used methods. In the first case most of the eluant above the gel surface is removed by suction. The column outlet is opened and the remaining eluant is allowed to flow into the bed. The outlet is then closed and the sample is carefully pipetted onto the top of the bed. To prevent disturbance of the surface, a pipet with a bent tip may be used. The column outlet is now opened and the sample is allowed to drain into the bed. The gel surface is then washed with several small portions of eluant. The space above the bed is then filled with eluant and the top cap is connected to the eluant reservoir.

With the porous Sephadex gels it may be advantageous at times to keep an eluant layer a few centimeters deep on top of the bed and to apply the sample beneath this layer. This can be done by means of a syringe or a pipet. The sample must, of course, have a higher density than the eluant. If it is not dense enough, a suitable amount of sucrose should be added.

The third and most convenient way of applying the sample is with the use of a flow adaptor. The flow adaptor stabilizes the bed surface and insures uniform sample application with large or small diameter columns.

The flow adaptors are recommended for downward flow as well as upward flow experiments. Since they are adjustable, they can be used with beds of various lengths. The two adaptors should be used with upward flow experiments. The bottom adaptor allows observation of the bottom of the bed and can be adjusted to correct for any tendency of the gel to lift off of the adaptor. The top adaptor is required to hold the gel in place and allows the fractions to be removed with a minimum of dilution.

Sample Volume and Concentration

When conducting a gel filtration experiment, there are always two questions that must be answered. How much sample volume should be used and what should the sample concentration be? In general, the smaller the sample volume the greater the resolution, but the dilution of the eluted components is also greater. A sample volume must, therefore, be selected which will give the desired resolution with a minimum of dilution. Experience has shown that for fractionation of compounds with similar molecular size, a sample which represents 1–4% of the total bed volume should be used for a preliminary experiment. For desalting experiments or in cases where the elution volumes are widely separated, sample volumes which represent 10–25% of the total bed volume may be used.

Due to the linear partition isotherms, gel filtration is remarkably independent of sample concentration. However, the viscosity of the sample often limits the concentration that can be used. A high viscosity of the sample causes instability of the sample zone and an irregular flow pattern [11]. This leads to very broad and skewed zones. The critical variable is the viscosity of the sample relative to the eluant. In general, we can say that for good separation the viscosity of the sample should never be more than twice the viscosity of the eluant. This rule is somewhat dependent upon the sample size because with a small sample the sample is rapidly diluted and its viscosity is correspondingly decreasing.

EXPERIMENTAL PROCEDURE FOR PROTEIN FRACTIONATION

Packing of G-200 Column

(a) Preparation of Sephadex G-200 (omit steps 1–6 if prepared gel is available).
  (1) With gentle mixing, slowly add required amount of Sephadex (7 g) to 500 ml buffer.
  (2) Allow gel to swell for 72 hr at room temperature or 5 hr on a boiling waterbath.
  (3) Resuspend gel and allow to settle for 20 min.
  (4) Remove excess buffer and fine particles by suction or decanting.
  (5) Resuspend gel in fresh buffer and repeat setting and decanting procedure three times.
  (6) Degas gel slurry in a suction flask with a water aspirator or vacuum pump.

(b) Bed packing.
  (1) Install bottom flow adaptor 5 cm into the column.
  (2) Connect a LV-3 valve to the capillary tubing from the flow adaptor.
  (3) Mark a bed height of 35 cm on the glass tube with tape or marking pen. Erect and plumb column on ringstand.
  (4) Fill the column to marked height with buffer and measure column volume (V_t).
  (5) Attach gel reservoir to top of column.
  (6) Connect a 90 cm long capillary tubing to LV-3 valve.
  (7) Fill column with fresh degassed buffer to a height of 5–10 cm.
  (8) Remove any air bubbles that might be trapped under the net of the flow adaptor by letting buffer flow through or by suction from above net.

GEL FILTRATION

(9) Suspend swollen gel in approximately twice the column volume of buffer.
(10) Carefully pour all slurry into reservoir.
(11) Allow gel to settle for 5 min.
(12) Establish a hydrostatic pressure of 15 cm and open column outlet. (For convenience an eluant reservoir can be connected to the gel reservoir.)
(13) Stabilize bed by letting 1 column vol of buffer pass through the bed. It might be necessary to remove some gel to produce the desired bed height.
(14) Empty and remove gel reservoir leaving approximately 2 cm of buffer above bed surface.
(15) Carefully insert top flow adaptor and connect eluant reservoir.
(16) Adjust hydrostatic pressure to 15 cm and allow column to equilibrate (if time allows, two columns of buffer).
(17) Reverse direction of flow by connecting the eluant reservoir to the LV-3.
(18) Adjust the hydrostatic pressure to achieve a flow rate of 30–35 ml/hr. (Do not exceed 15 cm water pressure.)

Fractionation of Serum on G-200 Column

(1) Set up fraction collector to collect 3.0 ml fractions.
(2) Draw 3.0 ml reconstituted serum into a syringe.
(3) Attach syringe to luerport on LV-3 (vent air bubbles).
(4) Apply the serum carefully at a flow rate lower than the equilibration flowrate (approximately 0.5 ml/min).
(5) Start eluting the column and collecting fractions.

Assay of Fractions for IgG and α-Amylase

A total of 55–60 fractions will contain an eluted volume equal to V_t. The first third of the fractions will not contain anything but buffer (V_o) fractions 1–19.
  Assay for IgG in fractions 20–36. (Assay every other fraction.)
  Assay for α-amylase in fractions 37–60. (Assay every other fraction.)

(a) Assay for IgG.
  (1) Spot 10 μliter of antihuman serum IgG in centerwell of two agar plates.
  (2) Spot 10 μliter of fractions to be assayed in outer wells. In one well also spot 10 μliter of the whole serum sample run on the column.

(3) Incubate plates in a humid atmosphere (covered beaker containing moist filter paper) for at least 4 hr at room temperature.
(4) Look for precipitin lines formed by antihuman IgG and serum IgG.
(5) Plot fraction number versus relative concentration of IgG on graph.

(b) Assay for α-amylase.
  (1) Put one Phadebas* tablet into each test tube to be assayed. (Be careful not to touch the tablet with your fingers.)
  (2) Shake tubes on Vortex mixer or invert until tablets are disintegrated completely.
  (3) Incubate at room temperature for 1 hr.
  (4) Add 1 ml of 0.5 M sodium hydroxide solution to stop the reaction.
  (5) Centrifuge tubes or filter through Whatman 1 filter paper.
  (6) Read adsorbance of supernatants at 620 nm or inspect visually the blue color. α-Amylase will liberate blue dye from the substrate; maximum color means a maximum amylase activity.
  (7) Plot fraction number versus adsorbance on graph paper.

Note: To determine V_e, zone width and K_{av} values, consult the Pharmacia Calibration Kit booklet or other pertinent literature.

APPLICATIONS

Let us now consider a few of the many and varied applications for gel filtration. Sephadex and Sepharose gels have been employed for the separation, fractionation, and purification of a wide variety of biological compounds including proteins, peptides, carbohydrates, and nucleic acids [12,13,14,15]. Many of these compounds such as hormones, enzymes, vitamins, antigens, serum globulins, toxoids, and transfer ribonucleic acids have specific biological activities. Gel filtration is a powerful separation technique and is widely used because it is an exceedingly mild method which does not tend to alter labile biological materials. It also utilizes the parameter of molecular size for separation and can be performed on a very small or a very large scale.

Column Desalting

Sephadex is extremely effective for the desalting of polymers, that is, the separation of molecules which are excluded from a gel from those which can penetrate a large fraction of the internal gel volume. Such separations include removal of salts from proteins or peptides, phenol from nucleic acids, unreacted fluorescein

*Phadebas anylase diagnostic kit, Pharmacia Laboratories Inc.

GEL FILTRATION

from fluorescent tagged antibodies, and unbound drugs from protein-bound drugs. Gel filtration with Sephadex is such a mild technique that some enzyme substrate complexes which have more than a transient existence may also be separated from free substrate.

Centrifugal Desalting

A centrifugal technique employing Sephadex has been devised for the desalting of large or small volumes of highly viscous polymer solutions. A slurry of swelled Sephadex gel is poured into a basket centrifuge and the void volume is removed by centrifugation. The polymer salt solution is then poured onto the rotating gel cake and allowed to equilibrate. Later the desalted polymer in the void volume is removed by increasing the centrifugal field.

Concentration of Polymers

The ability of a Sephadex gel to swell in aqueous solutions can be utilized to concentrate polymer solutions. By adding dry Sephadex to a diluted buffered protein solution, the protein may be concentrated severalfold. A change in the buffer ionic strength or pH does not occur because the buffer ions can penetrate into the inner volume of the gel and equilibrate with the water taken up by the gel. The polymer is recovered in the supernatant after removal of the gel by filtration or by centrifuging in a filter centrifuge tube.

Buffer Exchange

Sephadex gels may be used to change the buffer in which a protein or other polymer is dissolved. The Sephadex bed is equilibrated with the desired buffer. The polymer is placed on the bed in its existing buffer. The buffer ions being small are retarded, and the high molecular weight material is eluted in the desired buffer with which the column was preequilibrated.

Protein Fractionation

Gel filtration is a very popular technique for the purification of proteins. The fractionation of a typical mixture of proteins has been illustrated by the separation of serum proteins on Sephadex G-200. The use of a UV or refractive index monitor indicates the presence of three protein major peaks [19S (S = Svedberg units) globulins, 7S globulins, and albumin, respectively), and one peak containing the low molecular weight compounds such as amino acids (see Figure 4).

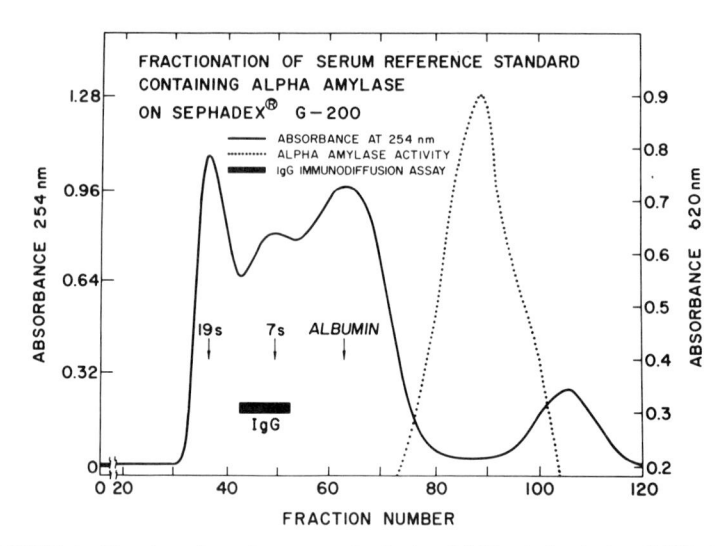

FIGURE 4. Fractionation of serum on Sephadex G-200 gel: Sephadex G-200; bed 2.5 × 35 cm; flow rate: 35 ml/hr; sample: 3 ml human serum; monitor: Pharmacia UV monitor 254 nm; range: NL1.28; amylase activity determined with Pharmacia Laboratories Phadebas Amylase Diagnostic Kit; IgG determined by Ouchterlony immunodiffusion technique with antihuman IgG.

Molecular Weight Determination

Gel filtration is an established chromatographic technique for the separation of molecules according to size. A number of investigators have reported that for a homologous series of compounds, a linear relationship exists between the various elution volume parameters and the logarithm of molecular weight [16–20]. By measuring the elution volumes of several standard globular proteins of known molecular weights, the corresponding K_{av} values can be calculated. The K_{av} value is a constant for a given compound when chromatographed on a specific Sephadex gel and is similar to a distribution coefficient as used in partition chromatography. A plot of K_{av} values versus the logarithm of the molecular weight of each substance is called a selectivity curve, and is linear within the fractionation range of the Sephadex gel employed. If the K_{av} value is determined for a protein of unknown molecular weight, then the molecular weight of that protein can be estimated directly from the selectivity curve.

The use of gel filtration for the determination of molecular weights offers several advantages:

GEL FILTRATION

(1) The substance of unknown molecular weight need not be pure if its elution volume can be determined selectively, for example, by enzyme activity, radioactivity, photometric absorption, etc.
(2) Only very small amounts of substances are required.
(3) The sample can almost always be recovered with little or no denaturation.
(4) The molecular weight determination can often be combined with a gel filtration purification step.
(5) Either column or thin-layer chromatographic techniques may be employed.
(6) The procedure is highly reproducible and rapid.

Elution data from the fractionation of standard proteins on a Sephadex G-150 SF column monitored continuously with a Pharmacia Refractive Index Monitor, as shown in Figure 5, was used to plot a selectivity curve for the estimation of molecular weights of globular proteins. (See Figure 6.)

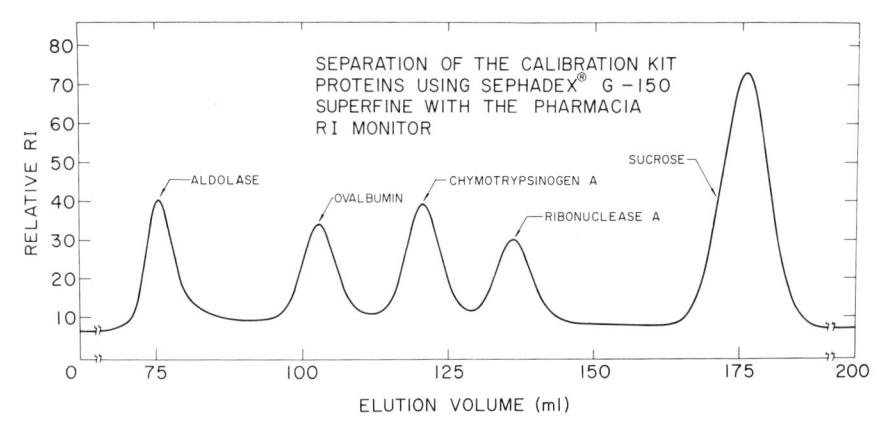

FIGURE 5. Separation of Calibration Kit proteins. Gel: Sephadex G-150; column: K25/45, bed; 2.5 × 35 cm; flow rate: 15 ml/hr; sample: 1 ml containing ribonuclease A 15 mg/ml, ovalbumin 15 mg/ml, chymotrypsinogen A 15 mg/ml, aldolase 15 mg/ml; monitor: Pharmacia RI Monitor, range 64.

The use of a Refractive Index Monitor for continuous monitoring of chromatographic columns is extremely useful since compounds need not absorb UV radiation or visible light in order to be detected. Such instruments are almost universal monitors and for most biological compounds give responses which are all within one order of magnitude, that is, the response to a 1% solution of sucrose is similar to that for a 1% solution of protein.

Sephadex also offers a convenient way of determining the molecular weight distribution of polymers such as dextran, inulin, and polyethylene glycol.

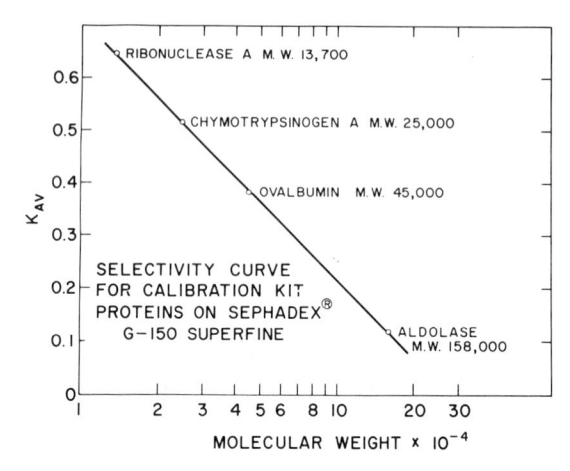

FIGURE 6. Selectivity curve for standard proteins calculated from data in Figure 5.

The average molecular weight of several fractions is determined by independent means. Placing these molecular weight values in their proper place on the effluent axis of the elution diagram will give a logarithmic scale from which the average molecular weights of the other peak fractions may be read directly.

THIN-LAYER GEL FILTRATION (TLG)

A useful analytical procedure utilizing Sephadex gels is TLG, which was introduced independently by Determan [21] and Johansson and Rymo [22] in 1962. The advantages of the technique are that chromatography of many samples at one time under identical conditions is possible; that only small quantities of sample are required; that permanent records of runs can be made; and that two different gels can be run simultaneously in the same apparatus. In addition, TLG experiments, unlike many TLG procedures, can be scaled up easily to column experiments.

The usefulness and simplicity of TLG can be illustrated by the separation of certain common food dyes (McCormick red, yellow, blue, green dyes) and standard proteins (aldolase, chymotrypsinogen A, ovalbumin, ribonuclease A) on Sephadex G-50 SF and G-75 SF, respectively. The TLG apparatus shown in Figure 7 is ideal for this technique and is referred to in the following experiment.

Gel Preparation

The superfine grades of Sephadex are used for TLG and because they have an affinity for glass do not require the addition of binders. The gels are spread

GEL FILTRATION

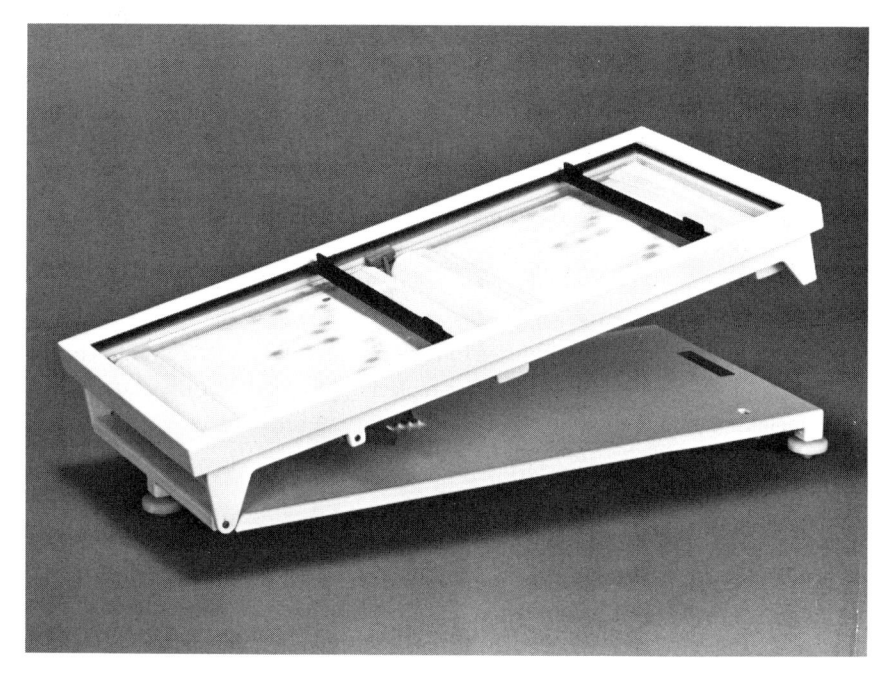

FIGURE 7. Pharmacia TLG apparatus.

wet and the consistency of the gel slurry is important for the preparation of a good layer. The gels (G-75 SF and G-50 SF) are swollen in the desired buffer (phosphate 0.05 M, pH 6.9, containing 0.1 M NaCl, 0.02% NaN_3) according to the figures in Table IV to give the proper gel slurry density.

TABLE IV. Gel Slurry Densities for TLG

Type of Sephadex SF	Amount of gel, g/100 ml
G-50	10.5
G-75	7.5
G-100	6.5
G-150	4.8
G-200	4.5

Spreading of Plates

The glass plates (20 × 20 cm or 20 × 40 cm) are washed carefully and dried. The plate is placed on a board or plastic sheet so that the excess gel can be collected.

An appropriate amount of gel (25 ml slurry for a 20 × 20 cm plate) is poured across the end of the plate. A Teflon-coated rod with blocks on the ends to provide a gel layer of 0.25–1.0 mm is used to spread the gel. The spreader is grasped in both hands and in one smooth motion the gel is spread from one end of the plate to the other. Be sure to continue the spreading motion beyond the plate so as to remove all excess gel. The plate is then placed in the TLG apparatus chamber and the cover is put on (see Figure 7). Make sure the apparatus has been leveled. Wet the filter paper wicks (Whatman 3 M filter paper 4 × 18 cm) with buffer and use them to connect the gel layers with the buffer troughs. Be careful not to disturb the gel layer or to trap air between the gel and wick. Add an appropriate amount of buffer to each trough (60 ml and 25 ml for top and bottom troughs, respectively). After replacing the cover, set the plate at an angle of 20° and allow to equilibrate for several hrs.

Sample Application

Return the chamber to the horizontal position for sample application. Remove the rubber slit cover above the G-50 SF plate and carefully apply five 5 μliter samples at even intervals (one sample of each McCormic Food dye and one of a mixture of the four). Remove the slit from above the G-75 SF plate and apply seven 5 μliter samples (one of each protein, one containing all four proteins, and two of Blue Dextran 2000). The Blue Dextran should be spotted near the edge of the plate as a reference marker. Protein and Blue Dextran concentrations of 15 mg/ml and 2 mg/ml, respectively, should be used.

TLG Development

The plates are developed at an angle of 20° which should correspond to a migration rate of approximately 2 cm/hr. After the Blue Dextran spots have migrated 12–15 cm, stop migration by returning the plate to the horizontal position. Visually inspect the migration and separation of the food dyes. With colored materials the plate may be dried and measurements of migration distance can be determined directly from the plate. Visualization of the proteins is usually accomplished by the replica technique.

After removal of the G-75 SF plate from the chamber, the origins are marked on the back of the glass plate with a felt marking pen. A 20 × 20 cm sheet of Whatman 3 M filter paper is then carefully placed on top of the gel layer. The origins and Blue Dextran spots are circled with a soft lead pencil. After 5–10 min the filter paper is removed and dried. Staining of the filter paper replica for 10 min in 1% Coomassie Blue in methanol:acetic acid:water (80:10:10, v/v) followed by destaining in methanol:acetic acid:water (70:15:15, v/v) gives good visualization of the protein spots.

TLG has been used for molecular weight determinations with a procedure analogous to that used for columns. The inverse migration distance relative to a compound moving in the void volume is plotted versus the log molecular weight for the protein standards to obtain a selectivity curve.

The technique has also been employed to determine the best gel for column experiments, as a support for isoelectrofocusing, and for clinical analysis of blood and urine proteins [23]. The TLG technique with Sephadex has also been employed in conjunction with electrophoresis and immunodiffusion [24,25,26].

REFERENCES

[1] Deuel, H., and H. Neukom. 1954. Hydrocolloids 11:51.
[2] Lathe, G. H., and C. R. J. Ruthven. 1955. Biochem. J. 60:XXXIV.
[3] Lathe, G. H., and C. R. J. Ruthven. 1956. Biochem. J. 62:665.
[4] Ayres, J. A. 1947. J. Amer. Chem. 69:2879.
[5] Bauman, W. C., R. M. Wheaton, and D. W. Simpson. 1956. In Nachod and Schubert (ed.), Ion exchange technology. Academic Press, New York.
[6] Porath, J., and P. Flodin. 1959. Nature 183:1657.
[7] Araki, C. 1956. Bull. Chem. Soc. Japan, 29:543.
[8] Pharmacia Fine Chemicals Inc. 1970. Sephadex gel filtration in theory and practice, p. 7.
[9] Laurent, T. C., and J. Killander. 1964. J. Chromatog. 14:317.
[10] Flodin, P. 1962. Dextran gels and their application in gel filtration. Meijels Bokindustri, Halmstad, Sweden.
[11] Flodin, P. 1961. J. Chromatog. 5:103–115.
[12] Pharmacia Fine Chemicals Literature References. 1959–68; 69–71.
[13] Determan, H. 1967. Gelchromatography. Springer-Verlag. Berlin, Heidelberg, New York.
[14] Fischer, L. 1969. In T. S. Work and E. Work (ed.), Laboratory techniques in biochemistry and molecular biology, vol. 1. North-Holland Publishing Co., Amsterdam, London.
[15] Pharmacia Fine Chemicals Inc. 1970. Sephadex gel filtration in theory and practice, p. 14.
[16] Ackers, G. K. 1967. J. Biol. Chem. 242:3237.
[17] Andrews, P. 1964. Biochem. J. 91:222.
[18] Andrews, P. 1965. Biochem. J. 96:595.
[19] Determan, H., and W. Michel. 1966. J. Chromatog. 25:303.
[20] Whitaker, J. R. 1963. Anal. Chem. 35:1950.
[21] Determan, H. 1962. Experientia 18:430.

[22] Johansson, B. G., and L. Rymo. 1962. Acta Chem. Scand. 16:2067.
[23] Pharmacia Fine Chemicals Inc. 1971. Thin-layer gel filtration with the pharmacia apparatus.
[24] Hanson, L. A., B. G. Johansson, and L. Rymo. 1966. Clin. Chem. Acta. 14:391.
[25] Williamson, J., and A. C. Allison. 1967. Lancet 2:123.
[26] Agostonic, A., C. Vergani, and B. Lomanto. 1967. J. Lab. Clin. Med. 69:522.

A Test for de novo Synthesis of Enzymes in Germinating Seeds: Density Labeling with D_2O

MAARTEN J. CHRISPEELS
J.E. VARNER

INTRODUCTION

Development is characterized by the ordered appearance (and disappearance) of a succession of enzymatic activities. The cellular mechanisms involved in the regulation of the appearance of new enzymatic activities have been the subject of a great deal of experimentation and speculation. Presumably an understanding of these regulatory processes will greatly contribute to an understanding of development itself. An important step in elucidating such a regulatory mechanism is to find out if the appearance of the enzymatic activity is accompanied by the de novo synthesis of the protein with which the enzymatic activity is associated, or alternatively, if the appearance of the enzymatic activity is the result of the activation of a preexisting enzyme (zymogen). Several methods are available to distinguish between these two possibilities.

METHODS FOR DETECTING de novo SYNTHESIS

1. Peptide Mapping or Fingerprinting

The tissue is incubated with a radioactive amino acid (preferably lysine) while the enzymatic activity is increasing. The tissue is homogenized and the enzyme is purified to homogeneity. The pure enzyme is denatured, digested with trypsin and the resulting peptides are separated by two-dimensional chromatography (on paper or thin-layer). The resulting peptide map is sprayed with ninhydrin to locate the peptides and an autoradiograph is made to locate the radioactivity. If the enzyme was synthesized de novo, most or all of the peptides should be labeled. If none of the peptides are labeled, the appearance of the enzymatic activity is most likely due to enzyme activation.

2. Immunology

This method is based on the specific interaction between an antigen (the enzyme under study) and its antibody. This means that it is necessary to first purify the enzyme to homogeneity, inject it into a suitable animal, and prepare an antiserum. This antiserum can then be used to look for zymogens, as well as to study enzyme synthesis and turnover. If the tissue in which the enzyme has not yet appeared contains a protein with antigenic determinants similar to the enzyme under study [so-called cross-reacting material (CRM)], one can tentatively conclude that this protein may be a zymogen and that the appearance of the enzyme may be due to enzyme activation. If no zymogen is found, one can measure the increase in enzymatic activity and the increase in CRM. If both increase in parallel, one can tentatively conclude that the polypeptide chain with which the enzymatic activity is associated is being synthesized de novo. By introducing a pulse of radioactive amino acid it is possible to measure under physiological conditions the half-life of the enzyme in the tissue and determine whether the accumulation of enzymatic activity is due to an enhanced rate of synthesis or a decreased rate of breakdown [9,15,16].

3. Density Labeling

The method is based on incubating the tissue or organism with a protein precursor carrying a stable heavy isotope (^{15}N, ^{13}C, ^{2}H, ^{18}O as ^{15}N-nitrate or ^{15}N-amino acids, ^{13}C-amino acids, ^{2}H$_2$O or H$_2$^{18}O) during the period that the enzymatic activity appears. The tissue is then homogenized (partial purification of the enzyme can be done, but is not necessary), and the buoyant density of the enzyme is determined by isopycnic equilibrium sedimentation in a CsCl gradient. This method, first used to study DNA replication in vivo [11,12], was first applied to the study of protein synthesis by Hu, Bock, and Halvorson [6]. Although the broadness of the bands on the CsCl gradient precludes the actual separation of proteins (as is achieved with DNA), mean densities can be measured and compared to a marker protein (either an enzyme or a radioactive protein). An increase in density of the enzyme is indicative of de novo synthesis during the time the tissue was incubated with the heavy isotope. Shifts from heavy isotope to light isotope (or vice versa) can be used to study enzyme turnover [17,18]. The method can also be used in conjunction with gel electrophoresis to study simultaneously the de novo synthesis of several specific isozymes [13,14]. In this laboratory exercise we demonstrate the de novo synthesis of acid phosphatase in the embryo portion of germinating barley seeds.

EXPERIMENTAL PROCEDURE FOR DENSITY LABELING

1. Germination and Extraction of the Tissue

Seeds of barley (Hordeum vulgare cv. Himalaya) are sterilized in 10% commercial bleach for 20 min and rinsed with sterile water. They are then allowed to germinate on sterile sand moistened with water (3 day germination) or with 80% D_2O (6 day germination). Germination in 80% D_2O is considerably slower than in water. When the seedlings (about 20) have reached a suitable size, separate the shoot and root axes from the endosperm and grind them in 1 ml of 0.01 M Tris pH 7.0 in a cold mortar and pestle. Use a total volume 5.0 ml of buffer to suspend the homogenate and pour it into a conical centrifuge tube. Spin 2 min at 3000 × g; decant the supernatant into a thickwalled Corex tube and spin 20 min at 15,000 rpm in a refrigerated centrifuge. Remove the layer of fat at the top by touching it with a piece of tissue paper and decant the clear extract. Assay an aliquot of the clear extract for acid phosphatase.

2. Setting Up the CsCl Equilibrium Sedimentation

The buoyant density of the proteins will be determined using CsCl isopycnic centrifugation. It is not necessary to preform a gradient and layer the enzyme on top, as is commonly done with a sucrose gradient, because a gradient will be formed as a result of centrifugation. All components (enzyme, CsCl solution, buffer) can be added to the centrifuge tube and mixed.

(a) CsCl. Most proteins have a density around 1.30 g/cm^3 (except glycoproteins and lipoproteins) and it is desirable to have a gradient which has a midpoint density of 1.30 g/cm^3. This can easily be achieved by mixing 1 vol of a saturated CsCl solution with 2 vol of water, buffer, or tissue extract. Saturated CsCl can be made by dissolving CsCl in water at room temperature until no more will go in solution and letting this sit for one day at room temperature. It is not necessary to use optically pure CsCl for this experiment.

(b) Cell extract. How much should be added? It is convenient if one can assay the entire fraction after the gradient has been collected, rather than an aliquot.

This means that enough enzyme has to be added to perform 50–100 assays since the enzyme can be expected to be spread out over 50 tubes if 80–100 fractions are collected. Alternately more enzyme can be added to the gradient, each fraction diluted, and an aliquot of it used to measure enzymatic activity. This has the advantage that each fraction can be assayed several times.

(c) Labeled Marker Protein. Any labeled protein can be used as a reference marker. It is not necessary to have a purified protein since the soluble proteins from a tissue labeled with a radioactive amino acid will do just as well. Labeled marker protein can be prepared by incubating some tissue with a radioactive amino acid, and preparing a 100,000 × g supernatant of the homogenate which is then dialyzed to remove the unincorporated radioactivity. Add 10,000–100,000 cpm to the mixture to be centrifuged.

(d) Water or Buffer. Water or buffer can be used to make up the total volume (4–6 ml depending on the size of the centrifuge tube). Add CsCl, labeled marker protein, tissue extract, and water to a total volume of 4.0 ml to a centrifuge tube and mix. Check the refractive index to make sure the density is around 1.3. Fill the centrifuge tube with mineral oil and assemble the SW 39 rotor of the Spinco ultracentrifuge. Centrifuge at 38,000 rpm for 65 hr.

3. Fractionation of the Gradient

The gradient can be collected with a variety of devices, but it is certainly not necessary to have an expensive gradient collector. A homemade device as shown in Figure 1 will do. Remove some of the mineral oil with a pasteur pipet. Be careful not to disturb the gradient. Insert the stopper with the plastic syringe into the tube. Puncture the bottom of the tube with a broken off #22 hypodermic needle. (You only get one try–no fumbling here–better practice first). The channel of the needle can be cleaned out with a thin wire to make sure that the solution will flow normally. If the flow has not yet started one should apply a small positive pressure. Collect six drops per fraction. Should you make a mistake, keep right on going. When the gradient is collected cover every eighth tube with a piece of parafilm and store all the tubes in the coldroom.

4. Assays

(a) Acid Phosphatase. Add 0.9 ml of p-nitrophenylphosphate (0.005 M of pNPP in 0.1 M acetate buffer pH 5.2 freshly made) to alternate fractions and incubate at 37°C until some fractions turn faintly yellow. Stop the reaction by adding 3 ml of 0.25 N NaOH and determine the optical density with a colorimeter set at 410 nM.

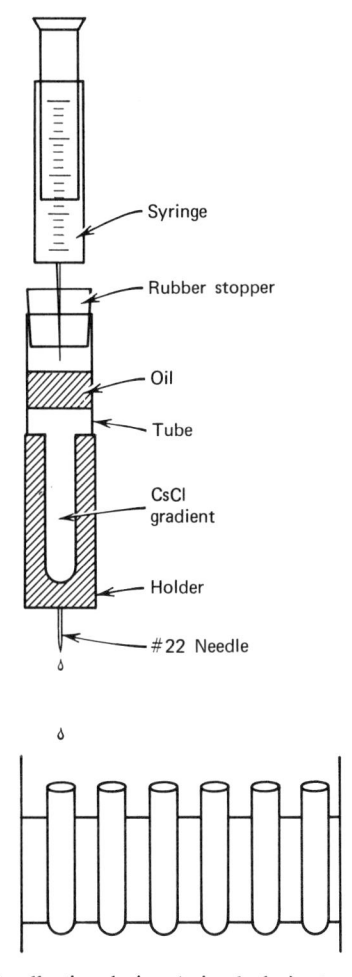

FIGURE 1. Gradient collection device. A simple device to collect density gradients consisting of a metal holder and a stopper with syringe. Pressure can be applied with the syringe. The dripping needle can be permanently welded in place, but this is not necessary.

(b) Radioactivity. Add 1 ml of water to alternate fractions to dilute the CsCl and then add 10 ml of a liquid scintillation solvent which mixes with water (Aquasol^T from New England Nuclear or Ready-solv^T from Beckman for example). Transfer to scintillation vials and determine the radioactivity.

(c) Refractive Index. It is necessary to determine the refractive indices of selected fractions (every eighth one) to determine the gradient of densities which established itself during the centrifugation. This is done by removing a drop from the tube with a pasteur pipet and placing it on the crystal of the refractometer. The refractive index can be read and converted to density using a refractive index table (see H. A. Sober (ed.), 1968. Handbook of biochemistry and molecular biology. The Chemical Rubber Co., Cleveland, Ohio).

RESULTS

The results of the experiment are shown in Figure 2. Results from the two gradients have been combined in one figure and normalized with respect to the marker

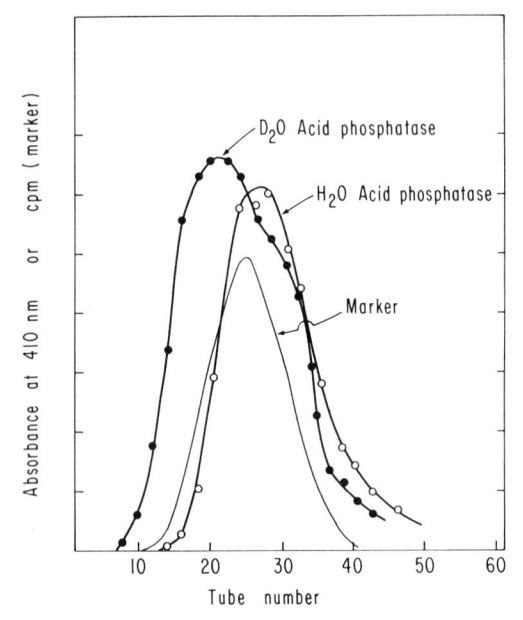

FIGURE 2. Distribution of acid phosphatase from H_2O grown and 80% D_2O grown barley on an equilibrium CsCl gradient. This graph is a composite of two separate gradients, one containing the extract of H_2O grown seedlings, the other of D_2O grown seedlings. The positions of the radioactive markers and the refractive indices were so closely matched as to be superimposable.

and the refractive indices. In both gradients the marker banded at a density of 1.3299 g/cm^3. The density of a protein is determined by calculating the midpoint of each peak. This can be done by averaging the midpoints of the peak at different peak heights (1/4, 1/2, 3/4 peak height). The data show that the acid phosphatase from D_2O-grown seedlings has a density of 1.3429 as compared to a density of 1.3212 for the enzyme from H_2O grown seedlings. This represents an increase of 0.021 g/cm^3 or 1.6%. The same data can be plotted on probability paper (Figure 3). This is a more accurate way to determine the midpoint of the peak.

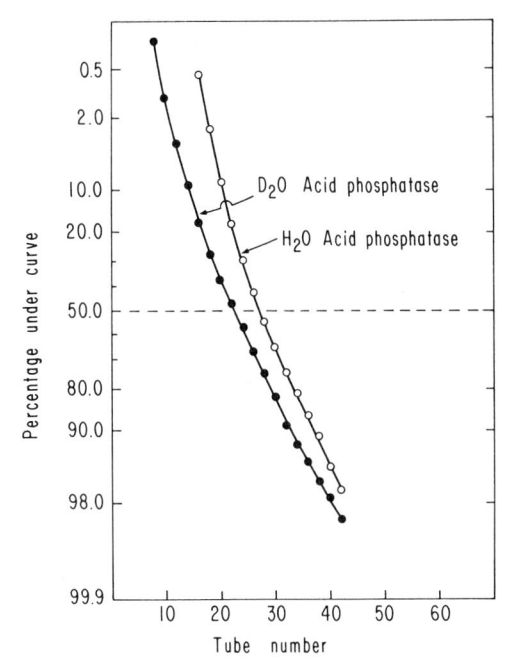

FIGURE 3. Distribution of acid phosphatase from H_2O grown and 80% D_2O grown barley seedlings on an equilibrium CsCl gradient. The data from Figure 2 are replotted on probability paper.

The D_2O–acid phosphatase peak (in Figure 2) is broader than the H_2O–acid phosphatase peak because the heavy leg of the curve is displaced much more than the light leg. This indicates the presence of mixture of heavy and light acid phosphatase. The light enzyme was probably already present in the seed before germination whereas the heavy enzyme was synthesized de novo during the incubation.

DISCUSSION

The reserve macromolecules (protein, carbohydrates, fats) present in the food storage tissues of seeds are hydrolyzed during germination. The products of this

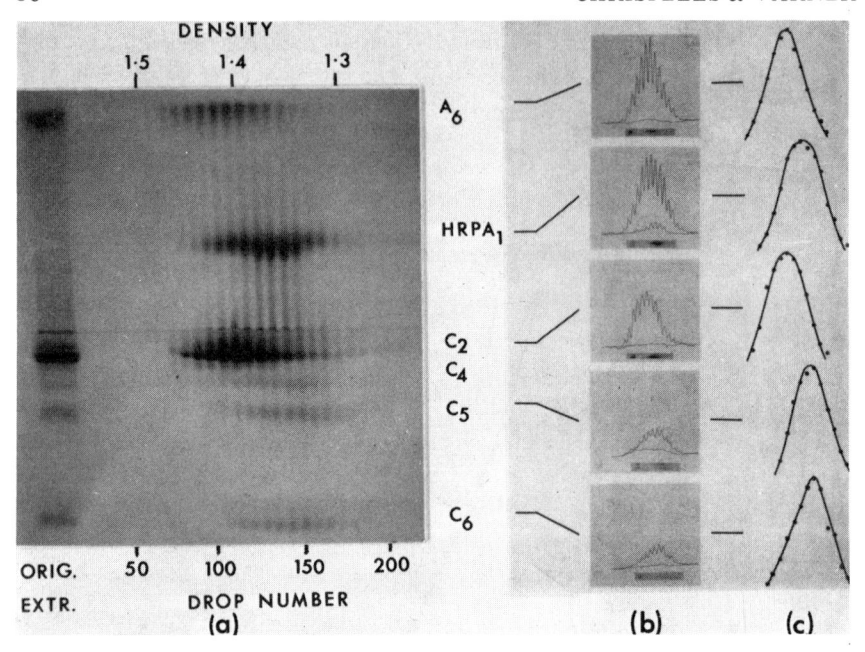

FIGURE 4. Examination of the density labeling of the individual isozymes of peroxidase by a combination of gel electrophoresis and isopycnic equilibrium centrifugation. Top lefthand panel: (a) Starch gel zymograms of barley root peroxidase following isopycnic equilibrium centrifugation of the enzyme in CsCl. A sample of the original extract without the HRPA, (horseradish peroxidase marker isozyme) is on the left for reference. A_6, C_2, C_4, C_5, C_6 denote various barley peroxidases. Density of the gradient decreases from left to right. Gel stained with benzidine and H_2O_2. Top righthand panel: (b) Densitometer tracings of the five major peroxidase bands on the zymogram taken from Polaroid color film used to photograph the stained gel. (c) Normalized Gaussian curves of the five major bands obtained from the densitometer tracings. Bottom panel: (d) Superimposed transparancies of peroxidase isozymes extracted from H_2O, $K^{14}NO_3$ and 50% D_2O, $K^{15}NO_3$ grown barley seedlings and separated by the combination gel electrophoresis–isopycnic equilibrium sedimentation method. The HRPA, marker isozymes have been aligned visually such that their peaks of activity coincide. The lower band of each pair of barley isozymes is the unlabeled ($H_2O^{14}NO_3^-$) control and the upper band of each pair is density labeled (D_2O, $^{15}NO_3^-$) [Quail and Varner 14].

hydrolysis usually undergo further modification before being used in the biosynthesis of macromolecules in the growing axis. The monosaccharides produced from the hydrolysis of reserve polysaccharides and the carbon skeletons of some of the amino acids are converted to sucrose; this sucrose is transported to the growing axis and then converted to a variety of small molecules. In the process there is ample opportunity to incorporate or exchange deuterium atoms for hydrogen atoms if the seeds are germinated in D_2O. Some deuterium atoms which are incorporated during the biosynthesis of the protein will be easily

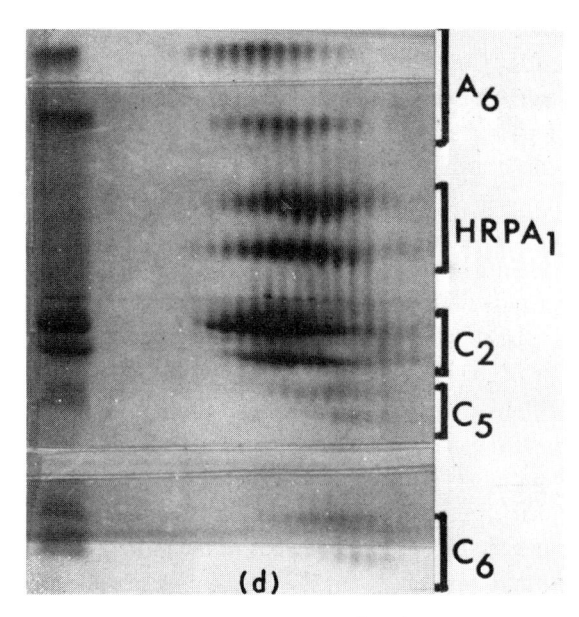

FIGURE 4. Continued.

exchangeable with the hydrogen atoms of water. This is the case for deuterium attached to atoms of oxygen, nitrogen, or sulfur. These deuterium atoms will be lost when the tissue is homogenized in water or subsequently during the centrifugation. This is just as well, since the fact that they are freely exchangeable also means that they may have been introduced in the protein during the incubation of the tissue with D_2O even though the enzyme was not being synthesized.

Deuterium atoms attached to carbon atoms are known to be quite stable (with the possible exception of the hydrogen atoms on the carbon atom bearing the α-amino nitrogen). Since we do not know the amino acid composition of acid phosphatase or the number of stable deuterium atoms incorporated in each amino acid it is impossible to estimate the density shift which should be expected for the enzyme if all of it were synthesized de novo. An increase in mass of 4–6% can be expected if every stable hydrogen atom is replaced with a deuterium atom. If there is no commensurate increase in the partial specific volume of the protein, this would result in a density shift of 4–6%. A 5.5% increase in the buoyant density of isocitratase was found when peanut cotyledons were incubated in 100% D_2O [10]. There is no linear relationship between the abundance of D_2O in the medium and the magnitude of the density shift. This is due to isotope discrimination. If H_2O is available (10 or 20%) it will be used preferentially. Little or no shift may occur if no more than 40% D_2O is in the medium. For all these reasons usually only qualitative conclusions can be drawn from the results. The results obtained in this experiment are consistent with the notion that acid phosphatase is synthesized de novo. It is not possible to say how much of the acid phosphatase present in the axis was synthesized de novo. Some conclusions may be drawn by carefully observing the shape of the acid phosphatase distribution curve on the CsCl gradient. If both light or H_2O-acid phosphatase and heavy or D_2O-acid phosphatase are present in the same extract the curve will be considerably broader than in the control sample containing H_2O-acid phosphatase only. The heavy leg of the enzyme curve of the D_2O-sample will be displaced towards the heavy side of the gradient when compared with the heavy leg of the H_2O-sample curve; however, the light legs of the two curves will be superimposed. When unequal amounts of light and heavy enzyme are present, the curve will be assymetrical. An additional consideration is that when the protein is synthesized and folded in its three-dimensional configuration some deuterium atoms attached to nitrogen, oxygen, or sulfur atoms or some D_2O may become trapped in regions of the proteins inaccessible to the solvent under normal conditions [7]. This could lead to erroneous positive results. Treatment of α-amylase with 8 M urea in the presence of 99.7% D_2O followed by removal of the urea by dialysis against D_2O showed that under these conditions little or no trapping on nonexchangeable deuterium atoms occurs in this protein [1]. If the protein which is being studied is a glycoprotein, one must consider the possibility that any increase in the buoyant density of the molecule is due to the attachment of newly synthesized and therefore density-labeled carbohydrates to a preexisting protein.

This method has been used by a number of investigators to simply show whether or not a protein is synthesized de novo [1-6,8,10,13,14,17,18]. More recently the method has been extended to look simultaneously at the multiple forms of a particular enzyme, [13,14], and to study enzyme turnover [17,18].

The technique developed by Quail and Varner [14] has been applied to the study of the isozymes of peroxidase [14] and catalase [13] in young seedlings. First, one localizes total enzymatic activity on the gradient by assaying every other fraction just as was done in the experiment described here. Then, 5 μliter aliquots are taken from the other gradient fractions (only from that portion of the gradient which contains enzyme activity) and applied at regular intervals to the origin of a large slab of starch gel. Electrophoresis is carried out to separate the isozymes in the gradient fractions and the gel is stained. Whether or not an increase in buoyant density of a particular isozyme occurred can be determined visually by superimposing the transparent photographs of gels made with enzyme from seeds germinated in normal and heavy isotope medium. This is shown in Figure 4. A quantitative determination of the distribution of each isozyme in the gradient can be made with the aid of a densitometer.

By shifting Escherichia coli cells from a growth medium made with 80% D_2O to one made with 100% H_2O, Williams and Neidhardt [17] were able to measure the turnover of several aminoacyl RNA synthetases in a variety of growth conditions. The density shift allowed them to measure the rates of disappearance of the old heavy enzyme and of appearance of the new light enzyme simultaneously (Figure 5 and Table I). Their results show that the cells are able to regu-

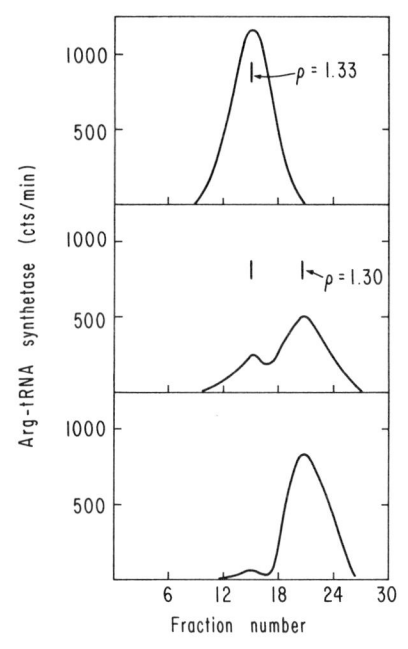

FIGURE 5. Banding in CsCl gradients of arginyl–tRNA synthetase from an arginine auxotroph after a shift from 80% D_2O to H_2O. The three panels concern a culture in a chemostat with limiting L-arginine and show the banding of enzyme in samples A, C, and E described in Table I (redrawn from Williams and Neidhardt [17]).

late the rate of synthesis of these enzymes over a 10- to 50-fold range. This regulation bears a superficial resemblance to repression of biosynthetic enzymes since manipulation of the amino acid supply affects the rate of enzyme formation.

Similar experiments were done by Zielke and Filner [18] who shifted cultured tobacco cells from a medium containing a ^{14}C-amino acid and $^{15}NO_3^-$ to a medium

TABLE I. Rate of de novo Synthesis of Arginyl-tRNA Synthetase by the Arginine Auxotroph, Strain HP1802, in Two Different Growth Conditions, as Revealed by Deuterium Labeling

Sample	Time after density shift, min	Protein in culture, mg/ml	Specific activity of extract, units/mg protein	Protein on gradient, mg	Heavy enzyme on gradient, units $\times 10^3$	Light enzyme on gradient, units $\times 10^3$	Total enzyme in culture, units/ml $\times 10^3$	Heavy enzyme in culture, units/ml $\times 10^3$	Light enzyme in culture, units/ml $\times 10^3$
Experiment									
A	0	0.018	0.130	0.090	3.51	0.00	2.34	2.34	0.00
B	0 to 60	0.021	0.100	0.090	1.65	0.97	2.10	1.33	0.77
C	60 to 120	0.028	0.090	0.100	0.90	2.29	2.52	0.71	1.81
D	120 to 180	0.039	0.090	0.100	0.30	2.96	3.51	0.31	3.20
E	180 to 240	0.053	0.080	0.108	0.14	3.40	4.23	0.16	4.07

A culture of the arginine auxotroph, strain HP1802, was grown for many generations in deuterium oxide medium supplemented with L-arginine (100 µg/ml). At 0 time the cells, which were in exponential phase of growth with k = 0.47/hr, were collected by centrifugation, washed once, and suspended in water medium lacking L-arginine in the growth chamber of a chemostat. One portion of the cells was retained as the 0 time sample. The flow of medium, containing L-arginine at a limiting concentration calculated to maintain the cells at their initial density, was begun with a dilution rate of 0.32/hr. The effluent culture from 0 to 60 min was collected and called sample B; from 60 to 120 min, sample C; from 120 to 180 min, sample D; and from 180 to 240 min, sample E. The samples were processed in the usual manner to produce extracts that were assayed for total arginyl-tRNA synthetase activity and then analyzed for heavy and light enzyme by CsCl centrifugation. Figure 5(a) shows the banding of samples A, C, and E. From Williams and Neidhardt [17].

containing an ^{3}H-amino acid and $^{14}NO_3^-$ or an ^{3}H-amino acid and casein hydrolysate. Their data indicate that turnover of nitrate reductase (synthesis and breakdown) occurs under conditions where the level of the enzyme stays constant and under conditions where the level of the enzyme drops exponentially.

REFERENCES

[1] Anstine, W., J. V. Jacobsen, and J. E. Varner. 1970. Deuterium oxide as a density label of peroxidases in germinating barley embryos. Plant Physiol. 45:148-152.

[2] Chrispeels, M. J., R. F. Boyd, L. S. Williams, and F. C. Neidhardt. 1968. Modification of Valyl tRNA synthetase by bacteriophase in Escherichia coli. J. Mol. Biol. 31:463-475.

[3] Chroboczek-Kelker, H. 1970. Activation of aspartate transcarbamoylase by purine nucleotides. Biochim. Biophys. Acta 198:20-30.

[4] Filner, P., and J. E. Varner. 1967. A test for de novo synthesis of enzymes: density labeling with H_2O^{18} of barley α-amylase induced by gibberellic acid. Proc. Nat. Acad. Sci. 58:1520.

[5] Gientka-Rychter, A., and J. H. Cherry. 1968. De novo synthesis of isocitratase in peanut (Arachis hypogaea L.) cotyledous. Plant Physiol. 43:653-659.

[6] Hu, A. S. L., R. M. Bock, and H. O. Halvorson. 1962. Separation of labeled from unlabeled proteins by equilibrium density gradient sedimentation. Anal. Biochem. 4:489-504.

[7] Hvidt, A., and S. O. Nielsen. 1966. Hydrogen exchange in proteins. Advance. Protein Chem. 21:287-386.

[8] Jacobsen, J. V., and J. E. Varner. 1967. Gibberellic acid-induced synthesis of protease by isolated aleurone layers of barley. Plant Physiol. 42:1596-1600.

[9] Kenney, F. T. 1962. Induction of tyrosine-α-ketoglutarate transaminase in rat liver. IV. Evidence for an increase in the rate of enzyme synthesis. J. Biol. Chem. 237:3495-3498.

[10] Longo, C. P. 1968. Evidence for de novo synthesis of isocitratase and malate synthetase in germinating peanut cotyledous. Plant Physiol. 43:660-664.

[11] Meselson, M., and F. W. Stahl. 1958. The replication of DNA in Escherichia coli. Proc. Nat. Acad. Sci. 44:671-682.

[12] Meselson, M., F. W. Stahl, and J. Vinograd. 1957. Equilibrium sedimentation of macromolecules in density gradients. Proc. Nat. Acad. Sci. 43:581-588.

[13] Quail, P., and J. G. Scandalios. 1971. Turnover of genetically defined catalase ioszymes in maize. Proc. Nat. Acad. Sci. 68:1402-1406.

[14] Quail, P. H., and J. E. Varner. 1971. Combined gradient-gel electrophoresis procedures for determining buoyant densities or sedimentation coefficients of all multiple forms of an enzyme simultaneously. Anal. Biochem. 39:344–355.

[15] Schimke, R. T. 1964. The importance of both synthesis and degradation in the control of arginase levels in rat liver. J. Biol. Chem. 239:3808–3817.

[16] Schimke, R. T., E. W. Sweeney, and C. M. Berlin. 1965. The roles of synthesis and degradation in the control of rat liver tryptophan pyrrolase. J. Biol. Chem. 240:322–331.

[17] Williams, L. S., and F. C. Neidhardt. 1969. Synthesis and inactivation of aminoacyl-transfer RNA synthetases during growth of Escherichia coli. J. Mol. Biol. 43:529–550.

[18] Zielke, H. R., and P. Filner. 1971. Synthesis and turnover of nitrate reductase induced by nitrate in cultured tobacco cells. J. Biol. Chem. 246:1772–1779.

Isolation of Multiple RNA Polymerases from Dictyostelium Discoideum

S.S. PONG
W.F. LOOMIS, JR.

Differentiation appears to result either directly or indirectly from differential expression of the genetic material. What are the mechanisms which determine that a specific subset of genes is expressed at a specific stage? Studies with model microbial systems have suggested two general mechanisms: (1) control of template activity by binding of specific repressor or activator proteins to operator sequences of the DNA, (2) control of RNA polymerase template range by binding of specific regulatory proteins to the catalytic core enzyme.

Studies on several bacterial genetic systems including the lac operon of Escherichia coli and the immunity system of phage λ [Jacob and Monod, 1961; Gilbert and Müller-Hill, 1966; Ptashne and Hopkins, 1968] have shown that purified repressor proteins are able to bind to DNA operator regions both in vivo and in vitro and limit RNA transcription. Although there is no such direct evidence for repressor control in higher organisms, recent studies on mammalian cell cultures indicate that similar mechanisms may be functioning in these systems [Klebe, Chen, and Ruddle, 1970; Tomkins et al., 1969].

Other microbial genetic systems appear to be controlled by the template range of RNA polymerases. For instances, when phage T4 infects E. coli, the bacterial RNA polymerase is modified, and as a consequence, the polymerase loses affinity to a protein factor, termed sigma, which is necessary for transcription from many bacterial genes [Burgess et al., 1969; Travers, 1969; Goff and Weber, 1970]. The infecting T4 phage then produces new binding factors which restrict the polymerase to different segments of the T4 genome [Hager, Hall, and Fields, 1970]. A similar control mechanism appears to determine which genes are active during differentiation of Bacillus subtilis. In this system, the β subunit of the polymerase appears to be cleaved by a protease at the onset of sporulation, and as a result, the enzyme loses affinity to the sigma factor [Losick et al., 1970]. It is thought that the vegetative factor may be replaced by a sporulation specific factor which directs binding and initiation of transcription at the subset of genes which is expressed during sporulation.

Since specific factors appear to determine which genes can be transcribed in a given cell by associating with RNA polymerase, it has been suggested that similar factors may control differentiation in higher organisms. This model has attracted considerable interest in recent years, although no case has yet been found where a specific differentiation can be attributed to a change in the properties of an RNA polymerase. The lack of direct supporting evidence may be attributed to the considerable technical difficulties encountered in the characterization of eukaryotic polymerases and the lack of specific mutations which can define gene function.

More than ten years ago, Weiss and Gladstone [1959] reported RNA polymerase activity in a crude nuclear preparation from rat liver. Difficulty was encountered in this and other systems when attempts were made to free the enzyme from the particulate nuclear material. Not until 1968 were methods developed which could extract the majority of the activity into the soluble fraction. A variety of techniques, including treatment of the nuclei in buffered isotonic solution [Liao, Sagher, and Fang, 1968; Keller and Goor, 1970; Sugden and Sambrook, 1970]; aging of the nuclei [Mertelsmann, 1969]; incubation of nuclei in an alkaline solution at 37°C [Jacob, Sajdel, and Munro, 1968; Goldberg and Moon, 1970]; and sonication of nuclei in high salt solution [Roeder and Rutter, 1969; Seifart and Sekeris, 1969; Mandel and Chambon, 1971; Chesterton and Butterworth, 1971b] are now used to extract the enzyme in a soluble form in which the activity is dependent on added DNA template. Isolation of RNA polymerase starting from whole cells has also been achieved [Furth and Austin, 1970; Stein and Hansen, 1970; Dezelee, Sentanae, and Fromageot, 1972].

The most generally useful solubilization technique appears to involve sonication which shears the chromatin and liberates the enzyme. Using this technique, Roeder and Rutter [1969] isolated polymerase activity from sea urchin embryos and rat liver. When the soluble enzyme preparation was chromatographed on DEAE–cellulose, the enzyme activity was clearly resolved into at least two fractions. It was subsequently found that the first enzyme (I) was resistant to the drug α-amanitin, while the second enzyme (II) was sensitive to the drug [Lindell et al., 1970]. Enzyme I is localized in nucleoli and directs predominantly the synthesis of ribosomal RNA, while the other polymerase forms are present in the nucleoplasm and direct the synthesis of DNA-like RNA

[Roeder and Rutter, 1970; Blatti et al., 1970; Zylber and Penman, 1971]. Thus, there appears to be specialization of template utilization among the eukaryotic polymerases. Different control of the polymerase forms might be involved in specific differentiations especially those which involve alteration in the rates of ribosomal RNA synthesis. However, when the relative abundance of the enzymes was measured in embryos of Xenopus laevis at stages when the rate of rRNA synthesis was changing rapidly, no corresponding change was found in the relative proportions of polymerase forms [Roeder, Reeder, and Brown, 1970; Tocchini-Vallentini and Crippa, 1970]. It was concluded that the activities must be controlled in vivo by factors not yet recognized.

There is now considerable interest in determining which factors can control the activity of specific polymerases on a variety of DNA templates [Stein and Hauson, 1970; Seifart, 1970; Dahmus and Lee, 1972]. The results to date have been encouraging but not conclusive. It has been difficult to demonstrate that various environmental conditions or protein fractions which affect polymerase activity, when measured in vitro, function in a similar manner in vivo and direct a changing pattern of RNA transcription. This problem would be greatly facilitated if one could focus on stage-specific gene products and could modify the pattern of RNA synthesis by genetic mutation. Correlations between changes in the polymerase activity, factor concentration, and gene expression could then be drawn.

Technical difficulties encountered in accumulating sufficient material for biochemical analysis and in isolating appropriate mutations have hampered this approach in many eukaryotic organisms. One of the few organisms which appears amenable to such studies is the cellular slime mold, Dictyostelium discoideum. For this reason, we have purified the RNA polymerase forms from exponentially growing cells of D. discoideum and compared them to the forms isolated from developing cells. The pattern of messenger RNA is known to change in a defined temporal pattern during development of D. discoideum [Sussman and Sussman, 1969; Loomis, 1969; Firtel, 1971] and it was thought that the pattern of transcription might result from changes in RNA polymerase. Since D. discoideum is a normal eukaryotic organism in which the DNA is associated in the chromosomes with histones similar to those of mammalian organisms, we felt that information derived from this developing system might be applicable to similar studies in higher organisms.

MATERIALS AND METHODS

Chemicals: Where possible, all chemicals were reagent grade. Ultrapure ammonium sulfate was purchased from Schwartz–Mann, Van Nuys, Ca. Spectral quality glycerol was the product of Matheson–Coleman and Bell Co., Los Angeles, Ca. α-amanitin, isolated from the poisonous toadstool, Amanita phalloides, was purchased from Henley Co., New York, N.Y. Actinomycin D was obtained from Merck, Sharp, and Dohme Co., Rahway, N.J. Rifampicin was purchased from Calbiochem, La Jolla, Calif.

Organism: D. discoideum strain A3 [Loomis, 1971] was used throughout this work. The cells were grown axenically in liquid broth medium containing 10 g protease peptone, 5 g yeast extract, 10 g glucose in 1 liter of 2×10^{-3} M potassium phosphate buffer pH 6.5. Cultures of 2 liters were vigorously rotated in 4 liter Erlenmeyer flasks at 22°C. Under these conditions, the cells grow exponentially with a doubling time of 12 hr to a titer of $1-2 \times 10^7$ amebae/ml. Cells in the exponential growth phase were harvested by centrifugation at 150 $\times$ g for 3 min, washed twice with cold distilled water and allowed to proceed through morphogenesis at 22°C on Whatman filters (#50, 12.5 cm). For this, 1.5 $\times 10^9$ washed amebae were spread evenly on each filter which was supported by eight absorbant pads (Whatman #3, 12.5 cm) saturated with a solution containing NaCl (9 mg/ml), streptomycin sulfate (0.5 mg/ml) and 10^{-3} M potassium phosphate buffer pH 6.5. Under these conditions, the amebae aggregate and form pseudoplasmodia during the first 12 hr, and then proceed synchronously through the stages in morphogenesis to form fruiting bodies each consisting of approximately 5×10^4 spores supported on a cellular stalk. The whole process requires 26 hr for completion. So as to avoid problems in the preparation of extracts from encapsulated spores, the cells were collected prior to culmination, after about 19 hr of development. The pseudoplasmodia were scraped off the filters with a stainless steel spatula and suspended in a 7% sucrose solution. Each filter provided about 1 g wet weight of differentiated cells.

Preparation of Nuclei: The cells were washed twice in cold 7% sucrose solution, collected by centrifugation, and suspended at 2×10^8 cells/ml in a 15% sucrose solution containing 0.04 M Tris HCl pH 7.8, 0.1 mM EDTA, 6 mM $MgCl_2$, 0.04 M KCl, 5 mM mercaptoethanol. The cells were broken by vigorous shaking for 50 sec following the addition of detergent Nonidet P40 to 0.8%. Nuclei were sedimented from the extract by centrifugation at 4000 $\times$ g in a Sorvall RC 2B for 10 min. The pelleted nuclei were suspended in the same buffer and resedimented before being suspended in sonication solution.

Assay of RNA Polymerase: RNA polymerase activity was estimated by measuring the rate of incorporation of ^{3}H-Uridine 5'-triphosphate (UTP) into polynucleotides. The standard assay contained guanosine 5'-triphosphate (GTP), cytidine 5'-triphosphate (CTP), and adenosine 5'-triphosphate (ATP) at 0.4 mM and UTP at 0.1 mM. It also contained 6 mM $MgCl_2$, 1.6 mM $MnCl_2$, 0.1 mM ethylene diaminetetra-acetic acid (EDTA), 5 mM 2-mercaptoethanol, 0.06 M $(NH_4)_2SO_4$ and 0.04 M Tris HCl pH 7.8. One µc of ^{3}H-UTP, 15 µg calf thymus DNA and enzyme were incubated in 0.15 ml of the above solution for 10 min at 25°C. The reaction was stopped by pipetting 0.10 ml of the reaction mixture onto Whatman DE81 filter disks (2.1 cm). Filters were dried and then washed six times for 5 min each in 5% Na_2HPO_4, followed by rinsing twice in water, twice in ethanol, once in diethyl ether. The filters were dried and counted in a Beckman Liquid Scintillation counter using a toluene scintillation fluor containing 4 g/liter 2, 5-diphenyloxazole (PPO) and 50 mg/liter p-bis-[2-(5-phenyloxazoyl)] benzene (POPOP). This procedure resulted in a background of 30–40 cpm. Sufficient enzyme was assayed to incorporate at least 500 cpm in 10 min. Alternatively the reaction was stopped by addition of 10% TCA containing 10 mg/ml pyrophosphate. When this procedure was followed, 100 µg bovine serum albumin and 100 µg yeast RNA were added as carrier to each sample and the precipitate collected on a glass fiber filter. The filters were washed with 5% TCA, followed by 95% ethanol and counted as described above. A unit of RNA polymerase activity is that amount which catalyzes the incorporation of 1 µmole uridine/min into polynucleotides. Specific activity is presented as units per milligram of protein. Protein was measured either by the technique of Lowry et al. [1951] or, in purified samples, by absorbance at 280 mµ or 210 mµ using bovine serum albumin as a standard.

Preparation of DNA Templates: Calf thymus DNA was purchased from Calbiochem, La Jolla, Ca. and utilized for routine assays without further purification. It should be realized that commercially available DNA often contains numerous single-stranded nicks and different batches may exhibit different template characteristics.

D. discoideum DNA was prepared from 2 to 4 × 10^{10} cells growing exponentially in liquid broth medium by a modification of the method of Firtel [1971]. The cells were collected by centrifugation, washed once in distilled water, and lysed by resuspending and stirring at room temperature in 40 ml of 10^{-2} M EDTA pH 8, 2% sodium N-lauroyl sarcosine. Solid CsCl was added to 0.25 g/ml and the mixture heated at 55°C for 5–10 min. Solid CsCl was then added to a final concentration of 0.95 g/ml. After cooling to room temperature, ethidium bromide was added to 0.33 mg/ml. The preparation was centrifuged at 40,000 rpm for 48 hr at 20–25°C in a Spinco Ti 50 rotor. The red protein cake which floated on top of the gradient was carefully removed, DNA was collected with a Pasteur pipet from the red band which was easily separated from the colorless band of glycogen. The DNA was resuspended in 10^{-2} M EDTA and CsCl was added to final concentrations of 0.95 g/ml. Ethidium bromide was again added to 0.33 mg/ml. After a second centrifugation, the

DNA band was collected as before, diluted 4-fold with water and the ethidium bromide was extracted with isopentyl alcohol until the solution was colorless. Two volumes of ethanol were added and DNA was wound out on a glass rod. The purified DNA was dissolved in 1/10 × SSC (1 × SSC:0.15 M NaCl, 0.015 M sodium citrate pH 7) and dialyzed against two changes of 1 × SSC for one day. DNA was then dialyzed overnight against 0.04 M Tris pH 7.8 buffer.

Lily microsporocyte DNA was the gift of Yasuo Hotta. E. coli DNA was provided by Bernard Weinstein. DNA from the B. subtilis phage SP01, as well as DNA from E. coli phage T4 and T7 were the gifts of E. Peter Geiduschek. The DNA was stored in 2 × SSC at 4°C.

SDS Gel Electrophoresis: Polyacrylamide gel electrophoresis in the presence of 0.1% SDS was carried out as described by Laemmli [1970]. The gels were prepared with upper and lower segments containing 3 and 7.5% acrylamide, respectively, cross-linked with N,N'-methylene bisacrylamide added to 2.6% of the acrylamide concentration. The upper gel was made in 0.125 M Tris HCl pH 6.8, 0.1% SDS while the lower gel was made in 0.375 M Tris HCl pH 8.8, 0.1% SDS. Polymerization was catalyzed by adding 1 µliter/ml of N,N,N',N'-tetramethylethylenediamine and 0.3 mg/ml of ammonium persulfate. The gels were placed so as to bridge two trays containing 0.1% SDS, 0.19 M glycine, 0.035 M Tris, pH 8.3. Bromophenol blue was added to mark the electrophoretic front. Electrophoresis was performed at 3 mA/gel for 5 hr at 22°C. The gels were fixed in 50% TCA overnight, stained with 0.2% Coomassie Blue in 50% TCA for 1 hr at 37°C and destained with a 5% methanol solution containing 7.5% acetic acid.

RESULTS

Solubilization of RNA Polymerase: Several procedures were explored to extract RNA polymerase activity from purified nuclei of D. discoideum. Treatment of the nuclei with the detergent, N-lauroyl sarcosine (0.5%) and incubation with 1 µg/ml deoxyribonuclease for 20 min at 25°C, resulted in quantitative release of the enzyme into the 43,000 × g supernatant. However, the activity so recovered was not dependent on added DNA template and gave very poor yields upon chromatography on DEAE–cellulose. Aging of the nuclei at 0°C gave only limited success in solubilizing the enzyme. Ultrasonic dissociation of nuclei in a solution of fairly low ionic strength resulted in solubilizing greater than 50% of the activity of whole nuclei in a form almost totally dependent on the addition of exogenous DNA template. The enzyme activity could be chromatographed on DEAE with excellent recovery and remained stable for weeks when stored at −70°C. We decided that sonication was the method of choice for solubilization of RNA polymerase from D. discoideum.

For large-scale purification, RNA polymerase was extracted from 2×10^{11} exponentially growing cells of D. discoideum and a similar number of developing cells. Washed nuclei prepared from these cells were suspended in sonication solution containing 0.04 M Tris HCl pH 7.8, 0.1 mM EDTA, 5 mM 2-mercaptoethanol, and 5% glycerol at a concentration of about 10^9 nuclei/ml. The nuclei were ultrasonically disrupted with a Branson sonifier adapted with a Microtip for 10 sec at 0°C at a tip energy of 40 w. The solution was adjusted to 1.6 mM $MnCl_2$, 6 mM $MgCl_2$, and 0.06 M $(NH_4)_2SO_4$ and centrifuged at 43,000 × g for 30 min. RNA polymerase activity was recovered in the clear supernatant.

Reaction Characteristics: The incorporation of ^{3}H-uridine by soluble nuclear extracts of both exponentially growing cells and developing cells was linear with time for 20 min and continued at a decreasing rate for up to 40 min. The reaction required the presence of all four nucleotide triphosphates and was stimulated 10- to 20-fold by the addition of exogenous calf thymus DNA template. Seventy percent of the TCA insoluble radioactive material could be converted to an acid-soluble form by hydrolysis with KOH or incubation with 10 μg/ml purified ribonuclease for 30 min at 30°C.

The template preferences of the enzymatic preparation were determined with DNA from a variety of organisms (Table I). Although homologous D. discoideum

TABLE I. Template Specificity of RNA Polymerases[a]

DNA source	Soluble enzyme source	
	Exponentially growing cells	Developing cells
D. discoideum	1.00	1.00
Calf thymus	0.85	0.90
Lily microsporocyte	0.68	0.71
Salmon sperm	0.52	0.58
E. coli	0.52	0.47
Phage SP01	0.24	0.18
Phage T7	0.15	0.16
Phage T4	0	0
D. discoideum-denatured DNA	1.20	1.54
Calf thymus-denatured DNA	0.99	1.23

[a]Six units of RNA polymerase solubilized from D. discoideum nuclei were incubated in the standard assay mixture with 100 μg/ml DNA from each of the various sources. This amount of D. discoideum DNA results in maximal incorporation of ^{3}H-UTP into polynucleotide which is set as 1.0. DNA was denatured immediately before the start of the reaction by heating to 98°C for 10 min followed by rapid cooling.

TABLE II. Purification of RNA Polymerase from D. discoideum

Step	Preparation
	Washed cells
Nuclear preparation	Cells broken with 0.8% NP-40 detergent in 15% sucrose, 6 mM MgCl$_2$, 0.04 M KCl, 5 mM mercaptoethanol.
	Preparation centrifuged 4000 × g for 10 min; nuclei collected from the pellet.
	Nuclei
Solubilization	Nuclei ultrasonically disrupted in 0.04 M Tris HCl pH 7.8, 0.1 mM EDTA, 5 mM mercaptoethanol, 5% glycerol.
	Soluble extract
DEAE ion exchange chromatography	Enzyme preparation made 25% (v/v) in glycerol and applied to a 2.5 × 35 cm DEAE–cellulose column. Activity eluted by a linear gradient of (NH$_4$)$_2$SO$_4$ from 0.06 M to 0.5 M, containing 0.04 M Tris pH 7.8, 25% glycerol, 0.1 mM EDTA, 6 mM MgCl$_2$.
	Enzymes I and II
Phosphocellulose chromatography	Enzyme I eluted from DEAE–cellulose column at 0.16 M (NH$_4$)$_2$SO$_4$ and stored at −70°C. Enzyme II eluted at 0.26 M (NH$_4$)$_2$SO$_4$. The preparation diluted 3-fold and adjusted to 40% glycerol and 0.1 M (NH$_4$)$_2$SO$_4$ before being applied to 1.5 × 13 cm phosphocellulose column. The enzyme eluted by a linear gradient of (NH$_4$)$_2$SO$_4$ from 0.1 M to 0.5 M in 0.04 M Tris pH 7.8, 0.1 mM EDTA, 0.5 mM dithiothreitol, 40% glycerol.

DNA was the most effective template, DNA from other cells functioned at least half as well. Bacteriophage DNA were markedly poorer templates for D. discoideum RNA polymerase. Although the enzyme exhibited clear template preferences, there were no significant differences between preparations from exponentially growing cells and those from developing cells with regard to the type of DNA that could be used as a template (Table I). The enzyme preparations utilized single-stranded DNA only slightly better than double-stranded DNA of D. discoideum or calf thymus.

TABLE II. Continued

Step	Preparation
	Phosphocellulose enzyme
Rechromatography on DEAE–cellulose	RNA polymerase eluted from PC column at 0.21 M $(NH_4)_2SO_4$ diluted and adjusted to 25% glycerol and 0.1 M $(NH_4)_2SO_4$ before being applied to a 1 × 12 cm DEAE–cellulose column. The enzyme eluted with a linear gradient of $(NH_4)_2SO_4$ from 0.06 M to 0.5 M.
	Enzymes II; forms a and b
Glycerol gradient	Polymerase activity eluted from DEAE–cellulose in two fractions at 0.17 M (form a) and 0.26 M (form b). Separate forms concentrated by vacuum dialysis against 0.04 M Tris pH 7.8; 0.3 M $(NH_4)_2SO_4$, 0.1 mM EDTA, 0.5 mM dithiothreitol, 6 mM $MgCl_2$ and applied to 10–30% linear glycerol density gradients prepared in the same buffered solution. The gradients centrifuged at 39,000 rpm in a Spinco SW41 rotor for 12 hr at 4°C.
	Purified RNA polymerase
	Glycerol gradients fractioned and the enzyme activity recovered from the region expected for a 15 S molecule. This preparation contains predominantly RNA polymerase.

Purification of RNA Polymerase: An outline of the approach we have used to purify RNA polymerase from D. discoideum is given in Table II. Nuclei from either exponentially growing cells or developing cells were sonically disrupted and the soluble fraction applied to a DEAE–cellulose column. Upon elution with a linear gradient of $(NH_4)_2SO_4$ the activity from both preparations was clearly separated into at least two fractions (Forms I and II) (Figure 1). The activity profiles consistently showed a shoulder eluting after Form II which might indicate the presence of a third form. However, the activity in these samples was not sufficiently stable for subsequent analysis. The relative proportions of the various forms did not change significantly during differentiation of D. discoideum; however, differences in the efficiency of extraction of the various forms could mask such changes.

RNA polymerase II was further purified from both preparations by chromatography on phosphocellulose, care being taken to avoid magnesium and

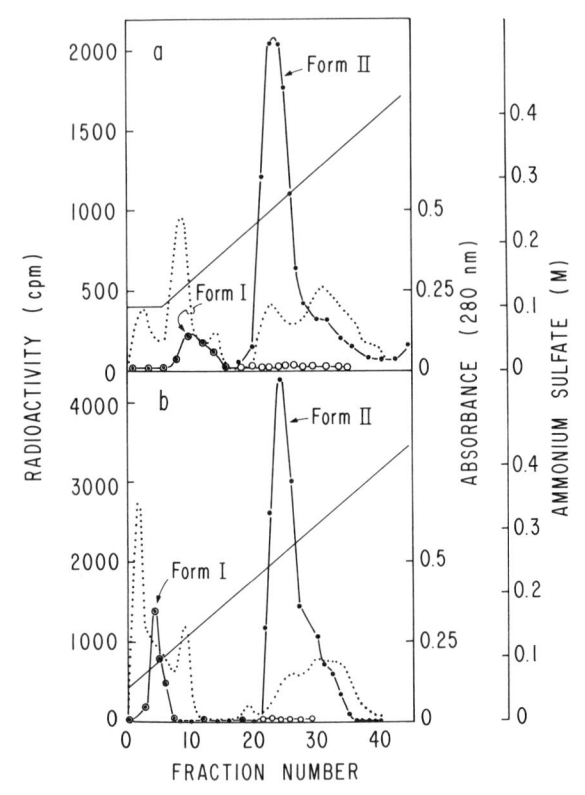

FIGURE 1. Multiple RNA polymerase forms from growing and developing cells of
D. discoideum. Soluble preparations from isolated nuclei were applied to 2.5 × 35 cm
DEAE–cellulose columns. The columns were washed and eluted as described in
Table II, and the absorbance at 280 nm was monitored in the fractions (........).
0.05 ml of each fraction was incubated in the standard polymerase assay
(materials and methods) and the radioactivity incorporated into polynucleotide was
determined (●————●). The fractions were also assayed in the presence of
6.6 μg/ml α-amanitin (○————○). (a) RNA polymerase activity of growing cells.
(b) RNA polymerase activity of developing cells.

manganese ions in the sample and elution buffers since these metals reduce the
capacity of the column [Burgess, 1969a]. The enzyme from both growing
and developing cells eluted from the phosphocellulose columns as a single symmetrical peak and was further purified by rechromatography on DEAE–cellulose (Figures 2 and 3). The enzyme activity separated into two fractions (forms
IIa and IIb) upon elution from DEAE with a gradient of $(NH_4)_2 SO_4$. Form
IIa predominated in the preparation from growing cells while form IIb predominated in the preparation from differentiating cells. It is not clear whether the

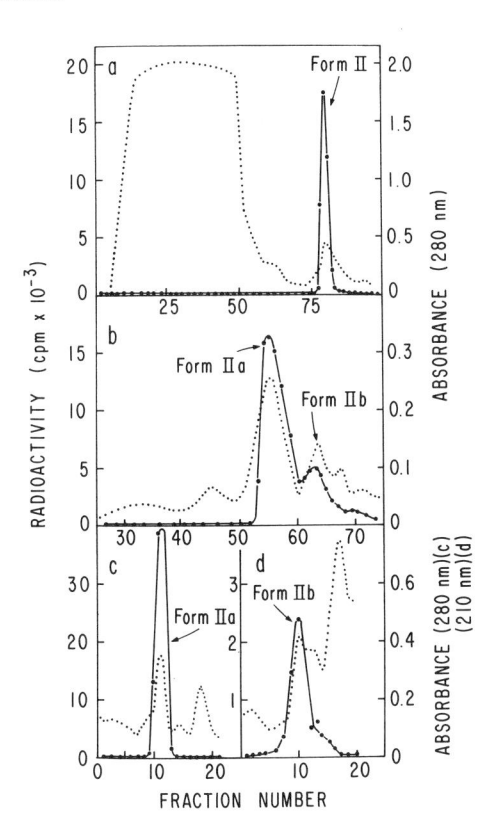

FIGURE 2. Purification of RNA polymerase II from growing cells. RNA polymerase II was isolated from growing cells of D. discoideum by chromatography on DEAE (Figure 1) and further purified as described in Table II. (a) Phosphocellulose chromatography. (b) DEAE–cellulose chromatography. (c) Sedimentation on glycerol gradient of polymerase form II$_a$. (d) Sedimentation on glycerol gradient of polymerase of form II$_b$. Absorbance was monitored in the fractions (........). 0.05 ml of each fraction was assayed for polymerase activity and the radioactivity incorporated into polynucleotide was determined (●————●).

different forms are distinct enzymes or result from modifications of a single enzyme. Preliminary evidence suggests form IIb may be spontaneously converted in vitro to form IIa. A similar conversion of polymerase II has been observed in enzyme preparations from Zea maize [Strain, Mullinix, and Bogorad, 1971]. Sedimentation analysis of the D. discoideum enzymes indicated that forms IIa and IIb were of similar size (about 15S) in preparations from both growing cells and developing cells (Figures 2 and 3).

The purification procedure resulted in about 4000-fold purification of the activity from total cell extract with an overall yield of close to 10% (Table III).

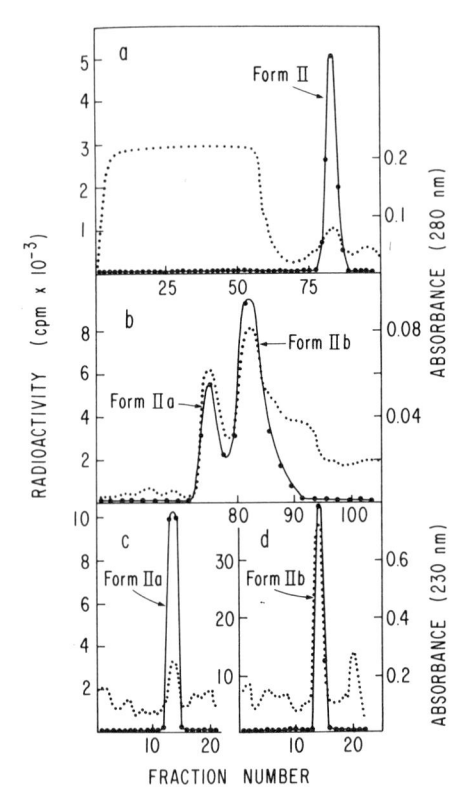

FIGURE 3. Purification of RNA polymerase II from developing cells. The techniques and procedures were the same as those described in the legend to Figure 2 except that RNA polymerase II was isolated from cells developing on filter supports. (a) Phosphocellulose chromatography. (b) DEAE–chromatography. (c) Sedimentation on a glycerol gradient of polymerase form II_a. (d) Sedimentation on a glycerol gradient of polymerase form II_b.

In the final step, protein concentration was found to parallel enzymatic activity in the region of 15 S suggesting that the preparation was essentially homogeneous.

The maximum specific activity achieved for RNA polymerase II from D. discoideum was 22,100 units/mg protein. This compares favorably with the maximum specific activity found in purified enzyme from E. coli, rat liver, and calf thymus of 50,000 units/mg protein [Burgess, 1969b; Weaver, Blatti, and Rutter, 1971]. The activity of the enzyme from these sources was determined at 37°C while that from D. discoideum was determined at 25°C, the physio-

TABLE III. Recovery of Purified RNA Polymerases

Fraction	Enzyme	Total activity, μμmole/min	Total protein, mg	Specific activity, units/mg protein	Percent initial activity
Growing cells					
Nuclear suspension		66,300	1,560	42	100
S-40		37,500	510	73	55
DEAE–cellulose	I	2,512	31	81	4
	II	35,052	108	325	53
PC column	II	16,872	7.2	2,316	26
DEAE–cellulose	II$_a$	7,159	2.0	3,579	11
	II$_b$	2,618	1.2	2,160	4
Glycerol gradient	II$_a$	5,940	0.60	9,900	9
	II$_b$	495	0.044	11,200	0.8
Developing cells					
Nuclear suspension		37,320	634	58	100
S-40		28,100	249	112	75
DEAE–cellulose	I	2,860	42	69	7
	II	23,160	84	273	62
PC column	II	9,288	2.412	3,820	25
DEAE–cellulose	II$_a$	2,314	0.378	6,132	6.2
	II$_b$	5,428	0.612	8,879	15
Glycerol gradient	II$_a$	1,210	0.058	20,850	3.5
	II$_b$	3,035	0.138	22,100	8

RNA polymerase was purified as described in the text and Table II from 2×10^{11} cells of D. discoideum A3 growing exponentially in broth medium or developing on filter supports.

logical temperature of this organism. If we assume a Q_{10} of about 2, the enzymes from these diverse organisms all appear to have similar turnover numbers.

The sedimentation velocity of the D. discoideum RNA polymerase enzymes was accurately determined by adding purified E. coli polymerase (13 S) as a marker during centrifugation of purified polymerase II on glycerol gradients. The polymerase activities were assayed separately by including either rifampicin or α-amanitin in the assays so as to specifically inhibit the bacterial or the eukaryotic enzyme respectively (Table IV). The sedimentation velocity of RNA polymerase from D. discoideum indicated a molecule of 15S. Assuming a globular configuration for the enzyme, the molecular weight of RNA polymerase appears to be about 450,000 dalton. We calculate that exponentially growing amoebae each contain 36,000 molecules of RNA polymerase II while developing cells each contain 8000 molecules. These values can be compared to

TABLE IV. Antibiotic Sensitivity of RNA Polymerases[a]

		Percent Inhibition			
		Polymerase from growing cells		Polymerase from developing cells	
Antibiotics	Concentration, μg/ml	I	II	I	II
Control		0	0	0	0
α-Amanitin	10	15	99	11	99
Rifampicin	150	0	0	0	0
Cycloheximide	150	0	0	0	0
Actinomycin D	30	84	89	87	85

[a]RNA polymerases I and II were partially purified as described in Figure 1 and assayed in the presence of various antibiotics which were added before the start of the reaction.

an estimated 3000 molecules per cell in E. coli, 10,000 molecules per cell in rat liver, and 800 molecules per cell in calf thymus [Weaver et al., 1971].

Subunit Composition of the Enzymes: RNA polymerase purified from either E. coli or B. subtilis has been estimated to be a large molecule of 360,000–440,000 molecular weight [Burgess, 1969b; Losick et al., 1970]. The E. coli enzyme is composed of two α chains (37,000–41,000 dalton), a β' subunit (150,000–180,000 dalton), and a β subunit (140,000–170,000 dalton) [Burgess, 1969b]. In addition, there is a protein of 85,000–90,000 molecular weight, termed sigma, associated with the bacterial enzyme which appears to be required for specific initiations [Burgess et al., 1969]. Many purified preparations also contain a low molecular weight subunit of 9000 dalton, the function of which is unclear. Polymerase preparations from rat liver and calf thymus have been shown to contain three subunits of about 190,000, 170,000, and 150,000 dalton, respectively [Kedinger, Nuret, and Chambon, 1971; Chesterton and Butterworth, 1971; Weaver et al., 1971]. Since the ratio of these subunits in different preparations of highly purified enzyme is constant, they are thought to be integral components of the enzyme. The highly purified calf thymus preparations may consist, however, of a mixture of two different forms of polymerase, one containing a 190,000 dalton and a 150,000 dalton subunit, and the other a 170,000 dalton and a 150,000 dalton subunit [Kedinger et al., 1971]. Recently, Weaver et al. [1971] suggested that the 170,000 dalton subunit was generated by proteolytic attack on the 190,000 dalton subunit during the purification process and thus the second form might be a laboratory artifact. Further study is needed to clarify this point. Purified liver and calf thymus polymerase also contained proteins of 35,000 and 25,000 dalton which may function as small subunits of the enzyme. However, in the absence of genetic analysis or reconstruction experiments, there is no direct evidence that the components are required for polymerase activity.

We have analyzed the subunit composition of purified polymerase II isolated from exponentially growing and developing cells of D. discoideum. Enzyme II forms a and b, purified through glycerol gradients as described in Table II, were dissociated into their polypeptide chains by incubating with 1% SDS and 1% 2-mercaptoethanol and applied to discontinuous, high pH acrylamide gels containing 0.1% SDS. The subunits were separated by electrophoresis at 3 mA/gel for 5 hr at 22°C. This technique separates proteins predominantly on the basis of molecular weight and the relationship between size and mobility can be calibrated using proteins of known molecular weight (Figure 4). Subunits of estimated molecular weight 190,000, 170,000, and 150,000 were found associated with each preparation of enzyme. The molecular weight determinations are subject to an uncertainty of ±10%. The molecular ratio of each of these large subunits was estimated from the gel tracings of several independent preparations. The proportions of the 190,000 and 170,000 dalton subunits varied from preparation to preparation, but the sum of the material always equaled that in the 150,000 dalton subunit. This suggests that the enzyme preparation contains two forms, one composed from the 190,000 and 150,000 dalton subunits and the other composed from the 170,000 and 150,000 dalton subunits as appears to be the case in polymerase preparations from calf thymus [Kedinger et al., 1971; Weaver et al., 1971]. It is not yet clear whether the 170,000 dalton subunit might be derived from the larger subunit during our purification procedure. However, McMahon and Seed [1972, personal communication] have preliminary evidence that when the purification of RNA polymerase from D. discoideum is carried out in the presence of the proteolytic inhibitor, phenylmethylsulfonyl fluoride, the proportion of the 170,000 dalton subunit is decreased and the proportion of the 190,000 dalton subunit is concomitantly increased. This suggests that the only large subunits of the native enzyme are the 190,000 dalton and the 150,000 dalton ones. Besides these large subunits, all of our preparations also consistently contained subunits of about 28,000, 21,000, and 15,000 dalton. Since polymerase II isolated from developing cells gave a pattern on SDS–acrylamide gels identical to that from enzyme isolated from growing cells, there appears to be no dramatic change in subunit composition of the enzymes during development of D. discoideum.

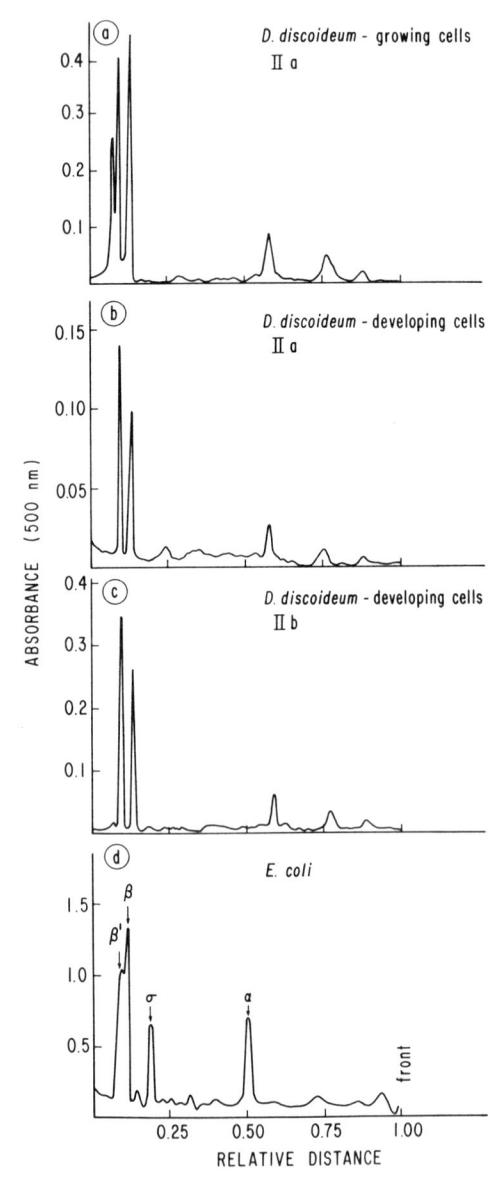

FIGURE 4. Densitograms of SDS acrylamide gels stained with Coomassie Blue after electrophoresis of purified RNA polymerase. (a) 20 μg of polymerase II_a from growing cells. (b) 5 μg of polymerase II_a from developing cells. (c) 15 μg of polymerase II_b from developing cells. (d) Partially purified E. coli polymerase was subjected to electrophoresis to provide protein markers of defined molecular weight. The front moved about 8 cm during the electrophoresis. The gels were analyzed on a Gilford Spectrophotometer equipped with a gel-scanning device.

Characteristics of Enzymes I and II: Enzymes I and II have been distinguished unequivocably from a variety of organisms by differential sensitivity to the drug, α-amanitin [Stirpe and Fiume, 1967; Lindell et al., 1970; Kedinger et al., 1970; Chesterton and Butterworth, 1971b; Jacob et al., 1970; Furth and Austin, 1970; Keller and Goor, 1970; Horgan and Griffin, 1971; Strain et al., 1971; Adman and Hall, 1971; Ponta, Ponta, and Wintersberger, 1971; Dezelle, Sentenae, and Fromageot, 1972]. The enzymes from D. discoideum, likewise, show greatly differing sensitivity to the drug (Table IV). Thus, it is clear that the enzymes differ in their functional characteristics. Moreover, it has recently been found that polymerase I in D. discoideum is preferentially associated with nucleoli, which suggests that enzyme I may be involved in ribosomal RNA synthesis [Miller and Loomis, 1973].

The activities of both enzymes I and II were inhibited in vitro as well as in vivo by actinomycin D (Table IV) [Sussman and Sussman, 1965]. The enzymes were not sensitive to rifampicin which blocks initiation by prokaryotic RNA polymerase [Hartmann et al., 1967].

Several studies both in vivo and in vitro have shown that the activity of RNA polymerase II is stimulated far more than that of polymerase I when Mn^{2+} ions replace Mg^{2+} ions [Windell and Tata, 1966; Roeder and Rutter, 1969]. However, the degree of stimulation appears to depend on the methods of enzyme extraction [Capobianco and Vescia, 1970] and the tissue of origin, such that often no differential stimulation by Mn^{2+} is found between the polymerase forms [Strain et al., 1971]. We found very little difference between the responses of enzymes I and II from either exponentially growing cells or developing cells to different metal ion additions (Figure 5). However, the general characteristics of the D. discoideum enzymes to Mn^{2+} and Mg^{2+} concentrations were similar to those of other eukaryotic enzymes, and indicated a preference for Mn^{2+}.

DISCUSSION

Differential gene expression has been found to be mediated by control of the template specificity of RNA polymerase in several bacterial systems [Travers, 1971; Dunn, Bautz, and Bautz, 1971; Losick et al., 1970]. In eukaryotes, two activities have been found associated with the nucleus: enzyme I, which appears to transcribe predominantly ribosomal RNA; and enzyme II, which transcribes other portions of the genome. A third form has also been seen on occasion [Roeder and Rutter, 1969]. Moreover, there are other polymerase forms associated with mitochondria and chloroplasts. Polymerase has been solubilized from Neurospora mitochondria and found to be a single polypeptide of 64,000 dalton [Tsai, Michaelis, and Criddle, 1971; Kuntzel and Schafer, 1971].

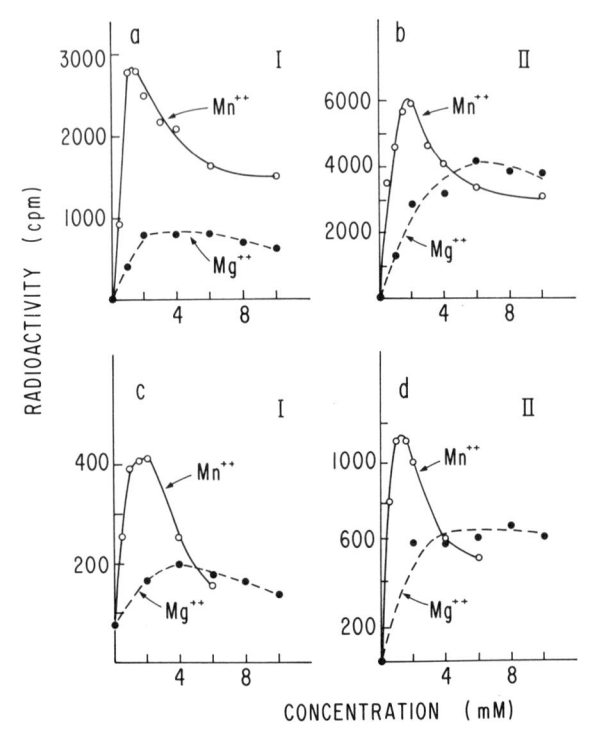

FIGURE 5. Effect of divalent metal ion concentration on the activities of D. discoideum RNA polymerases. Enzymes I and II were separated by chromatography on DEAE and dialyzed for 6 hr against 0.04 Tris HCl (pH 7.8), 0.06 M $(NH_4)_2SO_4$, 0.1 mM EDTA, 5 mM 2-mercaptoethanol and 25% glycerol at 0°C. Enzymatic activity was determined in assay mixtures lacking metal ions except for the indicated concentration of Mn^{2+} (o———o) or Mg^{2+} (●———●). (a) Form I of growing cells. (b) Form II of growing cells. (c) Form I of developing cells. (d) Form II of developing cells.

The enzyme from this organelle is resistant to α-amanitin and sensitive to rifampicin. A complex molecule of greater than 500,000 dalton appears to account for the polymerase activity of maize chloroplasts [Bottomley, Smith, and Bogorad, 1971]. This enzyme is not inhibited by either α-amanitin or rifampicin.

The specific localization of enzyme I and the organelle enzymes suggests that each transcribes a restricted portion of the total genome. However, it is not yet clear whether changing patterns of nuclear, ribosomal, and cytoplasmic RNA synthesis are mediated by changes in the relative proportions of RNA polymerase forms [Tocchini-Valentini and Crippa, 1970; Roeder, Reeder, and Brown, 1970].

Just as in other higher organisms studied, RNA polymerase I of D. discoideum appears to be localized in nucleoli and presumably directs rRNA synthesis. However, no significant change in the ratio of polymerase I and II was found during development (Figure 1) although the relative rate of rRNA synthesis decreases during this period [Firtel and Lodish, 1972]. Thus we must assume a mechanism other than availability of the enzymes is involved in directing this changing pattern. Although the proportions do not appear to change, both enzyme activities decrease severalfold during development (Table III). We were unable to find any change in the subunit structure of polymerase II during development. However, it is clear from DNA—RNA hybridization analyses as well as from determination of the transcriptive periods for various enzymes that the pattern of RNA synthesis changes during development [Sussman and Sussman, 1969; Loomis, 1969; Firtel, 1971]. If differential gene activity is controlled in this organism by specific polymerase factors, they must be lost during our purification procedure. Perhaps other purification techniques will uncover such factors.

A search for polymerase modifying factors in calf thymus has disclosed a protein fraction which stimulates RNA synthesis by purified polymerase when double-stranded DNA is used as a template [Stein and Hausen, 1970]. However, since the enzyme preparations in these studies utilized single-stranded DNA as a template to a much greater extent than double-stranded DNA when the factor was not added, it is possible that the addition of the factor stimulated the activity on double-stranded DNA by opening up the DNA duplex or inserting single-strand nicks. Whether similar processes occur in vivo is not clear. Dahmus and Lee [1972] have recently isolated one protein factor from rat liver which stimulates the activities of enzymes I, II, and III to different extents on native DNA. However, it is not yet clear whether this factor binds to the polymerase forms or affects the template directly.

The difficulties encountered in demonstrating control of template specificity in RNA polymerase may have resulted from the use of either nonphysiological conditions in the assay reaction or an inappropriate choice of templates. If the added DNA contains two equal subsets of genetic information which are differentially transcribed by two polymerase forms, no evidence for template specificity will be found among the enzymes when the overall incorporation of ^{3}H-uridine is followed although the products may be quite different. The only general technique presently available which can distinguish the products of RNA polymerase reaction on the basis of nucleotide sequence is DNA—RNA hybridization. This technique has been of inestimable value in the analysis of template specificity of RNA polymerase in bacterial systems but may not be as applicable in eukaryotic systems due to the greatly increased complexity of the eukaryotic genome. Thus, special techniques are required to measure most unique RNA species in eukaryotic systems.

Fairly high resolution has been reached by this technique in the analysis of ribosomal RNA species, since the high proportion of genes coding for rRNA facilitates the hybridization reaction. The technique has been used to show that in the presence of α-amanitin, nuclei transcribe predominantly rRNA [Blatti et al., 1970]. Similar analyses using purified enzyme I have inexplicably failed to demonstrate template specificity [Roeder et al., 1970]. It appears that the present in vitro assay conditions for purified polymerase using purified DNA as a template do not mimic the in situ conditions.

Control of specific gene activity in many cases of differentiation may not involve a change in RNA polymerase but a change in the chromosomal template. For this reason, several studies have been carried out to determine the ability of chromatin isolated from various organisms and tissues to direct the synthesis of RNA species in vitro [Huang and Bonner, 1965; Gilmour and Paul, 1969]. This work has shown that isolated chromatin can vary considerably in template activity but it was not clear whether the differences were the result of changes in the chromatin or variations in the isolation procedures. Moreover, it was not established whether the different patterns of RNA synthesized in vitro had a direct bearing on in vivo differentiations. For technical reasons, RNA polymerase isolated from E. coli rather than from the homologous tissue was used in these studies to direct the in vitro synthesis. It has recently been shown that RNA polymerase isolated from eukaryotic cells gives rise to quite different RNA products than does a bacterial polymerase when chromatin is used as the template [Butterworth, Cox, and Chesterton, 1971]. The purification of specific eukaryotic polymerases can provide enzyme for further analysis of chromosomal differentiation.

We thank Daniel McMahon, California Institute of Technology; William Summers, Yale University; and Maurice Sussman, Brandeis University for stimulating discussions and communication of unpublished results.

This work was supported by the National Science Foundation.

REFERENCES

[1] Adman, R., and B. Hall. 1971. Some properties of four RNA polymerase enzymes isolated from Saccharomyces cerevisiae. Federation Proc. 30:1301.

[2] Blatti, S. P., C. J. Ingles, T. J. Lindell, P. W. Morris, R. F. Weaver, F. Weinberg, and W. J. Rutter. 1970. Structure and regulatory properties of

eukaryotic RNA polymerase. Cold Spring Harbor Symp. Quant. Biol. 35:649.
[3] Bottomley, W., H. J. Smith, and L. Bogorad. 1971. RNA polymerases of maize: Partial purification and properties of chloroplast enzyme. Proc. Nat. Acad. Sci. 68:2412.
[4] Burgess, R. R. 1969a. A new method for large scale purification of Escherichia coli deoxyribonucleic acid-dependent RNA polymerase. J. Biol. Chem. 244:6160.
[5] Burgess, R. R. 1969b. Separation and characterization of the subunit of ribonucleic acid polymerase. J. Biol. Chem. 244:6168.
[6] Burgess, R. R., A. A. Travers, J. J. Dunn, and E. K. F. Bautz. 1969. Factor stimulating transcription by RNA polymerase. Nature 221:43.
[7] Butterworth, P. H. W., R. F. Cox, and C. J. Chesterton. 1971. Transcription of mammalian chromatin by mammalian DNA-dependent RNA polymerases. Eur. J. Biochem. 23:229.
[8] Capobianco, B., and A. Vescia. 1970. Some factors affecting DNA-dependent RNA polymerase solubilization from rat liver nuclei. Italian J. Biochem. 19:217.
[9] Chesterton, C. J., and P. H. W. Butterworth. 1971a. Selective extraction of form I DNA-dependent RNA polymerase from rat liver nuclei and its separation into two species. Eur. J. Biochem. 19:232.
[10] Chesterton, C. J., and P. H. W. Butterworth. 1971b. A new form of mammalian DNA-dependent RNA polymerase and its relationship to the known forms of the enzyme. FEBS Letters 12:301.
[11] Chesterton, C. J., and P. H. W. Butterworth. 1971c. Purification of the rat liver form B DNA-dependent RNA polymerases. FEBS Letters 15:181.
[12] Coccuci, S. M., and M. Sussman. 1970. RNA in cytoplasmic and nuclear fractions of cellular slime mold amoebaes. J. Cell. Biol. 45:399.
[13] Dahmus, D., and S. Lee. 1972. Multiple forms of RNA polymerase from their response to a purified stimulation factor. Fed. Proc. 31:428 (abstract).
[14] Dezelee, S., A. Sentenae, and P. Fromageot. 1972. Role of DNA−RNA hybrids in eukaryotes. I. Purification of yeast RNA polymerase B. FEBS Letters 21:1.
[15] Dunn, J. J., F. A. Bautz, and E. K. F. Bautz. 1971. Different template specificities of phage T_3 and T_7 RNA polymerase. Nature 230:94.
[16] Firtel, R. A. 1971. Regulation of development in the cellular slime mold Dictyostelium discoideum. Doctoral Thesis. California Institute of Technology, Pasadena, Calif.
Firtel, R., and Lodish, H. 1972. Massachusetts Institute of Technology, Cambridge, Mass. Personal communication.
[17] Furth, J. J., and G. E. Austin. 1970. RNA polymerase of lymphoid tissue: a preliminary characterization of the enzyme and the RNA it synthesizes. Cold Spring Harbor Symp. Quant. Biol. 35:641.
[18] Gilbert, W., and B. Müller-Hill. 1966. Isolation of the lac repressor. Proc. Nat. Acad. Sci. 56:1891.

[19] Gilmour, R. S., and J. Paul. 1969. RNA transcribed from reconstituted nucleoprotein is similar to natural RNA. J. Mol. Biol. 40:137.
[20] Goff, C. G., and K. Weber. 1970. A T4-induced RNA polymerase α subunit modification. Cold Spring Harbor Symp. Quant. Biol. 35:101.
[21] Goldberg, M. L., and H. D. Moon. 1970. Partial purification of RNA polymerase from bovine thymus. Arch. Biochem. Biophys. 141:258.
[22] Hager, G., B. D. Hall, and K. Fields. 1970. Transcriptional factors from T4-infected Escherichia coli. Cold Spring Harbor Symp. Quant. Biol. 35:233.
[23] Hartmann, G., K. O. Honikel, F. Knüsel, and J. Nüesch. 1967. The specific inhibition of the DNA-directed RNA synthesis by rifampicin. Biochim. Biophys. Acta 145:843.
[24] Horgan, P. A., and D. H. Griffin. 1971. Specific inhibitors of the three RNA polymerases from the aquatic fungus Blastocladiella emersonii. Proc. Nat. Acad. Sci. 68:338.
[25] Huang, R. C., and J. Bonner. 1965. Histone-bound RNA, a component of native nucleohistone. Proc. Nat. Acad. Sci. 54:960.
[26] Jacob, F., and J. Monod. 1961. Genetic regulatory mechanisms in the synthesis of proteins. J. Mol. Biol. 3:318.
[27] Jacob, S. T., E. M. Sajdel, and H. N. Munro. 1968. Altered characteristics of mammalian RNA polymerase following solubilization from nuclei. Biochem. Biophys. Res. Commun. 32:831.
[28] Jacob, S. T., E. M. Sajdel, W. Muecke, and H. N. Munro. 1970. Soluble RNA polymerases of rat liver nuclei: properties, template specificity, and amanitin responses in vitro and in vivo. Cold Spring Harbor Symp. Quant. Biol. 35:681.
[29] Kedinger, C., M. Gniazdowski, J. L. Mandel, F. Gissinger, and P. Chambon. 1970. α-amanitin: a specific inhibitor of one of two DNA-dependent RNA polymerase activities from calf thymus. Biochem. Biophys. Res. Commun. 38:165.
[30] Kedinger, C., P. Nuret, and P. Chambon. 1971. Structural evidence for two α-amanitin sensitive RNA polymerases in calf thymus. FEBS Letters 15:169.
[31] Keller, W., and R. Goor. 1970. Mammalian RNA polymerase: Structure and functional properties. Cold Spring Harbor Symp. Quant. Biol. 35:671.
[32] Klebe, R. J., T. R. Chen, and F. H. Ruddle. 1970. Mapping of a human genetic regulator element by somatic cell genetic analysis. Proc. Nat. Acad. Sci. 66:1220.
[33] Kuntzel, H., and K. P. Schäfer. 1971. Mitochondrial RNA polymerase from Neurospora crassa. Nature 231:265.
[34] Laemmli, U. K. 1970. Cleavage of structural proteins during the assembly of the head of bacteriophage T4. Nature 227:680.
[35] Liao, S. D., D. Sagher, and S. Fang. 1968. Isolation of chromatin-free RNA polymerase from mammalian cell nuclei. Nature 220:1336.

[36] Lindell, T. J., F. Weinberg, P. W. Morris, R. G. Roeder, and W. J. Rutter. 1970. Specific inhibition of RNA polymerase II by α-amanitin. Science 170:447.
[37] Loomis, W. F., Jr. 1969. Developmental regulation of alkaline phosphatase in Dictyostelium discoideum. J. Bacteriol. 100:417.
[38] Loomis, W. F., Jr. 1971. Sensitivity of Dictyostelium discoideum to nuclei acid analogues. Exp. Cell Res. 64:484.
[39] Losick, R., A. L. Sonenshein, R. G. Shorenstein, and C. Hussey. 1970. Role of RNA polymerase in sporulation. Cold Spring Harbor Symp. Quant. Biol. 35:443.
[40] Lowry, O. H., N. J. Rosebrough, A. L. Farr, and R. J. Randall. 1951. Protein measurement with the Folin phenol reagent. J. Biol. Chem. 193:265.
[41] Mandel, J. L., and P. Chambon. 1971. Purification of RNA polymerase B activity from rat liver. FEBS Letters 15:175.

McMahon, D. and Seed, B. 1972. California Institute of Technology, Pasadena, Calif. Personal communication.

[42] Mertelsmann, R. 1969. Purification and some properties of a soluble DNA-dependent RNA polymerase from nuclei of human placenta. Eur. J. Biochem. 9:311.

Miller, J. and Loomis, W. F. 1973. University of California, San Diego. Unpublished observations.

[43] Ponta, H., U. Ponta, and E. Wintersberger. 1971. DNA-dependent RNA polymerases from yeast. Partial characterization of three nuclear enzyme activities. FEBS Letters 18:204.
[44] Ptashne, M., and N. Hopkins. 1968. The operators controlled by the λ phage repressor. Proc. Nat. Acad. Sci. 60:1282.
[45] Roeder, R. G., R. H. Reeder, and D. D. Brown. 1970. Multiple forms of RNA polymerase in Xenopus laevis: their relationship to RNA synthesis in vivo and their fidelity of transcription in vitro. Cold Spring Harbor Symp. Quant. Biol. 35:727.
[46] Roeder, R. G., and W. J. Rutter. 1969. Multiple forms of DNA-dependent RNA polymerase in eukaryotic organisms. Nature 224:234.
[47] Roeder, R. G., and W. J. Rutter. 1970. Specific nucleolar and nucleoplasmic RNA polymerases. Proc. Nat. Acad. Sci. 65:675.
[48] Seifart, K. H. 1970. A factor stimulating the transcription on double-stranded DNA by purified RNA polymerase from rat liver nuclei. Cold Spring Harbor Symp. Quant. Biol. 35:719.
[49] Seifart, K. H., and C. E. Sekeris. 1969. Extraction and purification of DNA-dependent RNA polymerase from rat liver nuclei. Eur. J. Biochem. 7:408.
[50] Stein, H., and P. Hausen. 1970. A factor from calf thymus stimulating DNA-dependent RNA polymerase isolated from this tissue. Eur. J. Biochem. 14:270.
[51] Stirpe, F., and L. Fiume. 1967. Studies on the pathogenesis of liver necrosis by α-amanitin: Effect of α-amanitin on ribonucleic acid synthesis

and on ribonucleic acid polymerase in mouse liver nuclei. Biochem. J. 105:779.
[52] Strain, G. C., K. P. Mullinix, and L. Bogorad. 1971. RNA polymerases of maize: nuclear RNA polymerases. Proc. Nat. Acad. Sci. 68:2647.
[53] Sugden, B., and J. Sambrook. 1970. RNA polymerase from HeLa cells. Cold Spring Harbor Symp. Quant. Biol. 35:663.
[54] Sussman, M., and R. Sussman. 1965. The regulatory program for UDP-galactose polysaccharide transferase activity during slime mold cytodifferentiation: requirement for specific synthesis of ribonucleic acid. Biochim. Biophys. Acta 108:463.
[55] Sussman, M., and R. Sussman. 1969. Patterns of RNA synthesis and of enzyme accumulation and disappearance during cellular slime mold cytodifferentiation. Symp. Soc. Gen. Microbiol. 19:403.
[56] Tocchini-Valentini, G. P., and M. Crippa. 1970. RNA polymerases from Xenopus laevis. Cold Spring Harbor Symp. Quant. Biol. 35:737.
[57] Tomkins, G. M., T. D. Gelehrter, D. Granner, D. Martin, Jr., H. H. Samuels, and E. B. Thompson. 1969. Control of specific gene expression in higher organisms. Science 166:1474.
[58] Travers, A. A. 1969. Bacteriophage sigma factor for RNA polymerase. Nature 223:1107.
[59] Travers, A. A. 1970. Positive control of transcription by a bacteriophage sigma factor. Nature 225:1009.
[60] Travers, A. A. 1971. Control of transcription in bacteria. Nature 229:69.
[61] Tsai, M. J., G. Michaelis, and R. S. Criddle. 1971. DNA-dependent RNA polymerase from yeast mitochondria. Proc. Nat. Acad. Sci. 68:473.
[62] Weaver, R. F., S. P. Blatti, and W. J. Rutter. 1971. Molecular structures of DNA-dependent RNA polymerases (II) from calf thymus and rat liver. Proc. Nat. Acad. Sci. 68:2994.
[63] Weiss, S. B., and L. Gladstone. 1959. A mammalian system for the incorporation of cytidine triphosphate into ribonucleic acid. J. Amer. Chem. Soc. 81:4118.
[64] Windell, C. C., and J. R. Tata. 1966. Studies on the stimulation by ammonium sulfate of the DNA-dependent RNA polymerase of isolated rat liver nuclei. Biochim. Biophys. Acta 123:478.
[65] Zylber, E. A., and S. Penman. 1971. Products of RNA polymerases in HeLa cell nuclei. Proc. Nat. Acad. Sci. 68:2861.

The Isolation and Analysis of DNA from Eukaryotic Cells

STEPHEN H. HOWELL

This chapter contains a series of experiments which represent some of the current approaches to the study of DNA in higher organisms. The chapter is divided in six sections which are arranged in sequence. It is recommended but not required that the experiments be performed in the described order. Each section is self-contained. Basically, the sense of this sequence of experiments is to isolate subcellular fractions, extract DNA from those fractions and characterize the DNA in terms of its buoyant density, base composition, and chromatography characteristics on hydroxyapatite. Either animal cells (rat liver) or plant cells (spinach leaves or Chlamydomonas reinhardi) can be used as experimental material.

SECTION I CELL FRACTIONATION OF ANIMAL AND PLANT CELLS

Cell fractionation procedures are commonly used to identify enzyme activities or macromolecules such as nucleic acids, with certain organelles. The goal of such procedures is to purify an organelle with high yield and minimal damage. The procedures given here are for the fractionation of rat liver and spinach leaf cells in aqueous media. This fractionation yields nuclei, mitochrondia, chloroplasts, and microsomes from which nucleic acids will be extracted and analyzed. With certain modifications, these procedures can be applied to other tissues; however, different tissues often demand special techniques which cannot be included here.

All fractionation procedures begin by breaking the cell wall or membrane. This must be done in a way which causes minimal disruption to organellar components. With rat liver tissue, only gentle homogenization is needed to break cells. With plant cells, such as spinach leaves, cutting action (with blender or preferably with razor blades) accomplishes this task without extensive damage to organelles.

It is essential that broken cells release their contents into a suspending medium that will maintain organellar integrity. An important characteristic of that medium is its tonicity, usually maintained by sucrose. For animal cells, 0.25–0.30 M sucrose is commonly used and for plant cells, 0.40–0.50 M sucrose. To maintain nuclei, the presence of divalent cations (1–5 mM Ca^{2+} or Mg^{2+}) is a critical requirement. Other characteristics of a sucrose medium which are important for maintaining the integrity of selected subcellular fractions are listed in Table I. With discriminate use of the detergents, chelators, and enzymes

TABLE I. Additions or Conditions to Maintain Integrity of Subcellular Fractions in Isotonic Sucrose Solutions

Addition or condition	Sensitivity of fraction		
	Nuclei	Mitochondria	Chloroplasts
pH	7.0 (6.0–7.8)	7.6 (7.2–8.0)	7.2 (7.0–7.8)
Divalent cation	Required (1–5 mM Mg^{2+} or Ca^{2+})	Not required	Not required
Monovalent cation	(No general requirement, often helpful to disperse cytoplasm from nuclei at 10–20 mM K^+ or Na^+.)		
EDTA (5 mM)	Sensitive	Preserved	Preserved
Triton X100 (0.4%)	Preserved[a]	Sensitive	Sensitive
Nonidet P40 (0.5–0.05%)	Preserved[a]	Sensitive	Sensitive
Sodium dodecyl sulfate (0.5%)	Sensitive[a]	Preserved	Preserved
Sodium deoxycholate (0.1%)	Preserved[a]	Preserved	Sensitive
Pancreatic deoxyribonuclease (20–200 μg/ml)	Sensitive	Preserved	Preserved

[a]In the presence of 1–3 mM Ca^{2+}

shown in Table I, one can selectively destroy or remove contaminating material while maintaining the integrity of the subcellular material to be isolated. For example, nuclei isolated in the presence of 0.1% Nonidet P40 are preserved while other membrane organelles and the cytoplasmic tabs on the nuclei are solubilized.

Suspended organelles are subsequently isolated by differential velocity sedimentation (differential centrifugation) or by equilibrium density sedimentation (isopycnic centrifugation). It is important to monitor each fractionation step

ANALYSIS OF DNA

by cytological observation or by biochemical analysis. To do this, retain a small sample of each fraction at suggested steps in the procedure. Observe intermediate and final fractions in the light microscope using the cytological preparation listed in Table II. A small sample can be used for nucleic acid determination (section II) or the entire fraction used for DNA extraction (section III). In either case the sample or fraction can be processed immediately for nucleic acid isolation and analysis or kept overnight (or longer) in 70% EtOH at −20°C.

TABLE II. Identification and Characteristics of Subcellular Fractions

Subcellular fraction	Cytological preparation for unfixed sample	Nucleic acid content
Nuclei	Methyl green–pyronin[a]	High DNA, high RNA RNA:DNA = ~0.2:0.3 for rat liver nuclei
Chloroplasts	Unstained	—
Mitochondria	Janus green[b]	—
Microsomes	(Not visible by light microscopy—fraction should not be turbid)	High RNA

[a]Staining solution: 12.5 ml of 2% pyonin Y (aqueous solution, chloroform extracted), 7.5 ml of 2% methyl green (aqueous solution), and 30 ml distilled water.
[b]Stock solution: 1.0% Janus green B in neutral absolute alcohol. Dilute stock, 0.1 ml into 10 ml extraction buffer prior to use.

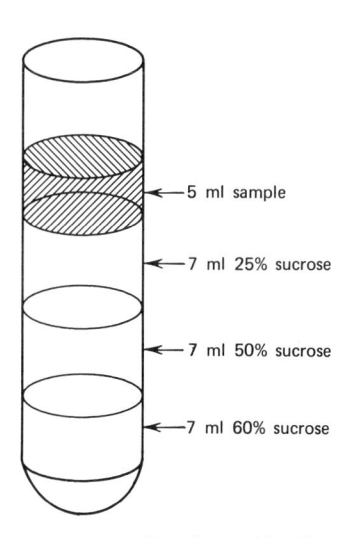

FIGURE 1. Discontinuous sucrose gradient for purification of spinach nuclei. All sucrose solutions are in 20 mM Tris HCl (pH 7.8), 10 mM NaCl, 1 mM $MgCl_2$, 2 mM $CaCl_2$, 2.5% Ficoll, and 5.0% Dextran.

Fractionation of Rat Liver Cells for Nuclei, Mitochondria and Microsomes

Sacrifice a rat (starved overnight) by cranial concussion. Surgically remove the liver lobes. Immerse liver in cold 0.3 M sucrose, 3 mM $CaCl_2$ solution. Remove connective tissue with forceps and scissors. All further procedures should be carried out in the cold (4°C) or on ice. Pour off excess solution and weigh out 5 g of tissue. Mince tissue with scissors in a petri dish or beaker.

Homogenize liver pieces with a Teflon pestle tissue grinder with 7.5 ml of 0.5 M sucrose, 3 mM ($CaCl_2$). (Use ~ 10 strokes at 400 rpm.). Observe one drop cytologically. Cells should be broken, nuclei intact. If cells are not broken, continue homogenization.

Add ~ 20 ml of 0.3 M sucrose, 3 mM $CaCl_2$ and filter through prewetted flannelette.

Adjust volume to 42 ml with 0.3 M sucrose, 3 mM $CaCl_2$. Use one drop for cytology. Retain 2 ml sample[a] in EtOH for nucleic acid determination.

40 ml
Centrifuge 1000 × g for 7 min.

Pellet

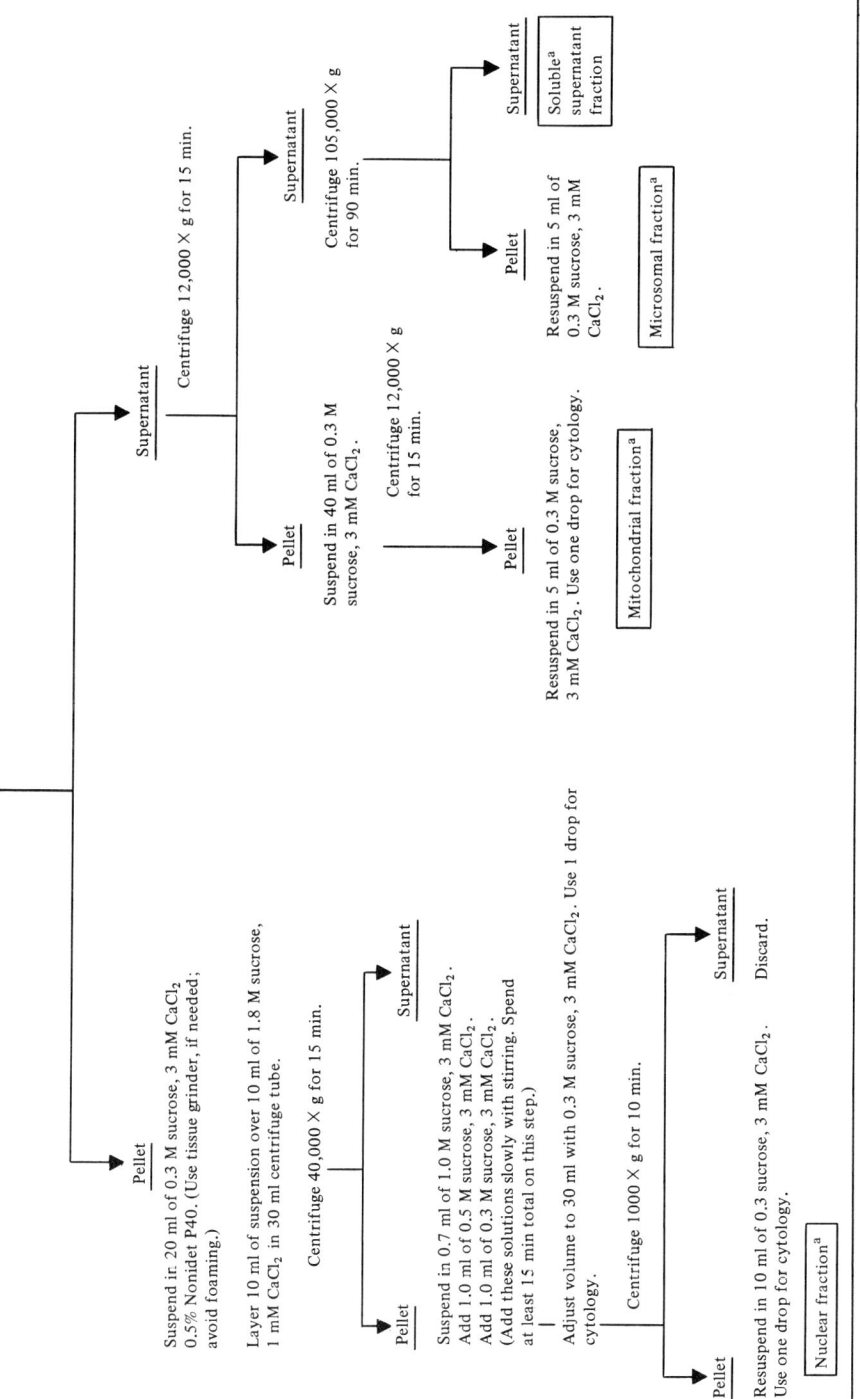

Suspend in 20 ml of 0.3 M sucrose, 3 mM CaCl$_2$, 0.5% Nonidet P40. (Use tissue grinder, if needed; avoid foaming.)

Layer 10 ml of suspension over 10 ml of 1.8 M sucrose, 1 mM CaCl$_2$ in 30 ml centrifuge tube.

Centrifuge 40,000 × g for 15 min.

→ **Supernatant**

→ **Pellet**

Suspend in 0.7 ml of 1.0 M sucrose, 3 mM CaCl$_2$.
Add 1.0 ml of 0.5 M sucrose, 3 mM CaCl$_2$.
Add 1.0 ml of 0.3 M sucrose, 3 mM CaCl$_2$.
(Add these solutions slowly with stirring. Spend at least 15 min total on this step.)
Adjust volume to 30 ml with 0.3 M sucrose, 3 mM CaCl$_2$. Use 1 drop for cytology.

Centrifuge 1000 × g for 10 min.

→ **Supernatant** Discard.

→ **Pellet**

Resuspend in 10 ml of 0.3 sucrose, 3 mM CaCl$_2$. Use one drop for cytology.

Nuclear fraction[a]

Supernatant

Centrifuge 12,000 × g for 15 min.

→ **Pellet**

Suspend in 40 ml of 0.3 M sucrose, 3 mM CaCl$_2$.

Centrifuge 12,000 × g for 15 min.

→ **Pellet**

Resuspend in 5 ml of 0.3 M sucrose, 3 mM CaCl$_2$. Use one drop for cytology.

Mitochondrial fraction[a]

→ **Supernatant**

Centrifuge 105,000 × g for 90 min.

→ **Pellet**

Resuspend in 5 ml of 0.3 M sucrose, 3 mM CaCl$_2$.

Microsomal fraction[a]

→ **Supernatant**

Soluble[a] **supernatant fraction**

---

[a] Sample to be used for nucleic acid determination (section II) or DNA extraction (section III). Precipitate appropriate sample volume with 2 vol of cold 95% EtOH. Store fractions at −20°C.

Fractionation of Spinach Cells for Nuclei and Chloroplasts

Wash spinach in chilled tap water. Select only the young, fresh leaves (yield of nuclei is low from older leaves). Remove the midribs from the leaves. Prepare 20 g of deribbed leaves. Carry out all further procedures in the cold (4°C) or on ice.

Place leaves in a Waring blender with 120 ml extraction buffer (0.25 M sucrose, 20 mM Tris HCl (pH 7.8), 10 mM NaCl, 1 mM $MgCl_2$, 2 mM $CaCl_2$, 2.5% Ficoll and 5% Dextran 40) and blend for 15 sec (at Variac setting ~ 50 volts). Filter homogenate through 2 layers of buffer-wetted flannelette. Adjust final volume to 120 ml. Use 1 drop for cytology. Retain 5 ml sample[b] for nucleic acid determination.

Centrifuge 2500 × g for 10 min.

→ Supernatant
   Discard.

Pellet

Resuspend in 10 ml extraction buffer. Layer onto a discontinuous sucrose density gradient built in a 30 ml Corex tube. See Figure 1.

Centrifuge at 8000 rpm in Sorvall HB-4 rotor for 30 min.

Green layer
50–60% sucrose interface (chloroplasts and nuclei).

Green layer
20–50% sucrose interface (chloroplasts).

→ Supernatant
   Discard.

Pellet

Resuspend in 4 ml of extraction buffer. Use 1 drop for cytology.

Nuclear fraction[b]

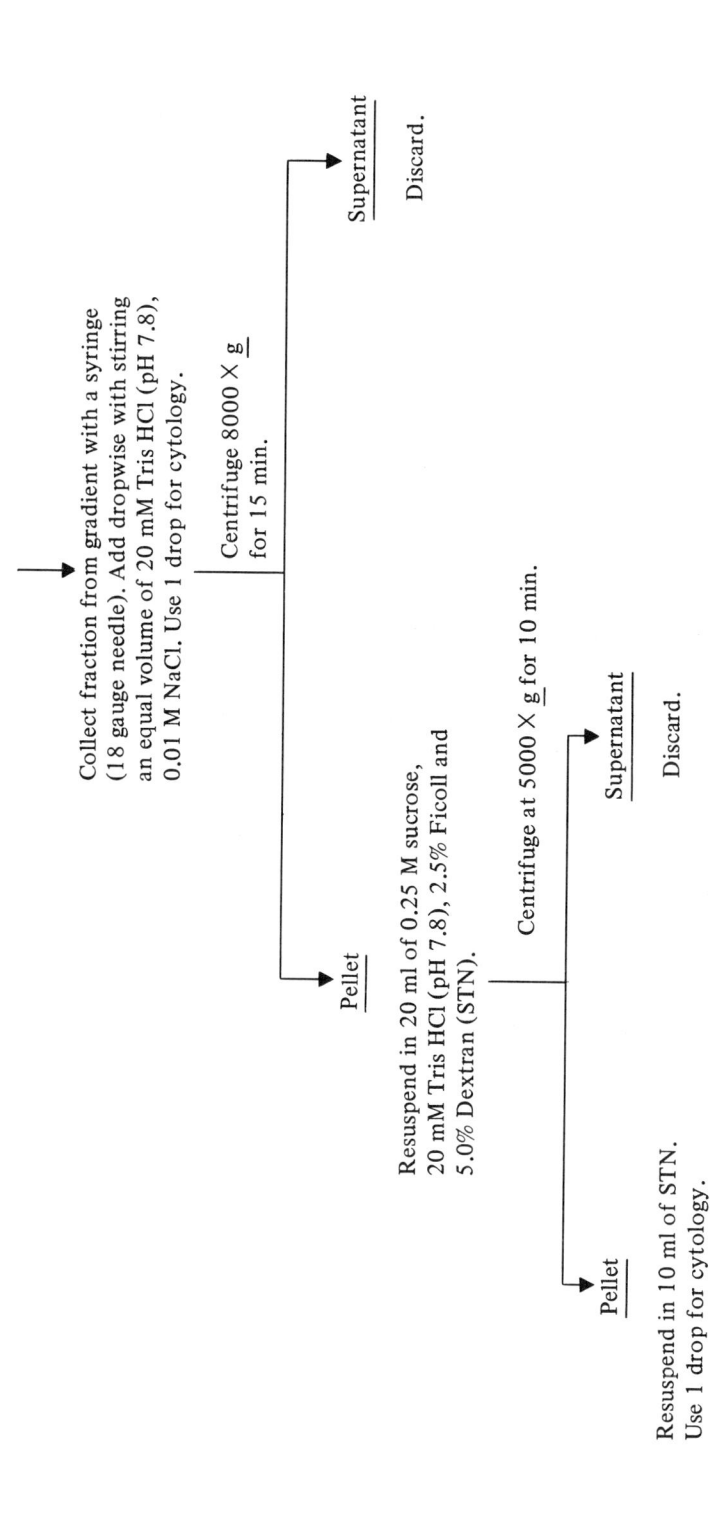

```
                                                    ┌─────────────────→ Supernatant
                                                    │                    Discard.
Collect fraction from gradient with a syringe       │
(18 gauge needle). Add dropwise with stirring       │
an equal volume of 20 mM Tris HCl (pH 7.8),         │
0.01 M NaCl. Use 1 drop for cytology.               │
                          │ Centrifuge 8000 × g     │
                          │ for 15 min.             │
                          ↓
                        Pellet

Resuspend in 20 ml of 0.25 M sucrose,
20 mM Tris HCl (pH 7.8), 2.5% Ficoll and
5.0% Dextran (STN).

              Centrifuge at 5000 × g for 10 min. ──→ Supernatant
                                                     Discard.
                  ↓
                Pellet

Resuspend in 10 ml of STN.
Use 1 drop for cytology.

   ┌──────────────┐
   │ Chloroplast  │
   │ fraction[b]  │
   └──────────────┘
```

[b]Sample to be used for nucleic acid determination (section II) or DNA extraction (section III). Precipitate appropriate sample volume with 2 vol of cold 95% EtOH. Store fractions at −20°C.

General References

Blobel, G., and Potter, V. R. 1966. Nuclei from rat liver: isolation method that combines purity with high yield. Science 154:1662–1665.
Busch, H. 1967. Isolation and purification of nuclei. In L. Grossman and K. Moldave (ed.), Methods in Enzymology. XIIA:421–448.
D'Allesio, G. and A. R. Trim. 1968. A method for the isolation of nuclei from leaves. J. Exp. Bot. 19:831–839.
Honda, S. I., T. Hongladarom, and G. G. Laties. 1966. A new isolation medium for plant organelles. J. Exp. Bot. 17:460–472.
Wang, T-Y. 1967. The isolation and purification of mammaliam cell nuclei. In L. Grossman and K. Moldave (ed.), Methods in Enzymology. XIIA:417–421.

SECTION II QUANTITATION OF DNA AND RNA

This procedure for the determination of RNA and DNA can be used to examine either the distribution of nucleic acids in subcellular fractions or the nucleic acid composition of unfractionated tissue. The procedure is based on the selective extraction of first RNA and then DNA from the tissue or fraction to be tested. Selectivity is achieved by the alkaline hydrolysis of RNA followed by the acid hydrolysis of DNA. Since the extraction involves degrative hydrolysis, the procedure obviously is not to be used for the preparation of nucleic acid components.

The extracted nucleic acid is roughly quantitated here by its UV absorption (A_{260nm} = 1.0 for 0.033 mg of hydrolyzed DNA or RNA). A more accurate determination can be achieved with diphenylamine determination of extracted DNA [Burton, 1968] and orcinol determination of RNA [Schneider, 1957]. The extraction procedure, of course, can also be used to determine the incorporation of an isotopically labeled precursor (for example, $^{32}PO_4$ or ^{3}H-adenine) into DNA or RNA. Besides nucleic acid, this procedure yields two other fractions in which the distribution of a radioactive precursor can be followed: (1) an alcohol ether soluble fraction (lipid fraction) and (2) a final residue (containing protein, among other things).

Since this procedure involves the successive washing and extraction of a precipitate, it is absolutely essential that at each step the precipitate is well dispersed and completely washed. This can be accomplished by resuspending the precipitate in a small volume (0.1–0.2 ml) of solvent or extraction solution, dispersing the precipitate by the homogenizing action of a glass rod and then adding the remainder of the solvent needed for that step.

ANALYSIS OF DNA

DNA and RNA Determination in Subcellular Fractions (or of ^{3}H-adenine labeled C. reinhardi)

Use 2 ml of each of the fractions noted in the cell fractionation procedure or the pellet from a 200 ml culture of ^{3}H-adenine labeled C. reinhardi.†

In a 15 ml glass centrifuge tube, precipitate sample by adding 2 vol cold 95% EtOH.

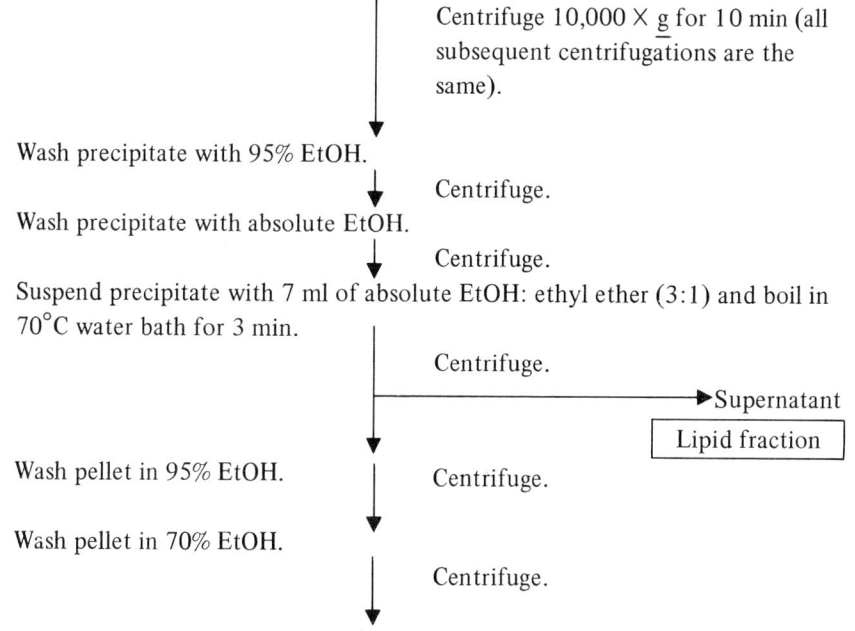

    Centrifuge 10,000 × g for 10 min (all subsequent centrifugations are the same).

↓

Wash precipitate with 95% EtOH.
↓ Centrifuge.

Wash precipitate with absolute EtOH.
↓ Centrifuge.

Suspend precipitate with 7 ml of absolute EtOH: ethyl ether (3:1) and boil in 70°C water bath for 3 min.

    Centrifuge.

→ Supernatant
    | Lipid fraction |

↓

Wash pellet in 95% EtOH.
↓ Centrifuge.

Wash pellet in 70% EtOH.
↓ Centrifuge.

Resuspend precipitate in 5 ml of 0.3 N NaOH and heat at 70°C for 30 min. Chill and add cold 5.0 N perchloric acid to final concentration of 1.0 N.

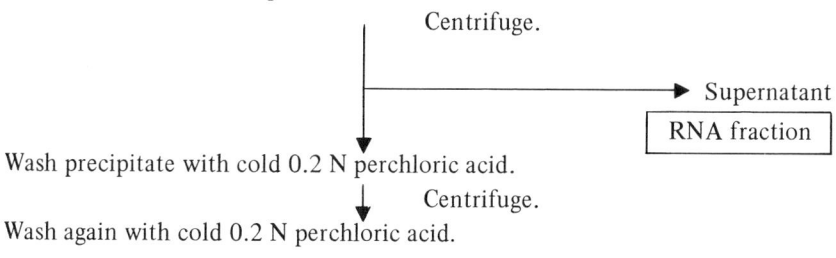

    Centrifuge.

→ Supernatant
    | RNA fraction |

Wash precipitate with cold 0.2 N perchloric acid.
↓ Centrifuge.

Wash again with cold 0.2 N perchloric acid.

†Conditions for the growth of C. reinhardi are described by Surzycki [1971]. Cells are grown under continuous illumination in the presence of 0.1–0.5 μc/ml ^{3}H-adenine. The pellet of cells for nucleic acid determination and DNA extraction can be derived from ~200 ml of cells harvested at late log phase growth (5–8 × 10^6 cells/ml). Cells are harvested by centrifugation at 10,000 × g for 5 min at 2–4°C. The cells are washed twice with 1 × SSC (saline sodium citrate–0.15 M NaCl, 0.015 M Na$_3$ citrate).

```
                    │
                    │  Centrifuge.
                    ▼
Resuspend precipitate in 2–4 ml of 1.0 N perchloric acid and heat at 70°C for
20 min. Chill mixture.
                    │
                    │  Centrifuge.
                    ├──────────────────────► Supernatant
                    │                         DNA fraction
                    ▼
                 Precipitate.
                   Residue
```

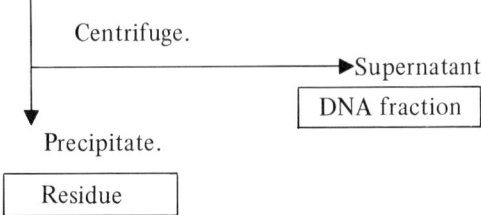

If you have elected to study the distribution of radioisotope from ^{3}H-adenine labeled C. reinhardi, then use 0.1–0.2 ml of each supernatant fraction to determine radioactivity. If you are analyzing unlabeled subcellular fractions, then read $A_{260\,nm}$ for the RNA and DNA fractions in perchloric acid. If necessary, dilute fraction with 1.0 N perchloric acid.

Sample Calculation

Amount of DNA in rat liver nuclear fraction (from section I).

(1) $A_{260\,nm}$ of a 1:20 dilution of DNA fraction = 0.818 Optical Density (OD) units.

(2) Total OD units in 3 ml DNA fraction = 49.1 OD units.

(3) Content of DNA in DNA fraction:

$$49.1 \text{ OD units} \times \frac{33 \, \mu g \text{ DNA}}{1.0 \text{ OD unit}} = 1.62 \text{ mg DNA}$$

(4) Total amount of DNA in rat liver nuclear fraction. A sample of 2 ml from the 10 ml nuclear fraction was used for DNA determination.

$$\text{Total amount of DNA} = \frac{1.62 \text{ mg} \times 10 \text{ ml}}{2.0 \text{ ml}}$$

$$= 8.1 \text{ mg}$$

(5) Amount of DNA in nuclear fraction based on fresh weight of rat liver. Nuclear fraction was derived from 5 g of fresh weight tissue.

$$\frac{8.1 \text{ mg}}{5.0 \text{ g}} = \frac{1.62 \text{ mg DNA}}{\text{g liver}}$$

ANALYSIS OF DNA

General References

Burton, K. 1968. Determination of DNA concentration with diphenylamine. In L. Grossman and K. Moldave (eds.), Methods in Enzymology. XIIB:163−166.

Ogur, M., and G. Rosen. 1950. The nucleic acids of plant tissues. I. The extraction and estimation of deoxypentose nucleic acid and pentose nucleic acid. Arch. Biochem. Biophys. 25:262−276.

Schmidt, G., and S. J. Thannhauser. 1945. A method for the determination of deoxyribonucleic acid, ribonucleic acid, and phosphoprotein in animal tissues. J. Biol. Chem. 161:83−89.

Schneider, W. C. 1957. Determination of nucleic acids in tissues by pentose analysis. In S. P. Colowick and N. O. Kaplan (eds.), Methods in Enzymology. III:680−684.

Surzycki, S. 1971. Synchronously grown cultures of Chlamydomonas reinhardi. In A. Sam Pietro (ed.), Methods in enzymology. XXIII:67−73.

SECTION III EXTRACTION AND PURIFICATION OF DNA

DNA must be extracted and purified from tissues, cells, or subcellular fractions before it can be characterized. The degree of DNA purification required for any characterization procedure may vary. For example, buoyant density analysis (section IV) often requires only a crude cell lysate while base composition analysis (section V) requires a purified product. The described procedure will yield either a crude lysate or, carried to completion, purified DNA. The crude lysate contains, among other things, high molecular weight DNA, while other components, RNA and protein, are enzymatically digested. DNA is purified from this lysate by phase separation and selective precipitation of the DNA.

Procedures for the extraction of DNA vary depending upon the material to be extracted. The first steps of all procedures, however, adhere to the general following principles: (1) The cells or organelles must be broken, disrupted, or lysed to extract DNA. This disruption, and all subsequent handling procedures, must be carried out without extensively shearing DNA. (2) The deoxynucleoprotein (DNP) must be solubilized and extracted from the disrupted material. This is usually accomplished by breaking cells in the presence of detergents and either low or high ionic strength solutions. DNP is less soluble in intermediate strength solutions (0.4−0.8 M). (3) Enzymatic digestion of the DNA must be avoided during both extraction and handling by a combination of preventatives. These preventatives include the use of chelating agents, high salt concentrations, detergents, heat or chemical denaturants (for example, phenol, chloroform) to inhibit endogenous nucleases and the addition of only deoxyribonuclease free enzymes (ribonuclease and pronase) during purification.

Failure to achieve a high quantity or quality of product can generally be laid to an error in the first steps of the extraction procedure. It is a common fault in an otherwise flawless DNA purification procedure that either the cells have not been completely lysed, the DNP has not been sufficiently solubilized, or the DNA has been enzymatically digested early in the extraction procedure.

There are also many variations in the later procedural steps of DNA purification—deproteinization and DNA precipitation. For deproteinization, phenol is used in this procedure. (Use care in handling phenol. It readily burns the skin.) Phenol is a superior protein denaturant and does not require vigorous shaking to mix phases. After shaking, chloroform is added to sharpen the phase separation between the organic solvent and aqueous phases. For DNA precipitation, ethanol is used here, but isopropanol can also be used to precipitate DNA. Isopropanol is more selective in the precipitation of DNA in the presence of contaminating RNA; however, isopropanol precipitation requires higher DNA concentrations for good yields.

Procedure

If you plan to characterize the DNA from one or more of the subcellular fractions from section I, then follow the extraction procedure in part A-I and B. If you plan to characterize the isotopically labeled DNA from C. reinhardi, then follow the steps in parts A-II and B. Continue on to part C only if you plan to purify DNA from the crude lysate.

(A) Extraction of DNA:
  (I) Extraction of DNA from subcellular fractions
    (1) Subcellular fractions from which DNA is to be extracted are either freshly prepared or stored in 70% ethanol at −20°C. The stored fractions are centrifuged at 8000 × g for 10 min at 2–4°C. The clear supernatant fluid is discarded and the centrifuge tube is briefly inverted to drain off the ethanol. Suspend the pellet by vigorous mixing with a glass rod in an equal volume of cold 1 × SSC.
    (2) The freshly prepared fraction or resuspended pellet is made 2.5% in sarkosyl and mixed until the suspension is reasonably dispersed.
    (3) Heat mixture at 70°C for 20 min. Centrifuge, if the solution has not completely clarified, at 8000 × g for 10 min at 2–4°C.

ANALYSIS OF DNA 129

Pour off supernatant fluid and pellet. Supernatant should be fairly viscous. Proceed to part B.

(II) Extraction of isotopically labeled DNA from C. reinhardi.
   (1) Use a frozen pellet from 200 ml culture of ^{3}H-adenine labeled C. reinhardi. (See footnote p. 125 for growth conditions.)
   (2) Thaw the frozen pellet and suspend it with a glass rod in an equal volume (~ 0.25 ml) of 50% sucrose in 1 X SSC. Add sarkosyl to make the final concentration 2.5%. Allow the cells to lyse at room temperature for 10 min. Lysis is indicated by a loss of turbidity and an increase in viscosity.

(B) **Enzymatic digestion of RNA and protein:**
   (1) Dilute mixture with 4 vol of 1 X SSC to give a final sarkosyl concentration of 0.5%. Add T_1 ribonuclease to 20 µg/ml and deoxyribonuclease-free ribonuclease A to 25 µg/ml. (Deoxyribonuclease-free ribonuclease A is ribonuclease A recrystallized five times at 2 mg/ml in 1 X SSC. The enzyme solution is heated to 90°C for 10 min and stored frozen.) Incubate at 37°C for 30 min.
   (2) Add slowly with mixing 0.2 vol of 5 M NaCl.
   (3) Add predigested pronase to 500 µg/ml. (Predigested pronase is B grade pronase at 2.5 mg/ml in 1 X SSC. The enzyme solution is incubated at 65°C for 20 min and stored frozen.) Incubate at 65°C for 1 hr.
   (4) The product at this point is the digested lysate which can be used for buoyant density analysis (section IV) or analysis on hydroxyapatite (section VI). If you wish to purify the DNA, then proceed to the deproteinization and DNA precipitation steps.

(C) **Deproteinization and Precipitation of DNA:**
   (1) Add an equal volume of freshly distilled water saturated phenol to the digested lysate. Tightly stopper the tube with Saran wrap and a rubber stopper. Mix phases by inverting tube about 30–60 times/min. After 15–30 min add an equal volume of chloroform and shake for another minute. Centrifuge mix at 8000 X g for 10 min. Remove top phase with a wide mouth pipet. Repeat phenol chloroform extraction until no precipitate is found at the interface.
   (2) Pipet top phase from the final phase separation into a centrifuge tube or small beaker. Carefully layer an equal volume of 95% ethanol onto the DNA solution. If you have a high concentration of DNA, then wind out fibers at the interface on a glass rod. If you have a

low concentration of DNA, then mix the phases, chill the solution, and centrifuge the barely turbid solution at 10,000 × g̅ for 10 min at 2–4°C. Wash pellet or fibers on the glass rod with 70% ethanol (to remove a̱ḻḻ phenol). Drain off excess ethanol.

(3) Dissolve DN̲A̲ in a small volume (2–4 ml) of 0.1 × SSC. Shaking overnight in the cold room is generally required to dissolve alcohol precipitated DNA.

(4) The purity of your preparation can be determined spectrophotometrically. Purified DNA has a 260:280 nm ratio of 2. Lower ratios usually indicate protein contamination (270 nm absorption maximum is seen if phenol has not been completely removed). Further purification requires that you repeat the ribonuclease, pronase, phenol chloroform extraction, and alcohol precipitation.

General References

Chiang, K-S, and N. Sueoka. 1967. Replication of chloroplast DNA in Chlamydo̲-̲ monas̲ reinhardi̲ during vegetative cell cycle: its mode and regulation. Proc. Nat. Acad. Sci. (U.S.) 57:1506–1513.

Kirby, K. S. 1968. Isolation of nucleic acids with phenolic solvents. In L. Grossman and K. Moldave (ed.), Methods in Enzymology. XIIB:87–99.

Marmur, J. 1963. A procedure for the isolation of deoxyribonucleic acid from micro-organisms. In S. P. Colowick and N. O. Kaplan (ed.), Methods in Enzymology. VI:726–738.

Stern, H. 1968. Isolation and purification of plant nucleic acids from whole tissues and from isolated nuclei. In L. Grossman and K. Moldave (ed.), Methods in Enzymology. XIIB:100–112.

SECTION IV BUOYANT DENSITY ANALYSIS OF DNA USING THE PREPARATIVE AND ANALYTICAL ULTRACENTRIFUGE

The determination of buoyant density from equilibrium sedimentation centrifugation is an important technique for characterizing DNA. Density analysis in CsCl can be used to identify DNA from different sources, to distinguish DNA components (for example, satellite DNA) from a single source, to separate single- from double-strand DNA and to analyze density-labeled DNA. Two important properties of DNA in CsCl solution are that (1) the buoyant density increases linearly with G + C content according to the relationship $\rho = 1.660 + 0.098 [GC]$ [Schildkraut, Marmur, and Doty, 1962] and (2) the density increases by a nearly constant increment (~ 0.015 g/cc) upon denaturation of native DNA.

ANALYSIS OF DNA

Density analysis in these experiments will be carried out in CsCl gradients formed during centrifugation. The gradients generated are relatively linear and the midpoint gradient density is the density of the starting CsCl solution. Centrifugation is carried out until DNA molecules equilibrate at their isodensity position in the CsCl gradient. The density of DNA in CsCl varies around 1.700 g/ml at pH 8.5.

The preparative ultracentrifuge is used if you wish to recover the separated DNA components or if you must analyze for the distribution of isotopically labeled DNA. The analytical centrifuge is used when the distribution of DNA in a gradient is to be determined optically and when no product recovery is required.

CsCl gradients are established in a fixed-angle rotor in the preparative centrifuge. Fixed-angle rotors are used because (a) such rotors can conveniently handle more samples, and (b) the gradient generated is less steep than in a swinging bucket rotor. The steepness of a CsCl gradient is governed by the effective column height of the gradient (the distance between the minimum and maximum radius of sample in the spinning rotor) and the speed of the rotor. The geometry of a sample in a fixed angle rotor reduces this column height when compared to a swinging bucket rotor. When using either preparative rotor or the analytical centrifuge, the column height of the gradient is kept to a practical minimum. A short column height reduces the time necessary both to generate a gradient and to allow DNA to move to its isodensity position in the gradient. The time needed to achieve equilibrium for high molecular weight DNA molecules in the analytical centrifuge at 44,770 rpm is 20–24 hr and in the preparative centrifuge with the Type 50 rotor at 35,000 rpm is 35–40 hr.

Buoyant Density Analysis of Chlamydomonas DNA Using the Preparative Ultracentrifuge

Before centrifugation, the density of the CsCl solution (with sample) must be adjusted to the desired midpoint gradient density. The proper density can be achieved by quantitative addition of solid CsCl to a DNA solution or by dilution of a stock CsCl solution with a small volume of a DNA solution. Precise adjustment of a final solution density should be made while monitoring refractive index. However, if the crude C. reinhardi lysate is used, the refractive increment of the sample may give a false density determination. Therefore, for crude lysates, densities will not be adjusted by refractive index measurements.

(1) In a graduated test tube, add 0.1–0.2 ml of the C. reinhardi crude lysate or a sample of purified ^{3}H-labeled C. reinhardi DNA that contains at least 10,000

acid-precipitable CPM. (Note: Perform all pipetting with a wide mouth pipet.) Also, add 2000–5000 acid-precipitable counts per minute (cpm) of a ^{32}P-labeled Escherichia coli DNA reference marker (ρ = 1.710 g/cc). Adjust volume to 4.34 ml with 20 mM Tris HCl (pH 8.5). Add 5.75 g of CsCl (optical grade, Harshaw Chemical Co.) and dissolve. Adjust refractive index to η = 1.404 for the purified DNA sample. Pipet 5.0 ml of the sample into a cellulose nitrate centrifuge tube. Fill the tube to the top with mineral oil and secure metal cap on the tube. (Make sure no air bubbles are trapped beneath the tube cap.) Tubes are placed in a fixed angle rotor (Type 40, 50 or 65) and centrifuged at 35,000 rpm for at least 30 hr at 20–25°C.

(2) After centrifugation, samples are collected by puncturing and dripping from the bottom of the tube. With a 5 ml gradient, 20 drops from a 24-gauge needle give 35–40 fractions.

(3) Take refractive index readings on at least 5 fractions spread through the gradient. Determine the density of CsCl in these fractions according to the relationship [Mandel, Schildkraut, and Marmur, 1968]:

$$\rho^{25°C} = 10.8601 \, \eta^{25°C} - 13.4974$$

A graph of $\eta^{25°C}$ vs $\rho^{25°C}$ is given in Figure 2.

(4) To each sample is added 0.1 ml of 2.5 mg/ml herring sperm carrier DNA solution followed by 0.5 ml cold 10% TCA. The chilled samples are individually filtered, washed 3 times with 5% TCA and finally once with 95% EtOH. Filters are counted in a scintillation counter. Plot CsCl concentration,

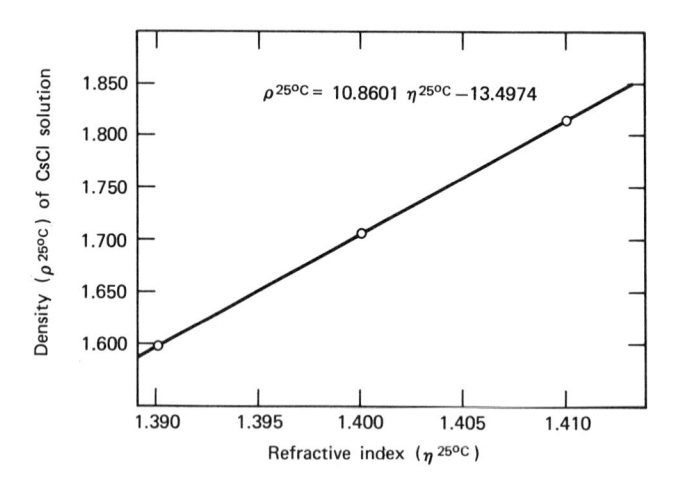

FIGURE 2. Plot of refractive index (η) versus density (ρ) of aqueous cesium chloride solutions.

ANALYSIS OF DNA

acid-precipitable CPM's and/or A_{260nm} vs fraction number. Compare that density to reported values in Table III. From the density of your sample, determine the G + C content.

TABLE III. Density of Selected Eukaryotic DNA's in CsCl[a]

Organism	Density of DNA in CsCl, g/cc		
	Nuclear	Mitochondrial	Chloroplast
Saccharomyces cerevisiae	1.700	1.685	
Neurospora crassa	1.712	1.701	
Chlamydomonas reinhardi	1.723		1.695
Spinacia oleracia	1.695		1.719, 1.705
Euglena gracilis	1.707	1.691	1.686
Ox	1.704 (1.715)[b]	1.703	
Rat	1.703	1.701	
Chick	1.701	1.708	

[a]from Borst et al. [1967].
[b]Density of satellite components found in nuclear DNA.

The reported density of the major component of C. reinhardi DNA is 1.723 g/cc [Sueoka, Chiang, and Kates, 1967]. This component accounts for 85% of the total DNA. The density of the minor satellite is 1.695 g/cc. This satellite represents from 7–15% of the total C. reinhardi DNA.

Buoyant Density Analysis Using the Analytical Ultracentrifuge

A description of the operation of the Beckman Model E analytical ultracentrifuge will not be provided here. All instrumentation procedures will be carried out by a qualified operator. You will be responsible for the preparation of your sample and the analysis of the UV absorption photograph.

You may use any DNA sample which you have purified from subcellular fractions (section III) or purified calf thymus DNA which will be provided.

(1) 5–10 µg of a purified DNA sample is pipetted into a graduated test tube. Add 5–10 µg of an appropriate reference marker—either poly dAT (ρ = 1.681 g/cc) or bromuracil hybrid E. coli DNA (ρ = 1.754 g/cc). Adjust the volume of the sample to ∼2 ml with 20 mM Tris HCl (pH 8.5). Add solid CsCl and adjust the refractive index to a density midway between that of the reference and the expected sample density.

(2) About 0.7 ml of this final solution is injected into the centrifuge cell with a syringe and a 22-gauge needle.

(3) Centrifugation is performed at 44,770 rpm at 25°C. DNA with a molecular

weight of $0.2-1 \times 10^7$ dalton will equilibrate at an isodensity position in ~20 hr. Ultraviolet absorption photographs will be taken of the samples during centrifugation.

(4) Make tracings of the photographs using the Joyce–Loebl microdensitometer. Calculate the density of your DNA sample from the midpoint density of the gradient and the position of the gradient marker (assume a linear gradient throughout the cell). Compare that density to those in Table III. From the density of your sample, determine the G + C content.

General References

Mandel, M., C. L. Schildkraut, and J. Marmur. 1968. Use of CsCl density gradient analysis for determining the guanine plus cytosine content of DNA. In L. Grossman and K. Moldave (ed.), Methods in Enzymology, XIIB:184–195.

Schildkraut, C. L., J. Marmur, and P. Doty. 1962. Determination of the base composition of deoxyribonucleic acid from its buoyant density in CsCl. J. Mol. Biol. 4:430–443.

Sueoka, N., K-S Chiang, and J. R. Kates. 1967. Deoxyribonucleic acid replication in meiosis of Chlamydomonas reinhardi. I. Isotopic transfer experiments with a strain producing eight zoospores. J. Mol. Biol. 25:47–66.

SECTION V BASE COMPOSITION ANALYSIS OF DNA

Base composition analysis provides an additional technique to characterize and distinguish DNA from various sources. In this experiment you will hydrolyze DNA with pancreatic deoxyribonuclease and venom phosphodiesterase. The product deoxynucleoside-5'-monophosphates will be separated by thin-layer chromatography and quantitated by UV absorption.

Procedure

(A) Preparation of DNA: If you have recovered sufficient DNA from the DNA isolation procedure, then you may use it here. If not, commercially prepared calf thymus DNA can be used. To detect nucleotides optically you must start with a DNA solution (preferably in $0.1 \times SSC$) that is at least 500 µg/ml. That concentration will yield a solution ~1 mM in nucleotides after hydrolysis.

If your sample contains RNA, it must be removed by hydrolysis in base. Dissolve the DNA sample in 0.3 N NaOH and hydrolyze at 37°C for 1–5 hr. Chill sample and precipitate DNA by the addition of cold 70% perchloric acid. Collect the precipitate by centrifugation, wash precipitate with 70% ethanol, and dissolve in $0.1 \times SSC$.

ANALYSIS OF DNA

(B) Enzymatic Hydrolysis of DNA: Both pancreatic deoxyribonuclease and venom phosphodiesterase will be used for hydrolysis. Pancreatic deoxyribonuclease degrades DNA into 5'-phosphoryl terminated oligodeoxynucleotides. Venom phosphodiesterase reduces these oligonucleotides to 5'-phosphoryl deoxynucleotides [Razzell and Khorana, 1959].

The reaction mixture for hydrolysis contains:
  0.25 ml of 0.5–2.0 mg/ml DNA solution
  0.025 ml of 1.0 M Tris HCl (pH 8.8)
  0.010 ml of 0.12 M $MgCl_2$
  0.010 ml of 0.25 M $CaCl_2$
  0.010 ml of ~ 1000 units/ml pancreatic deoxyribonuclease
  0.010 ml of 5 mg/ml venom phosphodiesterase

Incubate for 2 hr at 37°C in a small stoppered test tube. Add another 0.010 ml of venom phosphodiesterase and incubate an additional 2 hr (at least). Terminate the reaction by heating tube in a boiling water bath for 2 min. Immediately chill the reaction mixture and keep on ice until application of sample onto chromatograms.

(C) Thin-Layer Chromotography of Deoxynucleotides [Randerath and Randerath, 1967]: Apply hydrolyzed sample to strips of PEI cellulose thin-layer chromatography paper. Apply sample with a 2–5 λ pipet onto spots 2 cm from the lower edge of chromatogram (Figure 3). Apply 1 mM standards of the four deoxynucleoside-5'-monophosphates in similar spots next to the sample. (Use about 10 λ total of each sample.) Allow chromatogram to dry. Observe spots under a UV lamp (be careful to protect your eyes) to insure that each spot is easily visible.

Develop chromatogram by ascending chromatography in closed thin-layer chromatography tanks. Two solvent tanks will be used—the first containing 1 N acetic acid and the second containing 1 N acetic acid, 3.0 M LiCl (9:1, v/v). Adjust both tanks to a solvent depth of 8 mm. In the first tank, allow the solvent front to ascend 2 cm past the origin of the chromatogram (4 cm mark), and transfer the chromatogram without intermediate drying to the second tank. Develop front up to >15 cm past origin. Remove chromatogram and air dry.

Observe spots under UV light and circle with pencil. Approximate R_f values for deoxynucleotides:

| dCMP | 0.80 | dTMP | 0.54 |
| dAMP | 0.68 | dGMP | 0.37 |

Nucleotides can be eluted by scraping cellulose from marked spots with knife or spatula. Scrapings are carefully transferred to a glass centrifuge tube and

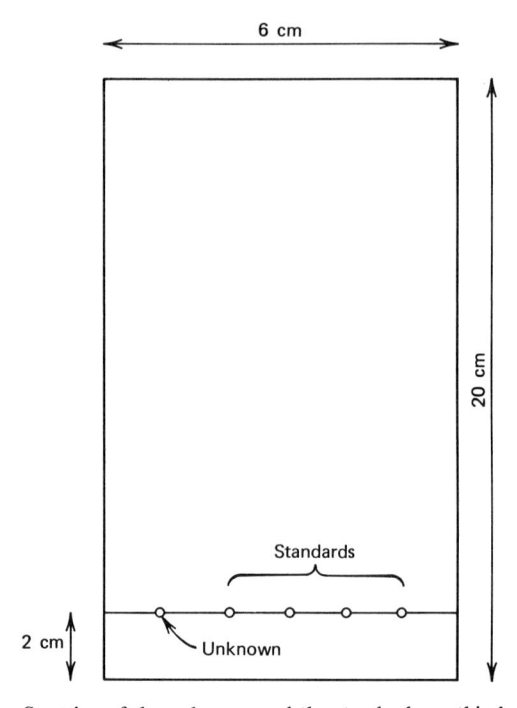

FIGURE 3. Spotting of the unknown and the standards on thin layer plates.

2 ml of 0.1 N HCl is added. The scrapings are shaken, allowed to sit overnight in the eluent and then are centrifuged out. The eluent is carefully drawn off each sample with a pipet. Spectral characteristics can be used to identify and quantitate the nucleotides (Table IV). Compare your results with selected data from the literature (Table V).

TABLE IV. Spectral Characteristics of Deoxynucleoside-5'-monophosphates

Nucleotide in acid[a]	$A_{max, nm}$	$E_{260\ nm}$
dCMP	280	6.5
dAMP	258	14.1
dTMP	267	8.4
dGMP	255	10.6

[a]From Volkin et al. [1951].

ANALYSIS OF DNA

TABLE V. Base Composition of Selected DNA's

Source of DNA	Base composition			
	A	G	C	T
Rat liver	28.4	24.4	20.7	26.4
Calf thymus	28.2	23.9	20.0	27.9
Human liver	30.3	19.5	19.9	30.3

Source: From Handbook of Biochemistry, table compiled by Herman S. Shapiro. Editors of the Chemical Rubber Co., Cleveland, Ohio, 1968.

General References

Laskowski, M. 1966. Pancreatic deoxyribonuclease. In G. L. Cantoni and D. R. Davies (ed.), Procedures in nucleic acid research. 85–101.

Laskowski, M. 1966. Exonuclease (phosphodiesterase) and other nucleolytic enzymes from venom. In G. L. Cantoni and D. R. Davies (ed.), Procedures in nucleic acid research. 154–202.

Randerath, K., and E. Randerath. 1967. Thin-layer separation methods for nucleic acid derivatives. In L. Grossman and K. Moldave (ed.), Methods in enzymology, XIIA:323–347.

Razzell, W. E., and H. G. Khorana. 1959. Studies on polynucleotides III. Enzymic degradation, substrate specificity and properties of snake venom phosphodiesterase. J. Biol. Chem. 234:2105–2113.

Volkin, E., J. X. Khym, and W. E. Cohn. 1951. The preparation of deoxynucleotides. J. Amer. Chem. Soc. 73:1533–1536.

SECTION VI ANALYSIS OF DNA ON HYDROXYAPATITE COLUMNS

Hydroxyapatite, $Ca_{10}(PO_4)_6(OH)_2$, columns are useful for the separation and purification of DNA components. The particular virtue of HA is its ability to discriminate between single- and double-stranded DNA and to be used over a wide range of temperature. For these reasons HA columns are extensively used for DNA reassociation experiments ($C_0 t$ analyses) and thermal denaturation analyses. Hydroxyapatite can also be used to purify DNA from a crude lysate. The inclusion of solubilizing agents in the crude extracts such as detergents or urea do not appreciably affect the binding of DNA to HA.

Here we will use an HA column to separate native ^{3}H-labeled C. reinhardi DNA (section III) from denatured ^{32}P-labeled E. coli DNA.

Procedure

(1) Pour a column (2 cm diam × 3 cm) from a slurry of HA (Hypatite C, Clarkson Chemical Co.). (The column will be run at room tempera-

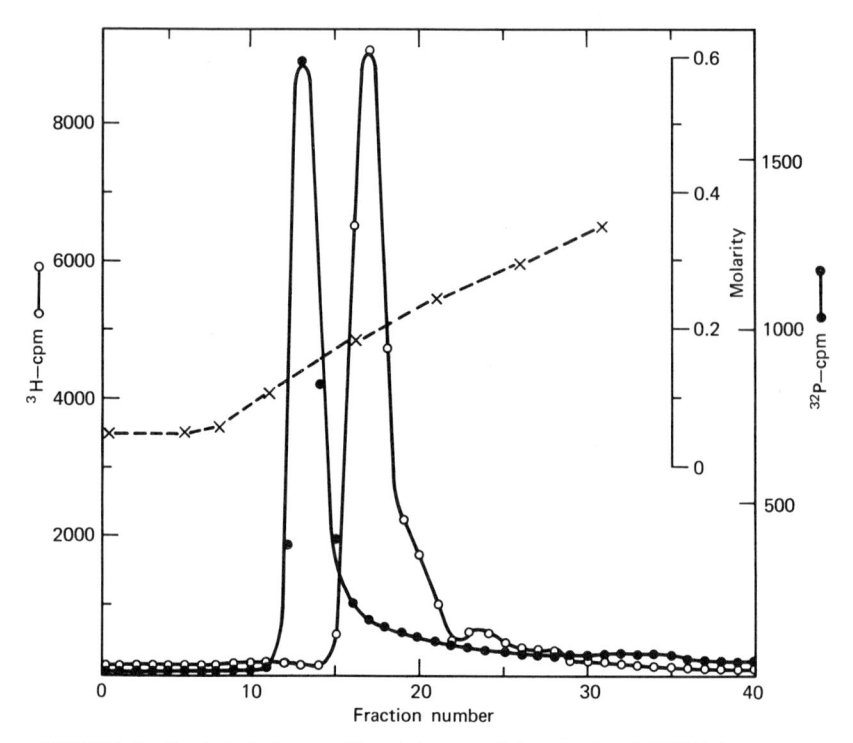

FIGURE 4. Typical elution profiles of single- and double-stranded DNA from HA column.

ture. Store slurry in refrigerator, but warm to room temperature before pouring.) Wash column with 40 ml of 0.05 M phosphate buffer (equimolar NaH_2PO_4 and Na_2HPO_4 buffers used throughout).

(2) Dilute to 10 ml with 0.05 M buffer ~ 50,000 acid-precipitable CPM of ^{3}H-labeled C. reinhardi DNA (either in a crude lysate or as purified DNA) and ~ 10,000 CPM of heat denatured ^{32}P-labeled E. coli DNA. Apply sample to column. Wash an additional 25 ml of 0.05 M buffer through the column. (Note: if a crude lysate is to be used, then both sample loading buffer and the first 5 ml of wash buffer should be made 8 M in urea.)

(3) Elute DNA in a continuous gradient. Use 100 ml each of 0.05 M and 0.35 M buffer and collect 5 ml fractions. After elution keep all fractions chilled.

(4) Read refractive index (η) of various fractions to determine salt con-

centration. Plot η vs buffer concentration for the stock buffer solutions (0.05 M and 0.35 M).

(5) Acid-precipitate each fraction by adding 0.2 ml of 2.5 mg/ml herring sperm DNA (carrier DNA) followed by 2.5 ml cold 40% TCA. The samples are individually filtered on glass fiber filters (Whatman GF/C), washed 3 times with a total of 15 ml of 5% TCA and once with 5 ml of 95% EtOH. Filters are dried and counted in a scintillation counter. Plot your results on graph paper (cpm vs fraction number and buffer concentration vs fraction number).

A typical elution profile is seen in Figure 4. ^{3}H-Adenine-labeled C. reinhardi and denatured ^{32}PO$_4$-labeled E. coli DNA are shown in this figure. NaCl concentration in elution buffer is expressed in molarity.

General References

Bernardi, G. 1971. Chromatography of nucleic acids on hydroxyapatite columns. In L. Grossman and K. Moldave (ed.), Methods in Enzymology. XXID:95−139.

Quantitative Measurement of RNA Synthesis

TOM HUMPHREYS

INTRODUCTION

Rates of incorporation of exogenous radioactive precursors are often used to study rates of synthesis of macromolecules. However, rates of incorporation are not equal to rates of synthesis. Rates of incorporation represent rates of flow of the radioactive precursor into the cell through various pools of intermediates into the macromolecules. Since the exogenous radioactive material is not the only source of precursor, indeed in higher cells it is seldom a significant source for synthesis of macromolecules, the added radioactive material is diluted during its flow through the pools. This dilution varies greatly depending on cell permeability, size of precursor pools, rate of turnover of the pools, expandibility of the pools, and other such factors. Thus the amount of radioactive precursor which becomes incorporated is usually much less than the total amount of precursor actually polymerized into macromolecules and cannot be used as a measure of synthesis.

To use incorporation as a measure of synthesis, the incorporation must occur under conditions where dilution of external isotope is insignificant or the actual dilution of the isotope is known. For example, it is sometimes possible with amino acids to add enough external radioactive amino acid to render the amount of endogenous amino acid insignificant [Berg, 1970]. When labeling RNA with exogenous precursors, however, this approach is seldom possible because the direct precursors of RNA, the nucleoside triphosphates, are at the end of a chain of organic phosphorylated intermediates. These are impermeable to the cell membrane and can, thus, remain well buffered from high concentrations of the permeable external precursors. This situation requires the measurement of the specific radioactivity of the direct precursor to the macromolecule in order to know the final dilution of the original external precursor added.

Direct measurement of the specific radioactivity of the nucleoside triphosphate precursor pools for RNA has been rare in experimental biology even though it is logically required in most studies of RNA synthesis. The major reason has been the technical difficulty of doing such measurements. Most techniques require considerable biological material which must be processed through rather tedious chromatography procedures. In this exercise, I will describe simple and sensitive techniques which have been worked out in my laboratory by Charles P. Emerson and Bruce P. Brandhorst to measure rates of RNA synthesis through determination of specific radioactivity of the nucleoside triphosphates.

The advantages of these techniques lie in the use of radioactive adenosine as an RNA precursor so that the ATP pool is the nucleoside triphosphate which has to be examined [Emerson and Humphreys, 1970]. This can be achieved using the very specific and sensitive luciferin-luciferase assay to measure ATP in a small partially purified extract of nucleotides obtained by simple thin-layer chromatography [Emerson and Humphreys, 1971]. Because the techniques are simple and sensitive, requiring as little biological material as 100 sea urchin embryos, extensive kinetic studies which provide a detailed view of RNA metabolism are possible [Brandhorst and Humphreys, 1971, 1972].

The accuracy and rigor of these techniques depend on the degree to which the ATP pool which serves as the precursor to RNA equilibrates with the total ATP pool in the cell. There are examples where the ATP pools serving as RNA precursor appear to be compartmentalized from the total pool. Such examples are usually derived from complicated labeling experiments with cells subjected to excessive concentrations of external nucleosides and often do not include direct measurement of the nucleotide pools or independent measurement of RNA synthesis in the cells so treated [Plagemann, 1972; Epstein and Daentl, 1971]. In our experience with sea urchins [Emerson 1970; Emerson and Humphreys, 1970, 1971; Brandhorst, 1970, 1971; Brandhorst and Humphreys, 1971, 1972; Humphreys, 1971, 1972], muscle cells in culture [Emerson, unpublished], and chick fibroblasts in culture [Emerson, 1970, 1971], we have seen no indication of compartmentalization of the ATP pool. These experiments include some rather direct tests for compartmentalization. The rate of ribosomal RNA synthesis as measured by pool analysis is equal to the rate of formation of new ribosomal RNA in growing chick fibroblasts [Emerson, 1970, 1971; Emerson and Humphreys, 1971] and in growing sea urchin larvae [Humphreys, 1972]. If there is a differential entry of radioactivity into the pools in the sea urchin embryos, this does not change between 4 min and 6 hr of labeling even though new radioactive adenosine ceases to enter the cells after 4 min. [Brandhorst and Humphreys, 1971, 1972]. In these same cells the specific activity of the dATP pool serving as precursor for DNA could be calculated from the rate of DNA synthesis, as determined from the rate of cell division, and the radioactivity incorporated into DNA. Even after a few minutes incorporation this specific activity was the same as the specific activity of the total ATP pool indicating rapid equilibration of the DNA precursor pool. The rate of RNA synthesis in sea urchin embryos has been estimated from the uridine pools [Roeder and Rutter, 1970] and the guanosine pools [Kijima and Wilt, 1969] as well as from adenosine pools. All of the measurements agree. Together these data argue rather strongly for the accuracy of the adenosine pool measurement procedures in the organism to which they have been applied. It remains to be seen if this generalization will remain valid as the techniques are applied to other systems.

EXPERIMENTAL

These techniques will be presented in the context of an experiment to measure RNA synthesis and turnover in sea urchin embryos [Brandhorst and Humphreys, 1971]. However, with slight adaptation they can be applied to most other biological material which will use exogenous adenosine as an RNA precursor. They also only deal with total RNA which in this case is rather unstable nuclear and messenger RNA [Brandhorst and Humphreys, 1972]. However, by adding a step for extraction and fractionation of the cell or of RNA, they could be applied to any defined class of RNA molecules [Emerson, 1971; Humphreys, 1971]. This exercise is organized as five flow sheets which present the experimental protocol for the various measurements necessary to calculate RNA synthesis. Each flow sheet has a number of footnotes which provide background information where further elucidation of technical details is appropriate.

FLOW SHEET A. Fertilization and Culture of Sea Urchin Embryos.[1]

Obtain ripe sea urchins.[2]

With a syringe and needle inserted into the visceral cavity through the soft area periferal to the oral opening inject 0.2–1.0 ml (depending on size of animal) 0.5 M KCl into each urchin.

When gametes appear on upper surface, ascertain if they are sperm (white) or eggs (yellow).

Invert females over 30 or 50 ml beakers filled with sea water.[3]

Leave males upright until 0.1 ml or more semen can be taken up with a pipet. Store pipet at 4°C and sperm will remain viable for hours.

When female has completed shedding (15–30 min) filter eggs through several layers of cheese cloth to remove debris (spines, feces, etc.) and put in 200 ml sea water in a 250 ml beaker.

FLOW SHEET A. (Continued)

Inspect eggs with compound microscope for homogeneity. Few or no immature oocytes with large nuclei or misshapen eggs should be evident.

Wash eggs by allowing them to settle to the bottom of beaker and aspirating. Wait only long enough for most eggs to settle; aspirate off slowly sedimenting eggs. Resuspend in 200 ml sea water.

Repeat wash 3 times.

Measure eggs by centrifuging an aliquot in a hematocrit tube or by counting the eggs in a given volume in a micropipet under the microscope. Resuspend eggs in 40 vol of sea water or at a concentration of 3.0×10^4 eggs per ml.

Fertilize with 1/100 vol of a sperm suspension of semen freshly (1–20 min) diluted 100- to 200-fold with sea water. Check sperm under microscope for motility. They should be very active.

Examine eggs for fertilization membranes; over 95% fertilization is desirable.

Wash zygotes as before by settling them in 200 ml sea water and resuspend again in 40 vol of sea water.

Incubate at 18°C with gentle agitation[4] to early mesenchyme blastula stage which will take about 15–16 hr.

FLOW SHEET B. Incubation of Embryos with Radioactive Adenosine and Preparation of Nucleotide Extract and Radioactive Nucleic Acid Precipitate.

Prepare in an ice bath:
  Six 12 ml conical tubes with 9 ml acid sea water[5]
  Twelve 12 ml conical tubes with 9 ml of a 3:1 mixture of acid sea water and 1.1 M sucrose[6]
  One 7 ml Dounce homogenizer (Kontes Glass, Vineland, New Jersey)
  Six 15 ml Corex round bottom centrifuge tubes

Set up for work with radioisotopes.[7]

Place 8 ml of the suspension of the embryos in a 50 ml flask.

When everything is prepared to start the experiment, add 20 microcuries (μCi) ^{3}H-adenosine.

Incubate, maintaining the cells in suspension.

Remove a 1 ml sample[8] using a disposal 2.5 ml syringe and 18-gauge needle at 10 min, 20 min, 40 min, 80 min, 160 min, and 320 min. Process each sample as soon as it is taken.

Squirt the sample into the tube of the acid sea water.

Centrifuge for 30 sec at 800 × g and aspirate the supernatant[9].

Resuspend embryos in 2 ml cold acid sea water and layer on to the sucrose sea water mixture in conical tube.

Centrifuge 30 sec at 800 × g and aspirate the supernatant from the top down[6].

Resuspend embryos in 2 ml cold acid sea water and layer onto a second tube of sucrose-acid sea water mix.

MEASUREMENT OF RNA SYNTHESIS 145

FLOW SHEET B. (Continued)

Centrifuge 30 sec at 800 X g and aspirate.

Resuspend in 2 ml 0.5 M PCA at 0°C[10] and homogenize by 20 strokes of the Dounce homogenizer (wash homogenizer between samples with 0.5 M PCA).

Transfer homogenate to 15 ml Corex round bottom centrifuge tube and centrifuge at 25,000 X g for 10 min (the glass tubes must be used with rubber cushions or they will break under this force).

Carefully remove the supernatant being sure not to remove any of the pellet[8] and place it in a 13 X 100 mm glass tube. This is your nucleotide fraction in PCA. It should be processed immediately according to flow sheet C.[11]

Resuspend the pellet in 2.5 ml 0.5 N PCA at 0°C using a 2.5 ml disposable syringe with an 18-gauge needle to break up the pellet.

Centrifuge 5 min at 25,000 X g and aspirate supernatant.

Wash pellet two more times with PCA as above to remove all free nucleotides.

The washed pellet is your nucleic acid sample. It should be processed immediately according to flow sheet D.

FLOW SHEET C. Thin-layer Chromatography of Nucleotide Sample[12]

Make up two standard samples in 13 X 100 mm tubes; one containing 0.5 mg each of GTP, ATP, and dATP; the other 0.5 mg each of GMP and ADP in H_2O.

Add 0.25 ml of a 100 mg/ml acid washed, activated charcoal suspension to each nucleotide extract and to the standard samples.[13]

Allow the tubes to sit on ice 5 min. Stir them several times during this interval.

Centrifuge 5 min at top speed on a clinical centrifuge at 0°C.

Aspirate the supernatant completely even if some charcoal is lost.

Resuspend the charcoal completely in 4 ml H_2O at 0°C.

Centrifuge again and aspirate.

Repeat above wash 4 more times.

Incubate the charcoal in 0.5 ml 0.1 N NH_4OH in 50% ethanol at 37°C for 30 min.[14]

Centrifuge for 15 min at top speed on a clinical centrifuge at room temperature.

Remove the supernatants with as little charcoal as possible and transfer them to 15 ml corex centrifuge tubes.

Centrifuge 10 min at 25,000 X g.

Transfer the supernatants without charcoal to 13 X 100 mm tubes.

Dry under a stream of air.[15]

Using a disposable, 10 μliter pipet, place 10 μliter of 0.1 N NH_4OH on the dried sample in the tube.

Scrub the bottom of the tube for a minute or so with the pipet and then let as much liquid as possible run back into the capillary pipet. Seven microliters can easily be recovered.

FLOW SHEET C. (Continued)

Spot the solution on a cellulose thin-layer plate.[16]

In a fume hood make up a fresh solution of developing solvent by mixing:
33 ml H_2O
66 ml isobutyric acid (stinks)
1 ml concentrated NH_4OH

Pour into a chromatographic tank and set the bottom of the thin layer plate in the solvent.[17]

Close the top and let the chromatogram develop 3 or 4 hr or until the solvent is about 3 cm from the top of the plate.

Remove and dry the plate in the hood for several hours.[18]

Observe the plate under UV light in a darkened room and mark the standard spots.[19]

Note the midpoint of the ATP spot on the samples.

Cut out the strip along which each sample migrated.

Remove the slower half of the ATP spot by cutting a 0.5 cm section from the midpoint of the ATP spot.[20]

Use for ATP assay described in flow sheet E.

FLOW SHEET D. Short and Long Term Alkaline Hydrolysis of PCA Precipitate[21] to Determine Radioactive AMP in RNA

A. Hydrolysis

Dissolve each pellet of PCA precipitate from flow sheet B in 2 ml 0.3 N NaOH.

Incubate at 37° for 90 min.

Remove 1 ml = short-term hydrolysis sample.

Cover remainder with parafilm and incubate overnight at 37°C for 18 hr[22] = long-term hydrolysis sample.

B. Processing of 1 ml short-term hydrolysis sample

1. Total counts.
    Remove 0.1 ml and determine the radioactivity by counting.[23]
2. Tritium exchange.[24]
    Remove 0.2 ml to a 13 × 100 mm tube with 0.2 ml 25% Dowex-1 formate w/v suspension.[24]
    Centrifuge at 800 × g for 2 min.
    Remove 0.2 ml supernatant and count[23] for Dowex-soluble cpm.
3. Alkaline stable radioactivity in DNA.
    Remove 0.3 ml to a 13 × 100 mm test tube.
    Add 0.3 ml 15% TCA.[25]
    Cool on ice for 10 min and collect on a 0.45 μ pore size millipore filter.
    Wash filter two times with cold 5% TCA.

MEASUREMENT OF RNA SYNTHESIS

FLOW SHEET D. (Continued)

Place in scintillation vial[26] and count for TCA-precipitable (TCA ppt) cpm.

4. Alkaline solubilized radioactivity and A_{260nm} in RNA.

   Remove 0.3 ml to 15 ml Corex round bottom centrifuge tube.
   Add 0.3 ml 1.5 M PCA[25] and cool on ice 10 min.
   Centrifuge 10 min at 25,000 × g.
   Remove supernatant and determine $A_{260\ nm}$.
   Take 0.1 ml supernatant and count radioactivity[23] for PCA-soluble cpm.
   Calculate percent exchange of ^{3}H and counts per embryo in RNA and in DNA.[27]

C. Processing of long-term hydrolysate for determination of radioactive AMP and GMP in RNA

Remove 0.1 ml and transfer to scintillation vial for total radioactivity.[23]

Remove 0.8 ml to 13 × 100 mm tube and add 0.2 ml 3.0 M PCA.[25]

Cool on ice for 10 min.

Centrifuge at 25,000 × g for 10 min.

Place 0.8 ml of the supernatant in a 13 × 100 mm tube and add 0.2 ml washed charcoal suspension.[13,24]

Let stand on ice for 5 min.

Centrifuge at 800 × g for 5 min.

Remove 0.1 ml of the charcoal supernatant to scintillation vial and count[23] to determine the fraction ^{3}H exchanged.[28]

Aspirate the remainder of the supernatant.

Wash the charcoal four times in cold H_2O.

Elute the nucleotides in 0.5 ml 0.1 N NH_4OH in 50% ethanol.

Centrifuge at 800 × g for 5 min.

Remove the supernatant to 15 ml Corex tube.

Centrifuge at 25,000 × g for 10 min.

Remove the supernatant and dry under a stream of air.[15]

Take up the nucleotides in 10 μliter of 0.1 N NH_4OH and spot on cellulose thin-layer plate.[16]

Develop with 33:66:1 H_2O, isobutyric acid, and conc NH_4OH as before for ATP chromatography.

Dry the chromatogram.

View with uv light and mark spots.[29]

Cut out AMP and GMP spots and count in scintillation counter.[26]

Calculate percentage radioactivity due to AMP.[30]

Calculate for each sample total radioactivity in AMP in the RNA using total radioactivity in RNA determined by the short-term hydrolysis and the percent radioactivity in AMP determined here. See Sample Calculations.

FLOW SHEET E. Luciferin-Luciferase Assay for ATP

A. Elution of the sample from thin-layer plate.

Place the ATP spots from the thin-layer sheet into 13 × 100 mm test tubes on ice.

Add 0.5 ml cold 0.04 M glycylglycine pH 7.4 buffer.

Shake or vortex vigorously several times over a 5 min period.

Remove the plastic strips.

Centrifuge at 800 × g for 1 min in cold.

Transfer the supernatant to new 13 × 100 mm test tube leaving behind most of the free cellulose from the plate. This is the ATP sample for assay.

B. ATP assay[31]

The samples should be run through the assay one by one. First run a sequence of standards. Make up a 10^{-6} M ATP solution in water and assay 10, 15, 20, 25, 35, and 50 µliter[32] (equal to 10, 15, 20, 25, 35 and 50 pmole ATP, respectively) of this solution. Then run assays of 5 µliter from each chromatographed preparation. If 5 µliter does not fall in the range of the standards, then use more sample or dilute the sample as may be appropriate to bring the sample within the range of the standards. Assay at least two samples of each unknown.

Prepare about 30 scintillation vials[33] with 0.9 ml glycylglycine buffer.

Pipet in ATP sample.

Pipet in 0.1 ml of firefly lantern extract.[34]

Swirl the vial and quickly put into the scintillation counter[35] with automatic printout and start counting immediately.

Take six consecutive 0.1 min counts from the vial.

Record the sample number on printout tape and on vials with unknown to use for determination of radioactivity.

Proceed to the next sample until all are run.

Draw a standard curve and determine the ATP in unknowns. See Sample Calculations.

C. Counting radioactivity in ATP samples.

Take the assay vials with the unknown radioactive ATP pool samples.

Add scintillation mix[36] and determine radioactivity.

Calculate the specific activity for each ATP sample $= \frac{\text{cpm in sample}}{\text{ATP in sample}}$. See Sample Calculations.

Draw a curve for the specific activity of the ATP during the incorporation period.

Calculate the average specific activity during the labeling period and the moles of ATP incorporated into RNA during the labeling periods. See Sample Calculations.

Plot the curve for accumulation of new RNA during the labeling period and determine the decay rate by plotting the data as a decay curve. See Sample Calculations.

MEASUREMENT OF RNA SYNTHESIS

SAMPLE CALCULATIONS

A summary of the data which might be obtained in these experiments and examples of the calculation and manipulation of the data necessary to determine rates of RNA synthesis and decay are presented below. Tables I, II, and III present sample results, respectively, for the luciferase assay for ATP, the short-term alkaline hydrolysis, and the long-term alkaline hydrolysis and chromatography.

To determine the ATP in the samples, plot a standard curve as shown in Figure 1 and then read off the ATP in the unknowns. Calculate the specific activity of each sample by dividing moles of ATP into cpm in the samples. Plot the specific activity of the samples to yield a curve as shown in Figure 2. The specific activity used to calculate the amount of RNA is the average specific activity of the RNA up to the time point in question. This is determined by integrating the curve over time and dividing by total time elapsed. The simplest method is to measure the area under the curve for the 10 min sample (this is the hatched area in the inset of Figure 2) and calculate the height of a level curve which

TABLE I. Data from Luciferase Assay of ATP

Sample	Second 0.1 min count of luciferase reaction, cpm	ATP, 10^{-12} mole	Radioactivity, cpm	Specific activity, cpm/10^{-12} mole ATP
10 μliter standard	14,600	10	–	–
15 μliter standard	48,200	15	–	–
20 μliter standard	88,600	20	–	–
25 μliter standard	138,000	25	–	–
35 μliter standard	256,000	35	–	–
50 μliter standard	641,000	50	–	–
5 μliter 10'	341,000	37	1368	37
5 μliter 10'	295,000	35	1086	31
5 μliter 20'	107,000	22.5	1102	49
10 μliter 20'	365,000	39	1834	47
5 μliter 40'	186,000	28.5	1593	54
5 μliter 40'	169,000	27.5	1431	52
5 μliter 80'	125,000	24	1211	50
5 μliter 80'	146,000	25.5	1352	53
5 μliter 160'	18,600	10.5	521	49
15 μliter 160'	249,000	31	1643	53
5 μliter 320'	3,450	–	259	–
15 μliter 320'	48,600	16	764	48
20 μliter 320'	99,700	22	1092	50

TABLE II. Data from Short-Term Alkaline Hydrolysis

Sample	A Radioactivity in 0.1 ml, cpm	B Dowex-soluble radioactivity, cpm	C TCA-precipatable radioactivity, cpm	D PCA-soluble radioactivity, cpm	E PCA-soluble A$_{-260nm}$
10'	623	48	275	259	0.49
20'	1354	88	708	569	0.43
40'	2351	153	1,857	881	0.46
80'	4141	244	3,530	1479	0.45
160'	5986	341	7,246	1823	0.41
320'	8318	504	14,078	2134	0.42

TABLE III. Data from Long-Term Alkaline Hydrolysis

Sample	A Total radioactivity, cpm	B Charcoal-soluble radioactivity, cpm	C Radioactivity in AMP spot, cpm	D Radioactivity in GMP and ATP spot, cpm	E Fraction of cpm in RNA in AMP
10'	651	375	179	46	0.80
20'	1,398	769	1089	129	0.89
40'	2,106	1221	1692	172	0.91
80'	3,619	2169	3036	315	0.90
160'	6,011	3364	1888	185	0.91
320'	7,255	5994	5124	593	0.90

would give a similar area (indicated by the stipled area in the inset of Figure 2). The average specific activity for all time points was determined by this method and are given in column D of Table IV.

Using the formulas presented in footnote 27, the data can be calculated to yield the results tabulated in Table IV. Such calculations for the 10 min sample are outlined here:

(a) Total cpm = 10 × cpm in 0.1 ml of short-term hydrolysis
= 10 × 623
= 6230 cpm

(b) ^{3}H exchange = 10 × Dower-soluble cpm
= 10 × 48
= 480

MEASUREMENT OF RNA SYNTHESIS

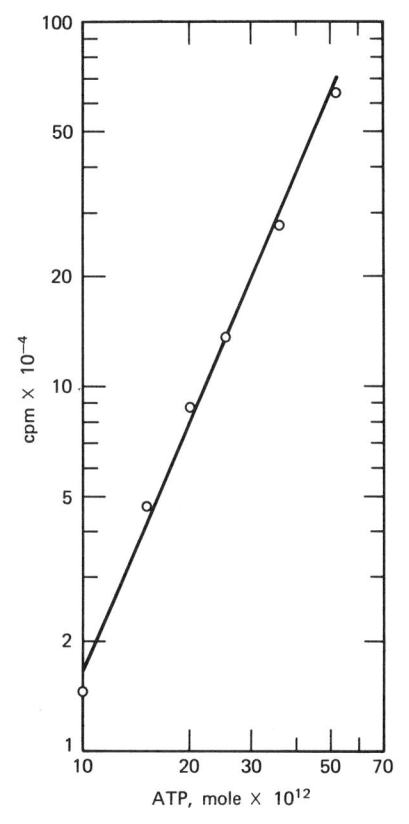

FIGURE 1. Standard curve from luciferase assay of ATP.

(c) $\text{DNA} = 3.3 \times \text{TCA ppt cpm} + \left(^3\text{H exchange} \times \dfrac{3.3 \times \text{TCA ppt cpm}}{\text{total cpm} - {}^3\text{H exchange}}\right)$

$= 3.3 \times 275 + \left(480 \times \dfrac{3.3 \times 275}{6230 - 480}\right)$

$= 981$

(d) $\text{RNA} = 20 \times \text{PCA-soluble cpm} - \left(^3\text{H exchange} \times \dfrac{3.3 \times \text{TCA ppt cpm}}{\text{total cpm} - {}^3\text{H exchange}}\right)$

$= 20 \times 259 - \left(480 \times \dfrac{3.3 \times 275}{6230 - 480}\right)$

$= 5103$

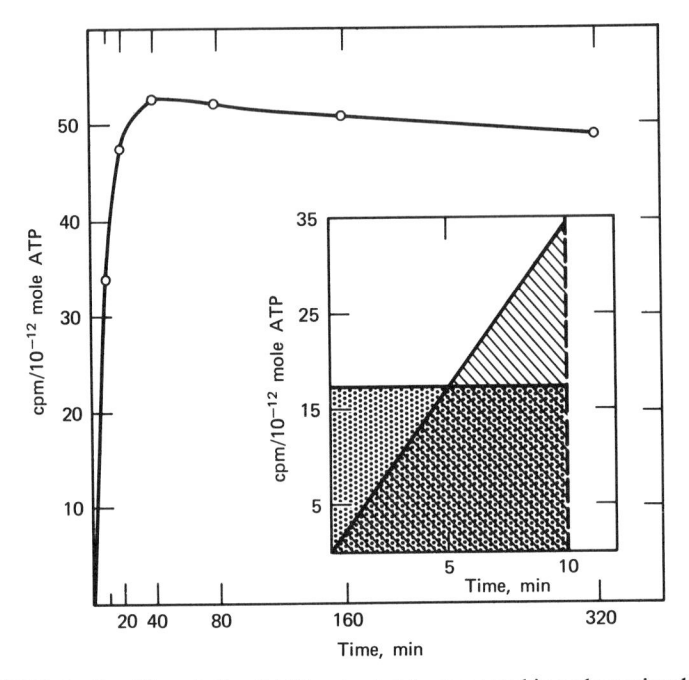

FIGURE 2. Specific activity of ATP extracted from sea urchin embryos incubated with radioactive adenosine. Inset: Illustration of a determination of the average specific activity of the ATP during the first 10 min of the incubation. The area under the actual curve (hatched area) is determined and a level curve with equal area (stippled area) is drawn. The height of the level curve is the average specific activity of the ATP during the 10 min incubation.

(e) Number of embryos $= \dfrac{A_{-260} \times 2}{1.2 \times 10^{-4} \, A_{-260}/\text{embryo}}$

$= \dfrac{0.49 \times 2}{1.2 \times 10^{-4}}$

$= 8170$

(f) Fraction of cpm in AMP $= \dfrac{\text{AMP cpm}}{\text{GMP cpm} + \text{AMP cpm}}$

$= \dfrac{179}{46 + 179}$

$= 0.80$

Using these values, the counts per minute in DNA and the counts per minute in AMP in RNA as shown in columns A and C of Table IV can be calculated by dividing the radioactivity in DNA and RNA by the number of embryos and

TABLE IV. Calculation of Incorporation into Nucleic Acids

Sample	A Radioactivity in DNA, cpm/embryo	B Radioactivity in RNA, cpm/embryo	C Radioactivity in AMP in RNA, cpm/embryo	D Average specific activity of ATP, cpm/10^{-12} mole	E 10^{-14} mole ATP in RNA per embryo	F Steady-state RNA radioactive, %	G Steady-state RNA nonradioactive, %
10'	0.120	0.623	0.498	17	2.9	28	72
20'	0.348	1.58	1.41	29	4.6	44	56
40'	0.863	2.24	2.36	40	6.0	58	42
80'	1.65	3.86	3.47	46	7.7	74	26
160'	3.73	5.13	4.67	49	9.2	88	12
320'	7.07	5.67	5.09	49	10.4	100	0

multiplying the latter by the fraction which is in AMP. The moles of A in RNA, a direct measure of the RNA accumulated from the time when the radioactive adenosine was added to the embryos, is calculated by dividing the counts per minute in AMP in RNA by the counts per minute per mole ATP. This is shown in column E of Table IV. This value can be converted to moles of nucleotides by dividing by 0.3, the proportion of nucleotides which are AMP in this DNA-like RNA [Emerson and Humphreys, 1970], and can be further converted to grams by multiplying by 330, the average molecular weight of a nucleotide.

The data for the accumulation of radioactivity in DNA and amount of radioactive RNA are plotted in Figure 3. The DNA is stable and to a first approximation accumulates at a linear rate. The RNA accumulates at a decreasing rate indicating it is unstable. At first, accumulation equals synthesis, but as radioactive RNA accumulates, it decays more and more rapidly until a steady state is reached. When it decays as rapidly as it is synthesized, accumulation ceases. The rate of decay can be determined by assuming that there is a constant steady-state level of RNA and that the nonradioactive RNA present when labeling was begun decays and is replaced by radioactive RNA. Thus, the accumulation curve of the radioactive RNA to a steady state is an inverse of the decay curve of the nonradioactive RNA from the steady-state level. The approach of radioactive RNA to a steady state, expressed as 100%, and the decay of nonradioactive RNA from

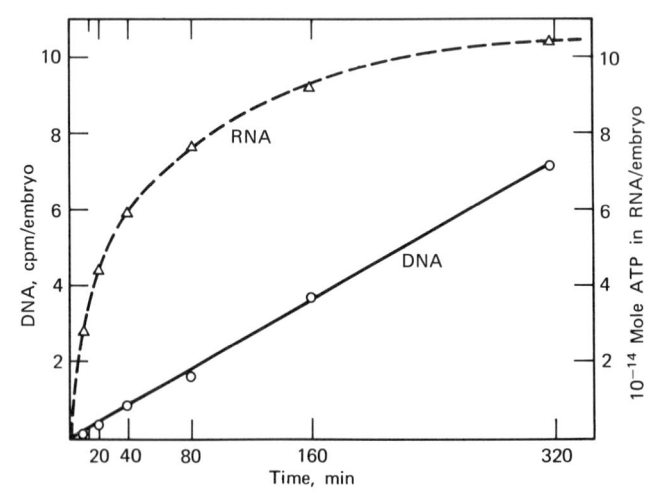

FIGURE 3. The incorporation of radioactive adenosine into DNA and the accumulation of total AMP in RNA during an incubation of sea urchin embryos with radioactive adenosine.

a steady state is given in columns F and G of Table IV. The decay of nonradioactive RNA is plotted as a first-order decay curve in Figure 4. Analysis of this curve into two components by standard procedures is shown on Figure 4 and is discussed in detail in recent papers [Brandhorst and Humphreys, 1971, 1972].

Acknowledgements

The original work from which these procedures were derived was supported by grant number HD 03480 and HD 06574 from NICHD.

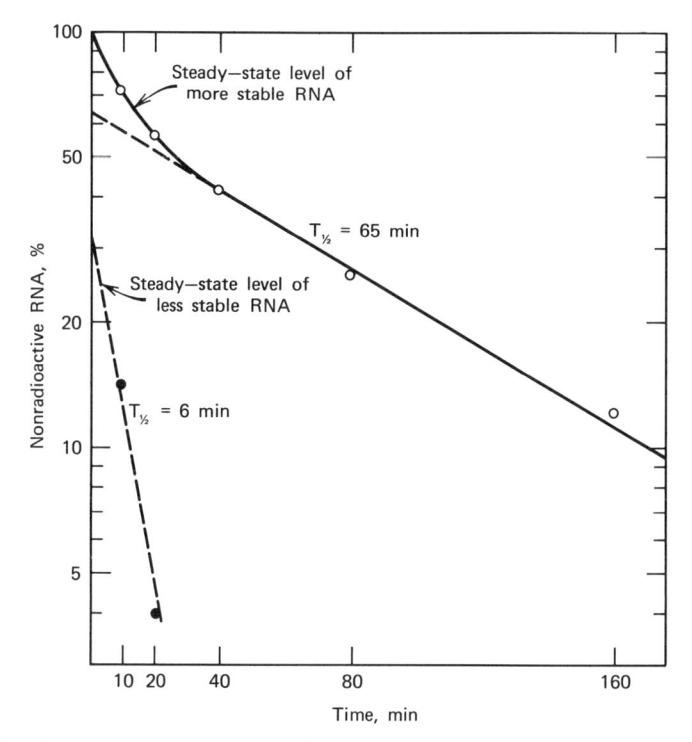

FIGURE 4. First-order decay plot of the accumulation of AMP in RNA as shown in Table IV and Figure 3. The steady state level of total AMP in unstable RNA is taken as the 320 min time point. When the radioactive adenosine is added, 100% of the RNA is unlabeled. The percent unlabeled at any time point is 100% minus the percent labeled as shown in Table IV giving a decay curve for the nonradioactive RNA from the time the isotope was added. The decay curve is resolved into two straight lines. One representing a more stable class with a 65 min half-life which makes up 65% of the steady state level of RNA. The other line, determined by extrapolating the decay curve of the more stable RNA and subtracting from the total curve, represents a less stable class of RNA. It represents 35% of the total RNA and decays with a half-life of 6 min.

FOOTNOTES

1. This procedure was designed for Lythechinus pictus. I believe it may be applied to Lythechinus variegatus without change; to Strongylocentrotus purpuratus if the semen is diluted from 2- to 4-fold more and the cell always kept below 20°C; and to Arbacia punctulata if care is taken to prevent contamination of the eggs and sperm by the toxic epidermal exudate which KCl sometimes causes this species to release. Both of the latter two species have smaller eggs and may be suspended at 5×10^4 eggs per ml.
2. Ripe sea urchins may be obtained most of the year by air from one of the following sources:

    Norris Hill
    P. O. Box 453
    Beaufort, North Carolina 28516
    919-728-4745

    Pacific Bio-marine
    P. O. Box 536
    Venice, California 90291
    213-397-7281

    Gulf Coast Specimen Company
    P. O. Box 237
    Panacea, Florida 32346
    909-984-2041

3. We normally use artificial sea water made up as two solutions mixed in equal portions when needed.

Solution I	g/liter	Solution II	g/liter
NaCl	46.4	$CaCl_2$ (anhydrous)	2.0
Na_2SO_4	7.3	$MgCl_2 \cdot 6H_2O$	19.8
KCl	1.4	pH of mixed sea water should	
$NaHCO_3$	0.4	be 7.5 to 8.4	

4. We achieve appropriate agitation by placing the suspension in an Erlenmeyer flask about 1/10 full and shaking on a rotatory shaker with a 3/4 in. diam of gyration at 80 rpm. Stirring slowly with a bent glass rod on a motor is also quite adequate.
5. The major defense against bacterial contamination is provided by washing with acid sea water. It is made by adding acetic acid to sea water to a final concentration of 0.02 M and adjusting the pH to 4.5. It dissolves the mucoid coat on the embryos and releases the bacteria which are then washed away in the sequence of washes. Most investigators also use penicillin and streptomycin in their cultures but we have found that most bacterial fauna associated with L. pictus are resistant to these antibiotics.
6. The addition of the isotonic (1.1 M) sucrose makes the bottom layer more dense and stabilizes the cell suspension layered on top of the tube thus

MEASUREMENT OF RNA SYNTHESIS

preventing mixing. The cells are then centrifuged into the denser layer producing an extremely efficient wash eliminating bacteria and external isotope. One wash removes over 99.9% of the external isotope from the cells. The second wash is repeated mainly for insurance. It should be noted that no wash is necessary in this experiment since the pool examined is ATP and external isotope is adenosine. All radioactive adenosine which is phosphorylated is within the cell.

7. The AEC has a manual of standard procedures for handling radioisotopes. Most institutions have a radiation safety officer who can provide instruction on appropriate safety measures.
8. Accuracy of pipetting or complete yields are not necessary at these points. The critical measurements are radioactivity per mole of ATP in the purified sample from the chromatogram and radioactivity per A_{260} of hydrolyzed RNA. It is only necessary that you have an adequately sized sample to make these measurements in the later parts of the experiment.
9. This is most easily done with a pasteur pipet on a hose connected to a vacuum flask. This efficiently removes the supernatant as well as safely collecting the radioactive solution without spills.
10. Macromolecular nucleic acids and most proteins (molecules larger than 5–15 nucleotides or amino acids) are precipitated by 0.5 N PCA or 0.5 N (5%) TCA. Both acids work much the same for precipitation but are preferable in various experiments for other reasons. For example, PCA is used when A_{260} or A_{280} is to be determined since it does not absorb at these wave lengths while TCA absorbs strongly. Perchloric acid precipitates with potassium ions and is used to remove these ions after an alkaline hydrolysis with KOH. Trichloroacetic acid is volatile and can be used when samples are to be dried while dry PCA is explosive; TCA is also used when there are potassium ions in the sample which one does not want to precipitate.
11. ATP, RNA, and DNA are slowly hydrolyzed in PCA (or TCA) even at $0°C$. An RNA sample will be almost completely degraded overnight. Thus, samples in PCA cannot be stored.
12. The luciferase reaction will generally measure ATP fairly accurately in the unpurified sample if the amount of ATP is an order of magnitude greater than that of the other nucleoside triphosphates. These latter can interfere with determinations due to production of ATP by kinases in the enzyme extract. However, radioactivity from adenosine enters a number of adenine and guanine nucleotides which must be purified from the ATP in order to measure the specific radioactivity of the ATP.

Since in early sea urchins, the ATP pool is apparently about three times as large as the combined pools of dATP, ADP, AMP, GTP, GDP, and GMP, this purification is easy. This thin-layer step will separate all of these nucleotides with the exception of GMP. GMP is present in sea urchins at only 0.1% of the ATP so it can be ignored. The contamination after chromatography of the ATP with GMP from other cell types can be determined by hydrolyzing the ATP to AMP and rechromatographing it to separate AMP from GMP. Hydrolysis may be achieved by binding the sample to charcoal and boiling for 30 min in 1 N HCl. Wash the charcoal, elute, spot, and run the sample as described in this protocol for separation of AMP and GMP from hydrolyzed RNA. The ratio of ATP to GMP in the original sample is given by the ratio of radioactivity in the AMP and GMP spots.

13. Nucleotides bind strongly to activated charcoal at acid and neutral pH. Many other organic molecules, including polynucleotides and salts, do not. Since salts interfere with the chromatography, they are removed from the nucleotide sample by binding the nucleotides to charcoal and washing. Before use, the charcoal is washed by low-speed centrifugation 3 times in 0.1 N HCl, 3 times for 30 min at 37°C in 0.1 N NH_4OH in 50% ethanol, and then 3 times with water. Since materials sometimes elute from the charcoal which effect the movement of the nucleotides on the thin-layer, the standards are carried through the charcoal wash to provide a better standard spot.

14. The nucleotides are partially removed from the charcoal by the alkali; yields of 50% can be considered maximal. ATP is quite stable in dilute alkaline solutions; for example, it is not measurably degraded in 0.3 N NaOH after 18 hr at 37°C. The ^3H in 8-^3H-adenosine exchanges with the ^1H in water under alkaline conditions but does not do so to a significant amount during the 30 min incubation in 0.1 N NH_4OH.

15. Drying usually takes 2–4 hr but can be left overnight. Be sure the air is oil-free and clean. We make a simple device for drying the eight samples at once. Eight 3/16 in. holes are cut at about 1 in. intervals into the side of 5/16 in. inside diam thin-walled tygon tubing. One end of the tubing is closed, the other is attached to the air source and eight pasteur pipet are inserted into the holes. The device is mounted so that the tip of a pipet blows into each tube.

16. We use the commercially available plates of cellulose prepared on plastic backing (Eastman Chromatogram #6064). Some batches of the plates are defective; they may have uneven or loosely attached cellulose or have UV-absorbing impurities and must be returned. Under humid conditions, it sometimes helps to dry the plates at 60°C for a while before spotting. Very lightly mark a line 2 cm from the bottom of the plate with a No. 1 (very soft) pencil. Make eight cross marks to position the three samples about 1 in. apart. Apply the sample by gently touching the tip of the capillary pipet to the spot, until a circle about 1/2 cm is wet. Lift the pipet and dry the spot with a steam of air. Repeat until the sample has all been applied. The thin-layer is very delicate and care must be taken at all times not to disrupt the layer while carrying out these manipulations. Do not touch the surface of the plate with fingers. Handle at top edge only.

17. It may be best to let the atmosphere in the tank become saturated with the solvent and to put the plate in a dry tray to equilibrate with the atmosphere before beginning development by pouring solvent into the tray. We have obtained good results, however, by ignoring these basic rules of chromatog-

MEASUREMENT OF RNA SYNTHESIS

raphy with the small tanks, 10 X 10 X 3 in., which we routinely use.

18. This drying step can be carried out at 60°C for 30 min. While the samples are drying a white frosty streak may appear for a while. This is an indication of excess salt or other material carried over with the charcoal.

19. The dark spots appearing under uv light on the samples from the embryos is ATP which is the most abundant nucleotide. There also may be streaks of fluorescent material. The appearance of the latter is variable and I do not know their source or nature. However, they do not seem to disturb the separation.

   This chromatography procedure separates the nucleotides on the basis of extent of phosphorylation with the nucleoside running the fastest and the trinucleotides the slowest. The guanine nucleotides run about 1/2 to 1/3 the rate of adenosine nucleotides. The pyrimidine nucleotides run between these two. Fortunately, the pyrimidine nucleotides can be ignored in this chromatography since they do not interact with luciferase or become labeled from radioactive adenosine. However, all purine nucleotides must be considered because radioactivity from adenosine enters them.

   The standards should show that both ADP and dATP run slightly ahead of ATP which has an RF of about 0.35–0.45 depending on the batch of TLC plates. The GTP runs well behind the ATP with an RF of about 0.1. GDP runs between GTP and GMP, which runs with ATP.

   Fortunately the GMP is not a significant contaminant of the ATP since it occurs at only 0.1% of the ATP concentration in these sea urchin embryos. Hypoxanthine nucleotides must also become labeled but we have not detected significant amounts of these.

20. The slower half of the ATP spot is selected to eliminate possible contamination by dATP which runs only slightly ahead of the ATP. It is interesting to cut up the rest of the strip into 0.5 cm sections and count them for radioactivity. The peaks of radioactive ADP and AMP will be evident. GTP might be detectable. If this nucleotide pool analysis is applied to another cell type, it is imperative to determine what percentage of the radioactivity is in ATP to prove that the single chromatography is adequate.

21. ^{3}H-Adenosine is precursor for both DNA and RNA. RNA is rapidly hydrolyzed in alkaline solutions while DNA is quite stable. This property is used to distinguish between the radioactivity incorporated into DNA and into RNA. RNA is hydrolyzed to PCA-soluble oligonucleotides in 15–30 min. However, the PCA precipitates we start with take longer to hydrolyze, presumably because they take a while to dissolve. During the short-term hydrolysis, very little protein becomes acid-soluble and does not interfere with measurement of absorbance of RNA at 260 nm.

   ^{3}H-Adenosine is converted to guanosine which is also incorporated into RNA. Since the specific activity of only the ATP pool is measured, only the radioactivity in adenosine in RNA must be included in the calculations. The radioactivity incorporated in guanosine is determined by hydrolyzing the RNA to mononucleotides, separating GMP from AMP, and counting each fraction.

22. This complete hydrolysis may also be achieved in 45 min at 80°C.
23. We count the sample in a scintillation counter after dissolving in 5 ml toluene with 0.4% PPO w/v (2,5-diphenyloxazole) and 0.005% POPOP [1,4-bis(2-(5-phenyloxazolyl))benzene] with 1.5% Beckman Biosolv-2 and 3% Beckman Biosolv-3.
24. 8-^{3}H-Adenosine, the cheapest radioactive adenosine available because it can be made by exchange at alkaline pH, exchanges ^{3}H with H_2O during the alkaline hydrolysis. The Dowex formate binds the mononucleotides and polynucleotides quantitatively leaving behind the ^{3}H which has exchanged with H_2O. This separation of exchanged ^{3}H will be achieved with charcoal after complete hydrolysis. However, charcoal does not bind the many oligonucleotides which are left after the short alkaline hydrolysis.

    The Dowex-1-x8 formate is made by washing Dowex-1-x8 chloride with 2 N formic acid until all chloride is removed (eluant does not precipitate with $AgNO_3$) and then washing with H_2O.
25. The extra acid in the 15% TCA, 1.5 N PCA, or 3.6 N PCA is to neutralize the base and bring the final concentration of acid to about 0.5 N.
26. To count a sample collected on a filter or on a piece chromatogram, we put the filter or strip in a counting vial, dissolve and elute it with 0.3 ml 0.3 N NaOH for about 15 min (do not leave the base on longer than 2 hr or the filter discolors and quenches), and count in 7.5 ml toluene with 0.4% PPO (2,5-diphenyloxazole), 0.005% POPOP [1,4-bis(2-(5-phenyloxazolyl))benzene], 3% Beckman Biosolv-2 and 7% Beckman Biosolv-3.
27. To make these calculations, one must account for the dilution of the various samples. The easiest way is to calculate back to the original volume of 1 ml. We are assuming equal efficiency of counting in all samples. The counting procedures we describe give such results.

    (a) Total cpm = cpm in 0.1 ml sample $\times$ 10
    (b) ^{3}H Exchange = Dowex-soluble cpm $\times$ 10
    (c) DNA = 3.3 $\times$ TCA ppt cpm
    $+ \left(^3H \text{ exchange} \times \dfrac{3.3 \times \text{TCA ppt cpm}}{\text{total cpm} - ^3H \text{ exchange}} \right)$
    (d) RNA = (20 $\times$ PCA soluble cpm)
    $- \left(^3H \text{ exchange} \times \dfrac{3.3 \times \text{TCA ppt cpm}}{\text{total cpm} - ^3H \text{ exchange}} \right)$
    (e) A_{260} = A_{260} reading of sample $\times$ 2

    There are 1.2 $\times$ 10^{-4} A_{260} units of hydrolyzed RNA per L. pictus embryo. 33 µg hydrolyzed RNA in PCA or 37 µg macromolecular RNA has one A_{260} unit, that is, gives A_{260} equal to 1.0 when dissolved in 1 ml.
28. As much as 60% of the ^{3}H may have exchanged during the 18 hr hydrolysis.
29. The four mononucleotides from the RNA hydrolysis will appear in three spots. The GMP will be closest to the origin with an RF of about 0.33. Next will be an elongate spot which includes UMP and CMP. Finally there is an AMP spot with an RF of 0.65.

MEASUREMENT OF RNA SYNTHESIS

30. The percentage of the total counts which are in adenine can be easily calculated directly from the counts in the two spots:

$$\% \text{ radioactivity in AMP} = \frac{\text{AMP cpm}}{\text{AMP cpm} + \text{GMP cpm}} \times 100$$

This is because the yields of AMP and GMP from charcoal are equal. Even though the ^{3}H in guanine exchanges at 0.6 the rate of ^{3}H in adenine, this difference can usually be ignored in sea urchins since conversion to guanine is very low. However, if it should be high, the correction is possible with the data from this experiment. The formula for the calculation is as follows:

$$\frac{\text{AMP cpm} + \text{GMP cpm}}{1 - \text{fraction exchanged}} = \frac{\text{AMP cpm}}{1 - X} + \frac{\text{GMP cpm}}{1 - 0.6X}$$

$$\text{fraction exchanged} = \frac{1.56 \times \text{cpm in charcoal supernatant}}{\text{cpm in total radioactivity sample}}$$

X = fraction exchange of A

$$\text{fraction of original radioactivity in AMP} = \frac{\dfrac{\text{AMP cpm}}{(1 - X)}}{\dfrac{\text{AMP cpm}}{(1 - X)} + \dfrac{\text{GMP cpm}}{(1 - 0.6X)}}$$

31. The assay is performed with a scintillation counter. When luciferase splits ATP in the presence of luciferin, light is emitted. The flashes of light are counted by the counter. The rate of flashes goes up exponentially with the concentration of ATP. Using 0.1 ml enzyme solution under these conditions, the 10 pmole ATP should give a flash rate of about 5000/min while the 50 pmole should give about 400,000. The rate of emission of light decays rapidly after reaching a peak soon after the enzyme is introduced. The peak is not usually seen in these experiments, since in practice 4–10 sec (depending on the make of counter) must elapse before the sample can be gotten into a scintillation counter for counting.

    To measure the ATP, we take sequential 0.1 min counts from each sample. The decay of counts should be smooth over the series of counts. Often the decay is not smooth indicating poor mixing of the sample, dirty vials, or other problems. If "bad" decay is observed, repeat the sample at least twice. Bad decay on chromotographed samples sometimes means that the peak of ATP was missed and another 0.5 cm section of the chromatogram, either above or below the original one should be eluted and assayed. For the actual assay we have found greatest reproducibility when we take the 0.1 min count which begins at about 20 sec after addition of the enzyme.

32. We have found the Drummond disposable microcaps the most convenient, reliably clean, and accurate pipets for dispensing these quantities.

33. These vials must be cleaned and well rinsed to remove detergent. We routinely boil ours in 7x, a tissue culture detergent, and rinse 10 times in hot water and two times in distilled water.

34. We purchase Sigma FLE-250 and make it up according to their directions. After dissolving for a day at 0°C we centrifuge at 1000 × g for 5 min, take the supernatant and dispense 2 ml aliquots into small tubes, and store frozen at −20°C. As we do this assay, the impure extract is satisfactory. Purified enzyme is available and can be used as the basis for an assay procedure with greater sensitivity and specificity.
35. The settings used for counting ^{3}H are adequate for this assay. We do not add a cap to the vial. Most counters will not accept an open vial unless the safety mechanism is overridden. This usually means covering a light or tripping a microswitch by hand.
36. Use 20 ml of 3 + 7% Beckman Bisolv-2 + 3 mix described in footnote 26.

REFERENCES

Berg, W. E. 1970. Further studies on the kinetics of incorporation of valine in the sea urchin embryo. Exp. Cell Res. 60:210–217.

Brandhorst, B. P. 1970. Kinetics of turnover of DNA-like RNA and its transport to the cytoplasm in sea urchin embryos. J. Cell Biol. 47:23–24a.

Brandhorst, B. P. 1971. Metabolism of DNA-like RNA in sea urchin embryos. Ph.D. thesis, Univers. California, San Diego.

Brandhorst, B. P., and T. Humphreys. 1971. Synthesis and decay rates of major classes of DNA-like RNA in sea urchin embryos. Biochemistry 10:877–881.

Brandhorst, B. P., and T. Humphreys. 1972. Stabilities of nuclear and messenger RNA molecules in sea urchin embryos. J. Cell Biol. 53:474–482.

Emerson, C. P. 1970. Analysis of the regulation of ribosomal RNA synthesis in animal cells. Ph.D. thesis, Univers. California, San Diego.

Emerson, C. P. 1971. Regulation of the synthesis and stability of ribosomal RNA during contact inhibition of growth. Nature New Biol. 232:101–106.

Emerson, C. P., and T. Humphreys. 1970. Regulation of DNA-like RNA and the apparent activation of ribosomal RNA synthesis in sea urchin embryos: quantitative measurements of newly synthesized RNA. Develop. Biol. 23:86–112.

Emerson, C. P., unpublished. Dept. of Zoology, Univ. of Virginia, Charlottesville, Va.

Emerson, C. P., and T. Humphreys. 1971. A simple and sensitive method for quantitative measurement of cellular RNA synthesis. Anal. Biochem. 40:254–266.

Epstein, C. J., and D. L. Daentl. 1971. Precursor pools and RNA synthesis in preimplantation mouse embryos. Develop. Biol. 26:517–524.

Humphreys, T. 1971. Measurements of messenger RNA entering polysomes upon fertilization of sea urchin eggs. Develop. Biol. 26:201–208.

Humphreys, T. 1973. RNA and protein synthesis during early animal embryogenesis. In S. J. Coward (ed.), Cell differentiation. Academic Press, New York (In press).

Kijima, S., and F. H. Wilt. 1969. Rate of nuclear RNA turnover in sea urchin embryos. J. Mol. Biol. 40:235–246.

Plagemann, P. G. W. 1972. Nucleotide pools in Novikoff rat Hepatoma cells growing in suspension culture. Ill effects of nucleotides in medium on levels of nucleotides in separate nucleotide pools for nuclear and cytoplasmic RNA synthesis. J. Cell Biol. 52:131–146.

Roeder, R. G., and W. J. Rutter. 1970. Multiple RNA polymerases and RNA synthesis during sea urchin development. Biochemistry 9:2543–2553.

DNA-RNA and DNA-DNA Hybridization, with Emphasis on Filter Techniques

DOUGLAS W. SMITH

I. INTRODUCTION

An amazing property of complementary single-stranded nucleic acid species is their ability to hybridize, that is, their ability to form stable duplexes, with each other. This property has led to the development of analytical biochemical assays for the immediate products of gene expression (RNA–DNA hybridization), for determination of redundancies and uniqueness of gene sequences (DNA–DNA hybridization), and for the cytological localization of gene sequences on chromosomes (for example, in situ DNA–DNA hybridization). In addition, hybridization properties have led to the development of preparative methods for RNA species and for DNA genes and types of DNA sequences. Hybridization techniques provide very powerful research tools for the developmental and molecular biologist.

The physical chemistry of nucleic acid hybrid formation has been extensively studied and reviewed [1–4]. The rate-limiting step in formation of a hybrid appears to be initial collision and formation of interstrand hydrogen bonds between a few complementary base pairs of the two single-stranded species [5]. Base-pairing of between 10 and 20 nucleotide pairs is necessary for formation of a stable complex [6]. A rapid "zippering" reaction then yields the final hybrid. Once formed, the stability of the hybrid duplex is due primarily to stacking forces rather than to hydrogen bond formation [1,7].

The rate of formation of the stable hybrid depends on many environmental factors, including temperature, salt concentration, viscosity of the solvent, and % (G + C) of the nucleic acid species. The temperature optimum for hybrid formation is about 25°C below the duplex melting temperature [5]. The reaction rate is proportional to the square root of the length of the single-stranded species [5], and second-order kinetics are obeyed. For DNA reassociation, such kinetics imply that the parameter of interest is the product $C_0 t$ of the DNA concentration C_0 and the time t of the reaction [4,8,9].

A. Types of Experiments

Hybridization experiments are of two basic types: kinetic experiments and saturation experiments. In practice, initial kinetic experiments are performed to characterize a new hybridization system and to establish the appropriate reaction conditions. Experiments involving reassociation of single-stranded DNA species usually determine the extent of hybridization as a function of the product $C_0 t$, resulting in a "Cot curve"; for a fixed DNA concentration, these represent kinetic experiments.

In any kinetic experiment, after a sufficient time of hybridization no further hybrid is formed; that is, saturation is reached. Saturation experiments determine the extent of hybridization as a function of concentration of one of the reactants. For RNA–DNA hybridization, the RNA concentration is usually varied. Such experiments can reveal information about the amount of a given source of DNA which is complementary to a given RNA species. For example, ribosomal RNA from Escherichia coli hybridizes to 0.3% of the E. coli genome [10]. This, however, is a particularly simple case, since the rRNA from E. coli can be easily purified free of other RNA species. Messenger RNA (mRNA) species are not so easily obtained. Preparations of mRNA often contain a high percentage of rRNA, and quantitative hybridization experiments are difficult to perform and interpret. Recently, the quantitative use of hybridization techniques has been questioned [11,12], and the difficulties involved have been recently reviewed [3,4]. Reactions with mRNA involve many mRNA species, each at a low concentration within a high concentration of RNA. These anneal with DNA samples containing a low concentration of the desired complementary DNA sequence among a high concentration of DNA sequences. Consequently, high RNA and DNA concentrations, long incubation times, and high temperatures are required with many nucleic acid reactions occurring at the same time.

Competition experiments are often performed to determine if two RNA species are identical in base sequence, that is, if they arise from the same DNA genes. Curves of relative hybridization versus concentration of nonradioactive "test" RNA are generally obtained. In most experiments, DNA is exposed to both nonradioactive and radioactive RNA simultaneously, although this procedure has disadvantages and alternative procedures have been used [13].

Quantitative interpretation of competition experiments is not always an easy task. For example, in many such experiments pulse-labeled RNA will be competed against a specific purified RNA species, for example, rRNA. The RNA molecules clearly will compete on a mass basis. But if the RNA molecules labeled during the pulse contain different amounts of the label, that is, if they have different specific activities, then the relationship between the label excluded by the competing rRNA to the mass of labeled RNA excluded is nearly impossible to determine. Further, the labeled RNA molecules under question, for example, pulse-labeled rRNA molecules, must be present in excess of the number of DNA sites, for example, rDNA genes. Otherwise, the degree of exclusion by adding competitor RNA will not be proportional to the mass of added competitor RNA. This means in practice that the relative amounts of labeled RNA, DNA, and competitor RNA must be chosen with great care, according to the experiment in question. These considerations with illustrative examples, together with further pitfalls, are admirably discussed by Kennell [4].

Hybridization of nucleic acids from eucaryotic cells presents further unique problems. The total genome content is greatly increased (up to 1000-fold) relative to that of a bacterium. Further, some DNA sequences are present more than once; that is, DNA redundancy in the genome exists, resulting in a "rapidly reannealing" fraction in DNA–DNA hybridization experiments. These factors taken together mean that annealing of RNA sequences to eucaryotic nonrepetitive DNA is very low under usual reaction conditions, for both thermodynamic (equilibrium) and kinetic reasons. Further, formation of "mismatched" hybrids between nucleic acids of similar but nonidentical sequence becomes a serious problem in studies of eucaryotes. Judicious choice of annealing temperature and salt conditions is required to yield a minimum of mismatched hybrids. Thermal elution profiles of the resulting hybrids should be performed to determine the extent of mismatching, since mismatched regions have a lower melting temperature, thus effectively broadening the melting region. "Presaturation" competition, that is, hybridization of the unlabeled RNA to the DNA prior to competition with the labeled RNA, has been used to avoid mismatching problems [14]. The above problems are also discussed by Kennell [4].

In spite of the severe problems related to quantitation mentioned above, hybridization has become one of the most important experimental techniques in studies of gene expression and nucleic acid relatedness. The following are a few specific examples of uses of hybridization methods in gene expression studies and in developmental biology: (1) the use of DNA carrying relatively few genes to synthesize RNA for studies of phage lambda gene expression [15] and expression of the genes for tryptophan biosynthesis in E. coli [16,17]; (2)

hybridization of 9 S messenger RNA for mouse globin to mouse embryo DNA [18]; (3) hybridization of rapidly labeled fetal mouse RNA to nonrepetitive DNA sequences [19]; (4) hybridization of total RNA from different mouse tissues to nonrepetitive mouse DNA sequences [20]; (5) the use of vast DNA excess to permit hybridization of cellular RNA to nonrepetitive DNA sequences [9]; (6) localization of highly repeated DNA sequences in Drosophila melanogaster via in situ hybridization to the chromocenter of the salivary gland chromosomes [21]; (7) distribution of the transcribing regions on the complementary strands of bacteriophage λ [22]; (8) hybridization of ribosomal RNA to the E. coli DNA genome [23]; (9) DNA–DNA relationships among vertebrates with evolutionary implications [24]; (10) cytological in situ localization of DNA complementary to ribosomal RNA in polytene chromosomes of Diptera [25]; (11) DNA–DNA hybridization to assay replication origin DNA in E. coli [26].

II. DNA–RNA HYBRIDIZATION

A. Introduction

Several techniques have been used to effect and assay the formation of RNA–DNA hybrid duplex molecules. In general, hybrids are formed when single-stranded or denatured DNA is exposed to an RNA solution under annealing conditions. The DNA may either be free in solution or immobilized on an appropriate matrix. Annealing conditions, in general, include (1) high cation concentration (0.01 M Na^+ or higher), (2) elevated temperatures, and (3) adequate concentrations and incubation times to permit hybridization to occur. In principle, any technique that distinguishes a bihelical nucleic acid species from a single-stranded species may be used to assay hybrid formation. When immobilized DNA is used, RNA bound to the matrix is assayed. When hybrid formation is permitted in solution, several methods which separate bihelical species from single-stranded species have been used. Such methods include banding in CsCl density gradients [27], isolation on methylated album kieselguhr (MAK) columns [28] or hydroxyapatite (HA) columns [29–31], and filtration on nitrocellulose filters [32,37,38]. Some assay methods, such as decrease in absorption of UV radiation (hypochromism) by the solution [1], have been used which do not involve separation of the hybrid from the single-stranded reactants.

Matrices which have successfully been used to immobilize single-stranded DNA include nitrocellulose columns [33], agar columns [34,35], acrylamide gel columns to which DNA is covalently bound using UV radiation [36], and nitrocellulose membrane filters [32,37,38]. The column methods require a separate column for each DNA species to be tested, and considerable experience is required for successful use. Filtration techniques are rapid, require only a separate filter for each DNA species, and little experience is needed for successful use.

The rate of hybridization depends on salt concentrations, temperature, base content of the DNA, and viscosity and nature of the solvent. The buffer most often used in hybridization studies is SSC (0.15 M NaCl, 0.015 M sodium citrate, pH 7.0) or some multiple thereof. A buffer of 2 times SSC, usually called "2 × SSC," containing 0.3 M NaCl, 0.03 M sodium citrate, pH 7.0, is convenient for most experiments. Sometimes 0.01 M Tris is used in place of 0.015 M sodium citrate. The temperature used must be high enough to remove any secondary structure in the RNA and must be chosen to yield the highest rate of hybrid formation to rate of RNA degradation. A temperature 15–30°C below the melting temperature (T_m) is usually used. For low molecular weight RNA species (less than 50 nucleotides), lower temperatures must be used. 55°C has often been used. More recently, formamide and other organic solvents have been used to reduce the T_m and permit hybridization at reasonable rates at low temperatures [4,39,40].

The rate of the overall hybridization reaction follows second-order kinetics, and varies inversely with the square root of the polynucleotide strand lengths [1, 5]. Thus, high concentrations and low molecular weights promote the reaction. In RNA–DNA hybridization, to decrease DNA–DNA renaturation, the DNA strands are usually relatively high molecular weight, whereas the RNA is sheared to low molecular weight.

Choice of formation of the hybrid on a filter or in solution depends on the experiment. At high RNA:DNA ratios, where a small fraction of the RNA will hybridize with the DNA, "sticking" of RNA to a blank filter is less of a problem when hybrid formation is permitted in solution. On the other hand, at low RNA:DNA ratios, DNA–DNA reannealing is less of a problem when hybrids are formed directly on the filter. Note that these ratios refer to the concentrations of nucleic acid species of interest. For example, in pulse-labeled RNA preparations from E. coli, the label appears mainly in a large number of mRNA species, and the concentration of each of these species is consequently a small percentage of the total RNA concentration.

To assay hybrid formation, CsCl density gradients are costly in time and equipment. Again, filter methods are rapid and inexpensive. However, the RNA–DNA hybrids cannot be separated from the remaining single-stranded DNA, and recovery of the RNA or RNA–DNA hybrid from the filter is difficult. Chromatography on HA columns separates single-stranded nucleic acids from bihelical species, and can be used over a wide range of temperatures and in the presence of many organic solvents [41,29–31]. Further, preparative amounts of nucleic acids may be obtained from such columns [8,42]. For these reasons, HA columns are often used in hybridization studies.

B. Hybridization in Solution

Labeled RNA and DNA are mixed in a convenient volume of 2 × SSC and incubated at the appropriate annealing temperature for the desired period of time. The temperature will vary between 23 and 67°C, as dictated by the absence or presence of formamide, and the RNA species under study. The tubes are then chilled, and the hybrids detected by one of the methods outlined in section II-D.

C. Hybridization with Immobilized DNA

1. Membrane Filters. The basic procedure is as follows: denatured DNA is bound to nitrocellulose filters, the RNA is hybridized to the bound DNA, and unpaired RNA and "imperfect" RNA–DNA hybrids, that is, RNA "noise," are removed.

a. Binding of DNA to Filters. Denatured DNA solutions are diluted to 5 ml with 2 × SSC, passed through a 25 mm Schleicher and Schuell B6 or a Millipore HA nitrocellulose filter, and washed with 100 ml of 2 × SSC. Before loading with DNA, the filter is presoaked in 2 × SSC for 1 min and washed with 10 ml of 2 × SSC. The loaded DNA filters are then thoroughly dried at room temperature, for at least 4 hr, and then at 80°C for 2 hr in a vacuum oven. This relatively simple procedure, essentially according to Gillespie and Spiegelman [38], assures immobilization of the DNA to the filter. Initial drying at room temperature helps prevent DNA renaturation. The filtration rate during loading of the DNA should be moderately low, ~ 5 ml/min, particularly with smaller DNA fragments or with synthetic polymers.

In some cases the above procedure is modified. Poly(dA) does not stick effectively to the filters and is loaded slowly in 6 × SSC. The helical secondary structure of poly d(A - T) necessitates loading in 6 × SSC containing 0.01 M KOH. Easily renatured DNA of higher % (G + C) base content may require higher KOH concentrations, although concentrations above 0.1 M should not be used. The filters are washed with 6 × SSC lacking the KOH. Fragmented DNA (as low as 10^4 dalton) can be loaded by increasing the salt concentration during loading, subsequent washing, and during the hybridization itself. 6 × SSC is often used. Also, low filtration rates should be used.

b. Hybridization. Hybrids are formed by immersing the 25 mm DNA filters in vials containing 5 ml of labeled RNA in either 2 × SSC or 6 × SSC as required. Annealing is carried out in water baths at controlled temperatures ranging from 23 to 67°C, in the presence or absence of formamide, as required by the RNA species and experiment. During the hybridization and all subsequent steps, the vials should be maintained in a tilted position to insure that the filters float free in solution. After hybridization, the vials are chilled in an ice bath. The volume of the RNA solution may be reduced by using smaller filters or by rolling up the filters.

c. Elimination of Nonspecific and Incomplete RNA–DNA "Hybrids." The filters are removed from the hybridization solution and each side is washed with 50 ml 2 × SSC by suction filtration. The hybrid present on the filter at this point is termed the "raw hybrid," and consists of an ribonuclease-sensitive part and an ribonuclease-resistant part. This latter part is the "true hybrid," and is purified by immersing the filter for 1 hr at room temperature in 5 ml 2 × SSC containing 20 µg/ml of heat-treated pancreatic ribonuclease; sometimes ribonuclease T1, at 15 units/ml, is also used. Pancreatic ribonuclease is heat-treated by incubation at 100°C for 10 min. After ribonuclease digestion, the vials are chilled, and the filters again washed on each side with 50 ml 2 × SSC. The conditions for pancreatic ribonuclease digestion are rather critical. Higher concentrations and temperatures above 37°C result in degradation of some true RNA–DNA hybrids, whereas milder conditions result in incomplete degradation of the nonspecific hybrids.

2. Other Methods for Immobilization of the DNA. Since the development of the agar column methods [34,35], the nitrocellulose columns and columns involving photochemical binding of DNA using UV radiation have not been used extensively. A brief discussion of such columns is presented by Gillespie [13].

For the DNA agar columns, high molecular weight single-stranded DNA is dispersed in 4% agarose and the resulting gel cut up into fragments. These fragments are extensively washed to remove nonimmobilized DNA. For DNA–DNA experiments, low molecular weight DNA is added to the DNA–agar fragments, followed by hybridization, washing, and assay. For RNA–DNA experiments, radioactive RNA in the absence or presence of varying amounts of nonradioactive RNA in competition experiments is incubated with the DNA–agar fragments under hybridization conditions, washed, and assayed.

Hybridized DNA or RNA can be recovered via transfer of the reaction mixture to a chromatography tube, with subsequent elution of the hybridized species with appropriate salt and/or temperature gradients. Fractionation according to %

(G + C) base content is possible using such methods [43].

Details of the DNA–agar method are discussed by Bendich and Bolton [44].

D. Detection of Hybrids

1. Membrane Filters. For experiments in which the DNA is initially immobilized on the filter, the hybridized RNA is detected simply by drying the filter containing the true hybrid, adding it to a scintillation vial containing an appropriate scintillation fluid, and counting the radioactivity in a liquid scintillation counter.

For hybridization performed in solution, the hybridization mixture is slowly passed through a nitrocellulose membrane filter by suction filtration. Denatured DNA and the RNA–DNA hybrids are retained by the filter; free RNA and renatured DNA duplexes pass through the filter. The filter is then washed with 100 ml 2 × SSC (or 6 × SSC). The retained raw hybrids are then converted into true hybrids by incubation of the wet filter in 5 ml 2 × SSC containing 20 μg/ml heat-treated pancreatic ribonuclease at room temperature with occasional shaking for 1 hr. The filters are removed from the vials, washed with 50 ml 2 × SSC on each side, dried, and placed in a scintillation counter.

2. Equilibrium Sedimentation in CsCl Density Gradients. Hybridization is done in solution, and the reaction is terminated by chilling to at least room temperature. CsCl and solvent are added, and the resulting solution centrifuged to equilibrium in an ultracentrifuge. As a typical example, 8.0 g CsCl is mixed with 5.5 ml 2 × SSC, and this solution is then mixed with a 0.5 ml hybridization reaction mixture. The resulting solution (about 8 ml) is added to a Spinco Ti 50 cellulose nitrate centrifuge tube. This centrifuge tube should be pretreated to prevent adsorption of RNA–DNA hybrid molecules to the tube sides, for example, by soaking the tube with a 100 μg/ml denatured herring sperm DNA solution. Mineral oil is layered over the sample to fill the tube, the tube is capped, and the solution centrifuged for 36 hr at 40,000 rpm in the Ti 50 rotor of a Spinco L3-50 ultracentrifuge at 20°C. After centrifugation, drops are collected from a hole punctured in the bottom of the tube, yielding about 25 fractions of 0.3 ml each. Aliquots from each fraction are assayed for radioactivity. Fractions containing the presumed hybrid are pooled, dialyzed extensively against 2 × SSC, treated with 20 μg/ml ribonuclease for 1 hr at room temperature to yield the true hybrid and then analyzed further as desired.

3. Chromatography on MAK Columns. RNA–DNA hybrids bind more tightly to a methylated albumin-kieselguhr (MAK) column than do oligoribonucleotides, permitting separation of the hybridized RNA from ribonuclease-digested free RNA [28]. Following hybridization, the reaction mixture is chilled to room temperature, and the raw hybrid is converted into true hybrid via treatment with heat-treated pancreatic ribonuclease at 20 μg/ml for 1 hr at room temperature. The ribonuclease-treated reaction mixture is diluted 10-fold into 0.5 M NaCl, 0.05 M NaPO$_4$, pH 6.8, containing 1% (w/v) kieselguhr. The mixture is then applied to a three-layer MAK column [45] of appropriate size, and the nucleic acids are eluted via a linear gradient of NaCl ranging from 0.5 M to about 1.2 M. Generally two peaks emerge, at about 0.6 M NaCl and at about 0.9 M NaCl. The first peak contains only RNA, and represents an ribonuclease-resistant RNA "core." The second, high salt peak contains the hybridized RNA and DNA.

4. Hydroxyapatite Column Chromatography At low concentrations of a phosphate buffer (0.035 M at 60°C), both DNA and RNA adsorb to HA. At higher concentrations (0.12 M), RNA and all double-stranded nucleic acid species adsorb to HA, whereas single-stranded DNA is eluted. At still higher buffer concentrations (0.4 M at 60°C), all nucleic species are eluted [8,29-31]. As developed by Kohne [42], HA column chromatography is used to detect and isolate RNA–DNA hybrids by assaying radioactive DNA bound to the column when eluted with 0.12 M phosphate buffer. The RNA bound to the DNA may also be detected using prior treatment with pancreatic ribonuclease to remove the free RNA [46,47].

Hydroxyapatite is obtained from Bio-Rad, Richmond, Ca., the Clarkson Chemical Co., Williamsport, Pa., or prepared in the laboratory [31] and used with water-jacketed columns able to permit temperatures of 100°C. Phosphate buffer at pH 6.8 is prepared at appropriate concentrations by mixing equimolar amounts of Na$_2$HPO$_4$ and NaH$_2$PO$_4$. Columns of the appropriate size are prepared and equilibrated at 60°C with 0.12 M phosphate buffer.

Hybridization is done in solution using appropriate RNA and DNA concentrations and time of hybridization to minimize DNA reannealing. The true RNA–DNA hybrid is prepared by treating the reaction mixture with 20 μg/ml heat-treated pancreatic ribonuclease for 1 hr at room temperature. The reaction mixture is then passed through an HA column. Extensive washing with 0.12 M phosphate buffer removes single-stranded DNA and the ribonuclease digestion products. The adsorbed RNA–DNA hybrid can then be eluted by washing with 0.4 M phosphate buffer. Alternatively, the DNA from the RNA–DNA hybrid can be eluted thermally by raising the temperature to 100°C and eluting with 0.12 M phosphate buffer.

III. DNA—DNA Hybridization

A. Introduction

The criteria and conditions necessary for DNA—DNA duplex formation, and the techniques used to effect and assay formation of these hybrids, are similar to those discussed above for RNA—DNA hybrid formation. With DNA—agar columns, DNA instead of RNA is loaded onto the column, and the DNA bound to the column is assayed. The filter methods used for RNA—DNA studies have been successfully modified to permit DNA—DNA hybridization studies, and are discussed here.

DNA—DNA reassociation, as with RNA—DNA hybrid formation, proceeds via second order kinetics, that is, the rate of reassociation is proportional to the concentrations of each of the reacting single-stranded DNA species. Solution of the rate equations shows that the important parameter in reassociation is $C_0 t$, where C_0 is the DNA concentration in moles of nucleotides per liter and t is the time of annealing in seconds [8,9]. Extensive studies with DNA from a variety of eucaryotic organisms and tissues have shown that some of such DNA reassociates at low $C_0 t$ values (rapidly reassociating fraction) and some only at very high $C_0 t$ values. In DNA from sources such as calf thymus, $C_0 t$ values of $10^3 - 10^4$ are required before all of the DNA sequences will reanneal. Sequences which anneal only at these high $C_0 t$ values have been shown to be unique DNA sequences. The $C_0 t$ value at which 50% of a given DNA sequence has reannealed (the "half-maximum" $C_0 t$) can be used to determine the length in nucleotide pairs of that DNA sequence. This value, together with the fraction of the total DNA sample composed of this sequence, leads to the degree of reiteration of this sequence in the total genome. For example, in calf thymus DNA, about 40% of the DNA rapidly reassociates with a half-maximum $C_0 t$ of about 0.03, indicating a length of about 300 nucleotide pairs. Since the calf genome contains about 3×10^9 nucleotide pairs, the 300 nucleotide pair segment must be repeated about $10^5 - 10^6$ times in a single cell!

The remaining 60% of the calf genome reassociates with a half-maximum $C_0 t$ of about 3000, indicating about 10^9 nucleotide pairs. Comparison with the genome size indicates that these are probably unique sequences, that is, present only once per cell [8].

Often in gene expression studies, the investigator is concerned only with the unique DNA sequences. Since the DNA from nearly all eucaryotes contains repeated sequences, and since very high $C_0 t$ values are required to observe reassociation of the unique sequences, considerable care is required in the design and execution of hybridization experiments. The methods to be used must be carefully considered. The reassociation conditions employed using the DNA–agar technique yield $C_0 t$ values of between about 1 and 100. For higher organisms, primarily only repeated sequences will have reannealed. Using DNA immobilized on filters, the rate of the reaction proceeds very slowly compared to the reaction in solution [48]. Thus, reassociation curves obtained from filter experiments yield higher apparent $C_0 t$ values for the same extent of reassociation. The method favored by most investigators involves reassociation in solution, with analysis of the reaction using the HA columns. The HA columns are stable over a wide range of temperatures and in the presence of many organic solvents. Different salt and temperature conditions permit binding of single- and double-stranded nucleic acid species, or binding only of double-stranded species. The latter conditions (0.12 M $NaPO_4$, pH 6.8; 60°C) effects quantitative separation of the reannealed DNA (bound to the column) from the single-stranded DNA. The bound DNA can be recovered via high salt elution (0.4 M $NaPO_4$, pH 6.8) or by raising the temperature, denaturing the bound double-stranded species.

Again, a separate HA column is used for each $C_0 t$ value, and these columns are water-jacketed for adequate temperature control. Analysis involves elution of the columns, with subsequent pooling of fractions and assay. Recovery and assay of the hybridized DNA species involves further steps. The filter methods again offer simplicity and ease of assay. For studies with genomes from procaryotic genomes, which contain little or no repeated sequences, but nevertheless anneal at $C_0 t$ values of between about 10^{-2} and 100, or with studies of the repeated sequences from eucaryotic organisms, filter methods are often very useful. The use of HA columns is discussed further in the article by R. Church of this volume.

To use filtration techniques in DNA–DNA hybridization studies, methods had to be found to remove the added single-stranded DNA which had not annealed with the DNA bound to the filter. Two techniques have been used: (1) preincubation of filters loaded with DNA in a solution which prevents binding of subsequently added single-stranded DNA to the filter [49], and (2) removal of single-stranded DNA by washing the filters containing the DNA–DNA hybrids with a buffer of low ionic strength and high pH [50].

B. Hybridization in Solution

The DNA is rendered as low in molecular weight as possible. Sonication or the use of a French Pressure Cell at $10-15 \times 10^3$ psi, followed by heat or alkali denaturation, yields single-stranded DNA fragments of about 500–2000 nucleotides in length. Pressures as high as about 50×10^3 psi have been used, to yield a relatively homogeneous population of fragments about 400–500 nucleotides in length; this pressure also denatures the DNA [8]. Hybridization is carried out in 0.12 M $NaPO_4$, pH 6.8, at 60°C for the desired period of time, at the desired concentration of DNA. For example, incubation for 1 hr at a concentration of 83 µg/ml (OD_{260} = 2) gives a C_0t value of 1. Thus, to obtain a C_0t of 10^4 with a DNA concentration of 8.3 µg/ml, incubation must proceed for 100 hr. Because of the long incubation times, samples are conveniently sealed in glass tubes prior to incubation. After hybridization, the tubes are chilled, the top of the tube is broken off, and the contents are analyzed on an HA column, for absorbance at 260 nm, and so on. If formamide is used in the hybridization mixture, the formamide concentration must be reduced to below 1% before application of the mixture to the HA column. Hybridization should also be carried out in the absence of sodium citrate to avoid incomplete separation of the nucleic acid species on the HA column.

C. Hybridization with Immobilized DNA.

1. Hybridization with Preincubation. The procedure is similar to that for RNA-DNA hybridization. Denatured high molecular weight DNA is bound to filters; the DNA filters are preincubated in a solution which prevents subsequent binding of denatured, or single-stranded, DNA; denatured, low molecular weight DNA is annealed to the bound DNA; and nonhybridized DNA is removed by washing.
a. Binding of Denatured DNA to Filters. DNA is denatured by heating to 100°C for 5 min in 6 × SSC and rapidly cooled in an ice bath. The DNA solution is passed through a filter prewashed with 6 × SSC. Suitable filters are Schleicher and Schuell B6 or Millipore HAWP nitrocellulose filters. The loaded DNA filters are washed with 5 ml 6 × SSC, dried thoroughly at room temperature, preferably overnight, and finally dried in a vacuum oven at 80°C and 29 in. Hg pressure for 2 hr. Usually, about 95% of the DNA is retained by the filter, and less than 1% is subsequently lost during 24 hr incubation at 65°C.
b. Preincubation of the DNA Filters. The filters are covered with 2 ml preincubation medium (PM), and incubated for at least 3 hr and preferably for 6 hr at 65°C. The PM contains 0.02% Ficoll (Pharmacia, average molecular weight 400,000), 0.02% polyvinylpyrrolidone (Sigma, average molecular weight 360,000), and 0.02% bovine serum albumin (Armour, fraction V), in 3 × SSC. After such treatment, less than 1% single-stranded DNA will stick to blank filters, while more than 50% will hybridize to appropriately loaded DNA filters.
c. Hybridization. Hybrids are formed by adding denatured DNA directly to

the vials containing the DNA filters in PM. Annealing results from incubation at 65°C for at least 12 hr. Denhardt [49] finds that there is a slow increase in the amount of radioactivity binding to both DNA filters and to blank filters if the incubation time exceeds 12 hr. However, other workers have used up to 25 hr incubation time.

Formamide and other organic solvents may be used to lower the temperature of incubation. In addition to increased retention of DNA bound to the filters and decreased degradation and depurination of the DNA species [40,51], formamide appears to promote higher reaction rates and greater specificity of hybridization, as well as to prevent microbial growth during incubation at reduced temperature [39]. These advantages are particularly important in studies with eucaryotic DNA species, because of the presence of nearly identical repeated sequences and the long incubation times required. The precise reaction conditions should be determined for each experiment. A concentration of formamide should be chosen to yield a T_m about 25°C above the desired incubation temperature. The T_m of native DNA or filter-bound duplexes is reduced about 0.72°C per 1% formamide added [39]. For DNA species of base content % (G + C) = 40%, incubation at 37°C in 5 × SSC containing 50% formamide closely mimics incubation in 1 × SSC at 60°C with no formamide [39], with the advantage of an increase of about 3-fold in reaction rate.

2. Hybridization with Low Ionic Strength, High pH Wash. The procedure is similar to that given above. A nitrocellulose filter is loaded with denatured DNA according to the procedure above (section III-C-1a). There is no preincubation of the loaded filters. Sonicated and denatured DNA is annealed to the DNA filters by incubating the DNA filters at 60°C with this DNA in 3.2 ml 1.25 × SSC, pH 7.0 buffered with 0.01 M Tris Cl. Incubation is permitted for at least 12 hr, and sometimes for as long as 50 hr. The filters are removed from the vials and briefly rinsed in 0.003 M Tris Cl, pH 9.4, and the nonhybridized DNA is removed by washing the filters by suction on each side with 100 ml 0.03 M Tris Cl, pH 9.4. After such a wash, the noise level of nonspecifically bound DNA could be reduced to less than 0.1% of the total sonicated, denatured DNA added to the annealing mix, while more than 40% will anneal to appropriately loaded DNA filters after long incubation times [50].

D. Detection of Hybrids

1. Membrane Filters. Using preincubated DNA-loaded filters, the filter is removed from the hybridization mixture after an appropriate period of time, and each side of the filter is washed with 40 ml SSC. The filters are dried, and the radioactivity is determined using a liquid scintillation counter. When filters are used with no preincubation, the filters are washed after hybridization with 40 ml 0.003 M Tris Cl, pH 9.4, on each side, dried, and counted in a liquid scintillation counter.

2. **Hydroxyapatite Column Chromatography.** The following procedure is that of Kohne and Britten [8,52]. Sheared, denatured DNA is reannealed in solution at 60°C for varying periods of time. A sample at each specified time is passed over a water-jacketed HA column previously equilibrated with 0.12 M NaPO$_4$, pH 6.8, at 60°C. The "useful capacity" of the HA is about 200 μg double-stranded DNA/ml of wet-packed HA. The "useful capacity" is defined to be the maximum amount of double-stranded DNA which can be adsorbed by a given amount of HA. Single-stranded DNA is washed from the column using 0.12 M NaPO$_4$, pH 6.8, and assayed for radioactivity. Following elution of all single-stranded DNA, the double-stranded DNA can be eluted by washing the column with high salt (0.4 M NaPO$_4$, pH 6.8). Alternatively, the temperature of the column can be raised to 100°C, denaturing the reassociated DNA. The denatured DNA can then be eluted by further washing with 0.12 M NaPO$_4$, pH 6.8.

The precision of nucleotide pairing in the adsorbed, reassociated DNA can be characterized by doing a thermal stability profile study. The temperature of the column is raised in discrete steps, and the DNA rendered single-stranded is removed by washing with 0.12 M NaPO$_4$, pH 6.8, at each step. The thermal profile so obtained is compared with the thermal denaturation profile (melting curve) of the initial double-stranded DNA species.

Some batches of HA will bind greater than 2% single-stranded DNA under the above conditions. New batches should be checked before use with a small quantity of freshly denatured bacterial DNA. Addition of 0.4% SDS to the hybridization mixture and to the washing buffers usually reduces the binding of single-stranded DNA to less than 1%. The presence of the SDS has no observable effect on the thermal stability or renaturation kinetics of the DNA [52].

IV. DETAILED PROTOCOL FOR A TYPICAL HYBRIDIZATION EXPERIMENT USING FILTERS

The following hybridization experiment will center on bacteriophage lambda DNA and RNA. Hybridization techniques have been used to answer questions concerned with the time of transcription of different genes, with which of the two DNA strands is transcribed, and with the direction of transcription of these genes [14]. DNA–DNA hybridization has been used primarily to

NUCLEIC ACID HYBRIDIZATION/FILTER TECHNIQUES

answer questions concerned with what percentage of a given DNA population is λ DNA [15].

In the experiments below, we will ask the following question: What fraction of the RNA and DNA synthesized at different times after infection of E. coli with phage λ consists of λ specific RNA and DNA, that is, hybridizes with λ DNA? To answer this question, RNA and DNA, pulse-labeled with ^{3}H-uridine and ^{3}H-thymidine for 2 min at times 0–2 min, 10–12 min, 20–22 min, and 30–32 min after infection, is first isolated and characterized. To characterize these species, absorption at 260 nm and assay of incorporated radioactivity using a liquid scintillation counter are used to determine the nucleic acid concentration and the specific activity in units of counts per minute per microgram of nucleic acid. Control RNA and DNA from pulse-labeled uninfected E. coli cells, as well as uniformly labeled ^{3}H-E. coli DNA and ^{3}H-λ DNA, are also isolated and characterized. These species are to be hybridized against ^{14}C-λ DNA, ^{14}C-E. coli DNA, and nonradioactive (cold) salmon sperm DNA; these DNA species are also prepared, or bought, and characterized.

A. RNA–DNA Hybridization Experiments

These experiments are to be done both by annealing in solution (see section II-B) and by annealing to DNA immobilized on the filter (see section II-C), with detection via filters (see section II-D-1).

1. Hybridization with DNA in Solution. Five concentrations of ^{14}C-λ DNA, three of ^{14}C-E. coli DNA, and one of nonradioactive salmon sperm DNA are incubated with ^{3}H-pulse-labeled RNA in 6 × SSC in screw-capped vials at 65°C for varying times. The data obtained will provide kinetics of annealing curves. At the given times, 0.5 ml aliquots are diluted into 5 ml cold 2 × SSC; the solutions are collected onto 25 mm Schleicher and Schuell B6 filters; and the filters are washed, treated with ribonuclease, dried, and counted. Details are provided on the flow sheet, Table I.

Percent of RNA hybridized for each time point is calculated by converting ^{3}H and ^{14}C counts present on the filter to micrograms of RNA and micrograms of DNA, via the specific activities. Correction should be made for any loss of DNA from the filter during hybridization, as seen by loss of ^{14}C. A plot of percent of RNA hybridized versus time of incubation provides kinetic curves. The percent of the pulse-labeled RNA hybridizable to λ DNA and the percent hybridizable to E. coli DNA is determined from the saturation levels, that is, maximum amount RNA hybridized, obtained from the kinetic curves

TABLE I. DNA–RNA Hybridization in Solution, Flow Sheet

Amount per time point

Substance		$\dfrac{\lambda}{1.0}$ 2 µg	3	8	$\dfrac{E.\ coli}{1}$ 2 µg	3	Salmon sperm 3 µg
^{14}C-DNA	0	0.4			0.4		
^{3}H-RNA							
6 point kinetics[a]		$\dfrac{\lambda\ DNA}{6}$			$\dfrac{E.\ coli\ DNA}{6}$		$\dfrac{\text{Salmon}}{\text{sperm DNA}}$
^{14}C-DNA	0	2.4	18	48	2.4	18	18 µg
^{3}H-RNA	12	12	12	12	12	12	12 µg
100 µg/ml DNA	0	—	0.18	0.48	—	0.18	0.18 ml
10 µg/ml DNA	—	0.24	—	—	0.24	—	—
10 µg/ml RNA	1.2	1.20	1.20	1.20	1.20	1.20	1.20 ml
6 × SSC	2.0	1.76	1.82	1.52	1.76	1.82	1.82 ml
	3.2	3.20	3.20	3.20	3.20	3.20	3.20 ml

Timetable

Type ^{14}C-DNA	Amount per time point DNA, µg	RNA, µg	DNA:RNA ratio	Times of annealing, hr
λ	8	2	4:1	0,1,2,4,8,15
	3	2	3:2	0,1,2,4,8,15
	1	2	1:2	0,1,2,4,8,15
	0.4	2	1:5	0,1,2,4,8,15
	0	2	0	0,1,4,8,15
E. coli	3	2	3:2	0,1,2,4,8,15
	1	2	1:2	0,1,2,4,8,15
	0.4	2	1:5	0,1,2,4,8,15
Salmon sperm	3	2	3:2	0,1,4,8,15

[a]Six times above amounts needed per annealing vial.

Protocol

Make up the annealing solutions given above, omitting the addition of the pulse-labeled ^{3}H-RNA (10 μg/ml preparation), until you are ready to initiate the experiment. Have 50 test tubes with 5 ml chilled 2 $\times$ SSC ready. Also, you will need 50 scintillation vials with 2.5 ml of 20 μg/ml heat-treated ribonuclease in 2 $\times$ SSC. Now add the ^{3}H-RNA.

Withdraw an 0.5 ml aliquot from each annealing vial. Dilute the 0.5 ml aliquots into separate tubes of the cold 2 $\times$ SSC you have ready. These are the 0 time points. Withdraw a second 0.5 ml aliquot from each annealing vial, place in a clean tube, and keep at 0°C. These will be for the 15 hr time points and should be placed at 65°C late in the day, to anneal at 65°C overnight. Place the annealing vials at 65°C. This is 0 time.

0 hr
1↓0 hr   Draw 9 0.5 ml aliquots; dilute each into 5 ml cold 2 $\times$ SSC.
2.0 hr   Draw seven samples; dilute each into 5 ml cold 2 $\times$ SSC. You should now be thinking about loading your collected samples onto 25 mm B6 filters. Do this slowly, as described. After you have loaded and washed the filters place them into the vials with the ribonuclease. Keep track of the time; they incubate for 1 hr at room temperature.
↓
4.0 hr   Draw nine aliquots, etc. Keep the filters flowing through the preparative procedure.

No more points for 4 hr. This is plenty of time to finish loading the collected samples, wash them with 6 $\times$ SSC, incubate with ribonuclease and wash them again, dry them under heat lamps, and load into scintillation vials containing 5 ml PPO–toluene for counting.
↓
8.0 hr   Last time point for today; draw nine aliquots into 5 ml chilled 2 $\times$ SSC, load, wash, ribonuclease, treat, wash, dry, and count.

Begin incubation of 15 hr aliquots overnight at 65°C.

Wash Procedure

After aliquots are diluted into 5 ml cold 2 $\times$ SSC, collect via slow filtration (5 ml/min or less) onto B6 filters, wash with 5 ml 6 $\times$ SSC, then with 5 ml 2 $\times$ SSC.

Incubate filter in scintillation vial containing 2.5 ml 2 $\times$ SSC and 20 μg/ml heat-treated ribonuclease for 60 min at room temperature.

Wash filter by immersing and stirring in beaker of 2 $\times$ SSC (100 ml or more). Dry under heat lamps; load into scintillation vials; count.

for each DNA:RNA ratio. A detailed protocol for such data reduction is given in Table II.

TABLE II. Detailed Analysis of the Data

Step 1. Subtract background from the raw counts per minute. Background is determined for your counter by counting a blank vial containing the PPO−toluene scintillation mixture and a loaded filter containing no DNA.

Step 2. Correct ^{3}H values for ^{14}C overlap, or "crosstalk." The overlap is determined for your counter from a sample which contains only ^{14}C, and will be about 15−20%. ^{3}H overlap into the ^{14}C channel is negligible.

Step 3. Determine the specific activities for the ^{14}C-labeled DNA species in your counter. This is done by counting a known mass, in micrograms, of ^{14}C-DNA in your counter.

Step 4. Normalize the ^{3}H values to the correct ^{14}C value. For example, for a minifilter from a filter containing 37.5 μg DNA of a ^{14}C specific activity of 250 cpm/μg, normalize to 3.0 μg or 750 cpm. This corrects for any loss of ^{14}C during the hybridization.

Step 5. For each RNA/DNA ratio, determine the ^{3}H values per microgram of DNA. Convert these ^{3}H values to microgram of RNA, using the specific activity of the ^{3}H-RNA, again determined in your counter.

Step 6. Plot μg RNA annealed per 100 μg DNA against time of annealing for each RNA:DNA ratio, and for the liquid and filter experiments. These are the kinetic curves.

Step 7. Assuming equal efficiency for annealing of λ RNA to λ DNA and for E. coli RNA to E. coli DNA, calculate the relative amounts of RNA annealed to lambda and to E. coli DNA. Do this from the saturation levels of the kinetic curves.

Data from a similar experiment using bacteriophage T7 is shown in Tables III and IV, and in Figure 1. RNA pulse-labeled with ^{3}H-uridine for 2 min was isolated from noninfected E. coli cells, and from E. coli cells infected with phage T7 and pulse-labeled 2−4 min, and 20−22 min, after infection. Table III illustrates data reduction for the case of hybridization of RNA from cells pulse-labeled 20−22 min after T7 infection against T7 DNA in solution, at a ratio of RNA:DNA of 2:3. The specific activity of the ^{3}H-RNA was 2.8×10^4 cpm/μg RNA, and that of the ^{14}C-DNA was 200 cpm/μg DNA, with a background of 13 cpm for both isotopes. Overlap of ^{14}C into the ^{3}H channel was 14%. Kinetic curves for several such hybridization experiments are shown in Figure 1.

In Table IV, the data from Figure 1 is used to calculate the percent E. coli RNA and percent T7 RNA found in the 2−4 min RNA, assuming that all RNA synthesized late during T7 infection is T7 specific RNA. Figure 1C shows

TABLE III. Example of Data Reduction

Experiment: RNA–DNA hybridization in solution at RNA:DNA ratio of 2:3. The RNA was isolated from E. coli cells pulse-labeled with ^{3}H-uridine from 20 to 22 min following infection with phage T7. The T7 DNA was isolated from purified T7 phage labeled with ^{14}C-thymidine during phage development.

Time, hr	^{14}C cpm on filter	^{3}H cpm on filter	^{14}C µg on filter	^{3}H µg on filter	^{3}H µg/ 100 µg DNA	^{14}C-DNA recovered, %
0	289	44	1.45	0.0016	0.108	48.2
1	230	2727	1.15	0.0974	8.47	38.3
2	480	7373	2.40	0.2633	11.0	80.0
4	339	7549	1.69	0.2696	15.9	56.5
12	286	4441	1.43	0.1586	11.1	47.7

Unpublished results of R. Tait and D. Smith [54].

TABLE IV. Calculation of Percent E. coli and T7 RNA Found in 2–4 Min Pulse-Labeled RNA

RNA type	RNA input, µg		RNA bound to DNA, µg		Fraction RNA bound to DNA	
	E. coli	T7	E. coli	T7	E. coli	T7
E. coli RNA	67	0	0.704	0.202	0.0105	0.00302
2–4 min RNA	x	y	0.620	2.72	–	–
20–22 min RNA	0	67	0.295	15.9	0.00441	0.237

Solving for x and y:
0.0105x + 0.00441y = 0.620
0.00302x + 0.237y = 2.72

	Amount	Percentage
	x = 55.6 µg	83.3
	y = 11.1 µg	16.7
	66.7 µg	100.0

Unpublished results of R. Tait and D. Smith [54].

that this is a reasonable approximation. A further assumption that is implicitly made is that E. coli and T7 RNA synthesized during the 2–4 min pulse hybridizes with the same efficiency as pulse-labeled E. coli RNA and pulse-labeled (20–22 min) T7 RNA. Since different RNA species may be present at different concentrations in each of these preparations [4], this assumption may not be strictly true. Values from the 4 hr time points are used, assumed to represent saturation values. Because of DNA:DNA reassociation in solution hybridization experiments, these values often decrease at later times. The calculations use values normalized to 100 µg DNA (Table III); the normalized amount of RNA is thus 66.7 µg for the ratio RNA:DNA = 2:3. This rather

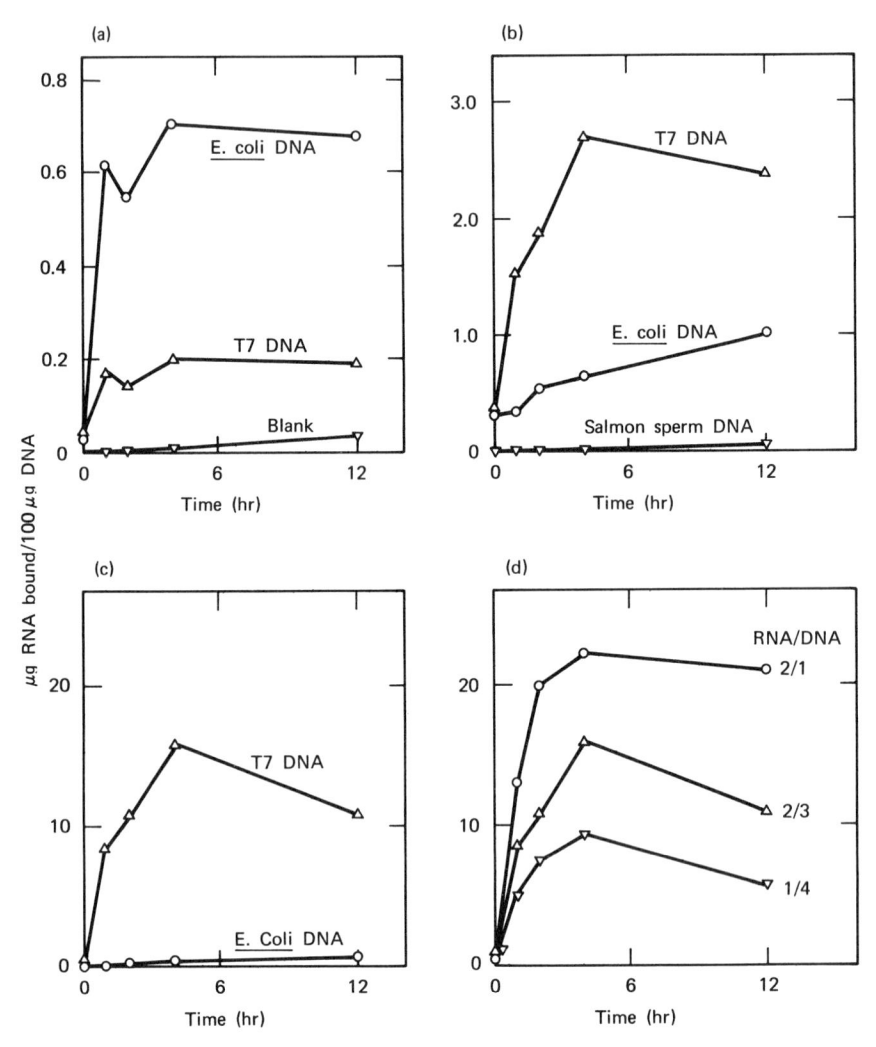

FIGURE 1. RNA–DNA hybridization in solution; kinetic curves. The experiment and procedure is given in the text. Specific activities: E. coli DNA: 200 cpm/μg; T7 DNA: 200 cpm/μg; E. coli RNA: 1.3×10^4 cpm/μg; 2–4 min RNA: 1.04×10^4 cpm/μg; and 20–22 min RNA: 2.8×10^4 cpm/μg. In each experiment, 12 μg RNA was hybridized against a DNA concentration to give the RNA:DNA ratios indicated. (a) E. coli RNA hybridized to E. coli and T7 DNA and to a blank filter (RNA:DNA = 2:3) (b) 2–4 min RNA hybridized to E. coli, T7, and salmon sperm DNA (RNA:DNA = 2:3) (c) 20–22 min RNA hybridized to E. coli and T7 DNA (RNA:DNA = 2:3) (d) 20–22 min RNA hybridized to varying amounts of T7 DNA, yielding the RNA/DNA ratios indicated. The values given are μg RNA hybridized per 100 μg DNA (see Table I). Unpublished results of R. Tait and D. Smith [54].

incomplete data shows that the 2–4 min pulse-labeled RNA contains about 16% T7 RNA and about 84% E. coli RNA.

2. Hybridization with Immobilized DNA. The same relative amounts of ^{14}C-λ DNA, ^{14}C-E. coli DNA, and salmon sperm DNA will be used as with the above experiments. As described in section II-C, 25 mm Schleicher and Schuell B6 filters are loaded with DNA. Hybridization and ribonuclease treatment are done in miniature as follows: "Minifilters" are punched out of the 25 mm loaded DNA filters using a hand paper punch. These minifilters are marked very gently with forceps or a soft pencil for later identification. Figure 2 illustrates the technique and provides a typical distribution of radioactivity among the minifilters. Hybridization takes place in small capped vials containing 0.2 ml 2 × SSC and the appropriate amount of ^{3}H-RNA, at 65°C, for the indicated times.

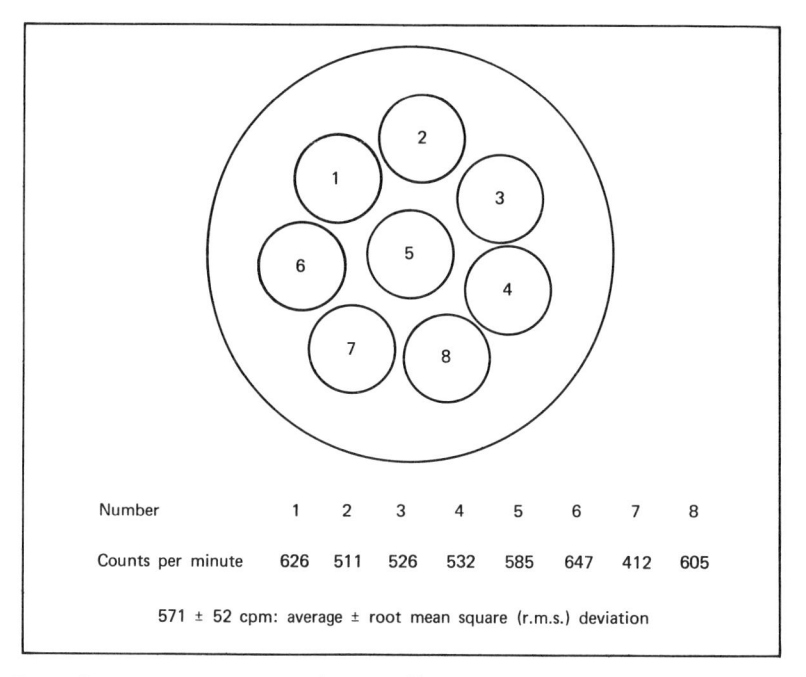

Number	1	2	3	4	5	6	7	8
Counts per minute	626	511	526	532	585	647	412	605

571 ± 52 cpm: average ± root mean square (r.m.s.) deviation

FIGURE 2. 0.25 ml of a 100 μg/ml stock ^{14}C-E. coli DNA solution, at 250 cpm/μg, was added to 5 ml 2 × SSC. A Schleicher and Schuell B6 filter was soaked for 1 min in 2 × SSC, mounted onto a filtration apparatus, and washed with 5 ml 2 × SSC. The DNA solution was applied at a flow rate of about 10 ml/min. The filter was washed with 100 ml 2 × SSC, dried overnight at room temperature, and then dried at 80°C and 29 mm Hg for 2 hr. Minifilters were punched according to the figure above, and ^{14}C counts assayed.

TABLE V. RNA—DNA Hybridization on Filters, Flow Sheets

Substance	Amounts
^{14}C-DNA	0, 5.0, 12.5, 37.5, 100 µg/filter (25 mm diam)
	0, 0.4, 1.0, 3.0, 8 µg/punched minifilter
^{14}C-E. coli DNA	0, 92, 250, 750, 2000 cpm/minifilter
	(specific activity: 250 cpm/µg)
^{14}C-λ DNA	0, 85, 213, 640, 1700 cpm/minifilter
	(specific activity: 213 cpm/µg)
^{3}H-RNA	2.0 µg/point (per minifilter)
DNA:RNA ratio	0, 1/5, 1/2, 3/2, 4/1

Timetable

Type ^{14}C-DNA	DNA, µg	DNA:RNA ratio	Times, hr
λ	8	4:1	0, 1, 2, 4, 8, 15, 24
	3	3:2	0, 1, 2, 4, 8, 15, 24
	1	1:2	0, 1, 2, 4, 8, 15, 24
	0.4	1:5	0, 1, 2, 4, 8, 15, 24
	0	0	0, 1, 4, 8, 24
E. coli	3	3:2	0, 1, 2, 4, 8, 15, 24
	1	1:2	0, 1, 2, 4, 8, 15, 24
	0.4	1:5	0, 1, 2, 4, 8, 15; 24
salmon sperm (nonradioactive)	3	3:2	0, 1, 4, 8, 15, 24

The minifilter is chilled, removed from the annealing mix, and washed by immersing and thoroughly shaking in 100 ml 2 × SSC. Such a filter contains the raw hybrid, and can be counted if desired. The true hybrid is purified by incubating the minifilter in 0.2 ml 2 × SSC containing 20 µg/ml heat-treated ribonuclease at room temperature for 60 min. If the true hybrid is to be purified on a minifilter which has been counted, the minifilter is removed from the PPO—toluene scintillation mix, washed again in 100 ml 2 × SSC, then incubated with ribonuclease as above. The minifilters are again washed by immersing and shaking in 100 ml 2 × SSC, followed by drying and counting. Data reduction is as described for hybridization in solution. Kinetic curves for these two hybridization methods may be compared. Details are provided in the flow sheets,

TABLE V. (Continued)

	Protocol
In brief:	anneal in scintillation vials, punch minifilters at times shown, wash, ribonuclease treat, wash, dry, count.
In detail:	Obtain one of each of the nine types of filters to be used (five types of λ, different in concentrations; three of coli; one of salmon sperm). Punch one minifilter from each of these nine, dry, count. This is 0 hr sample. Punch a second minifilter from each of these nine filters, place in a small capped vial, and save for later. These will be used for the 15 hr incubation time, done overnight.
0 hr	Place each type of filter in a separate scintillation vial and add 2.5 ml 10 μg/ml ^{3}H-RNA prep. Put the filled vials in the 65°C bath at 1–3 min intervals. Note the time you placed the first vial in the bath ; this is 0 time. Prepare shell vials containing 0.2 ml 20 μg/ml heat-treated ribonuclease in 2 × SSC. Keep them in a rack and note which filters will incubate in which vials. You will need 51 for this experiment.
↓	
1 hr	Nine samples; punch minifilters from the appropriate filters; remove them in the order they were put into the bath, to keep incubation times uniform. Wash the minifilters by immersing and shaking in 100 ml 2 × SSC, and placed in shell vial containing the ribonuclease solution. Incubate for 60 min at room temperature, wash again in 100 ml 2 × SSC, dry, and count.
↓	
2 hr	Seven samples; punch minis, etc., as above.
↓	Remove 1 hr samples from ribonuclease; wash, dry, count.
3 hr	Remove 2 hr samples from ribonuclease, wash, dry, count.
4 hr	Nine samples.
5 hr	Remove 4 hr samples from ribonuclease, etc. No more samples for 3 hr. This gives you time to get some of your filters into the scintillation counters.
↓	
8 hr	Nine samples; last batch for day 1. Add 0.2 ml ^{3}H-RNA solution to the small capped vials containing the minifilters for the 15 hr time point. Incubate for 15 hr overnight at 65°C.
↓	
24 hr 15 hr	Day 2, AM. Eighteen samples; treat as above.

Table V. Figure 3 compares RNA–DNA hybridization in solution with that on filters, using labeled stable E. coli RNA and E. coli DNA.

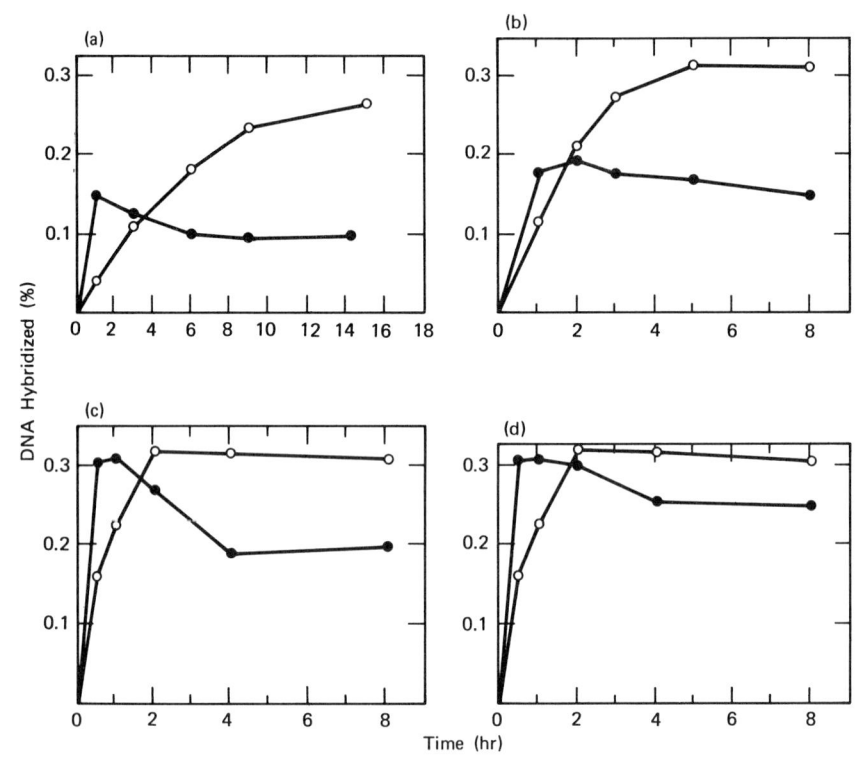

FIGURE 3. For the liquid experiments, reaction mixtures containing the amounts indicated of DNA and RNA were prepared in 1.5 ml 6 × SSC. The mixtures were held at 66°C, after which the hybrids were purified on filters as described in section II-D. Specific activities: DNA = 5000 cpm/µg; RNA = 100,000 cpm/µg. For the immobilized DNA experiments, DNA filters containing the indicated amounts of DNA were prepared using 6 × SSC and immersed in 5 ml 6 × SSC containing the indicated amount of RNA. Hybridization was carried out at 66°C without shaking. Purification of the hybrids was as described in section II-D. (a) 2 µg RNA and 50 µg DNA, DNA:RNA = 25:1; (b) 10 µg RNA and 50 µg DNA, DNA:RNA = 5:1; (c) 50 µg RNA and 50 µg DNA, DNA:RNA = 1:1; (d) 50 µg RNA and 10 µg DNA, DNA:RNA = 1:5; ○———○, immobilized DNA experiments; ●———●, liquid experiments. Adapted from Gillespie and Spiegelman [38].

B. DNA–DNA Hybridization Experiments

Filtration techniques, involving both preincubation of the loaded filters and no preincubation, are used in these experiments.

1. Hybridization after Preincubation of the DNA Filters.
^{14}C-λ DNA, ^{14}C-E. coli DNA, and salmon sperm DNA are immobilized to Schleicher and Schuell B6

filters as in the above RNA–DNA filter experiments. Three types of DNA are to be annealed to the loaded DNA: ^{3}H pulse-labeled DNA from λ-infected E. coli (mixture of E. coli and λ DNA), ^{3}H-λ DNA, and ^{3}H-E. coli DNA. The amount of DNA used relative to the above ^{14}C-DNA will be approximately 10^{-2}, in micrograms. The DNA filters are incubated in PM for 6 hr at 65°C, and the ^{3}H-DNA is then annealed to these filters for varying periods of time.

The experimental procedure is similar to the minifilter procedure used for the RNA–DNA hybridization done on filters. After the preincubation, minifilters are punched out of the 25 mm filters using paper punches, labeled for later identification, and placed into small capped vials containing 0.2 ml PM and the appropriate amount of ^{3}H-DNA. Following annealing at 65°C for the required time, the vial is chilled, the minifilter removed, washed by immersing and thoroughly shaking in 100 ml 2 × SSC, dried, and counted. Details are provided in the flow sheets, Table VI.

This data will provide kinetic curves for the 3μg minifilters for pulsed, λ, and E. coli DNA. Data from the time points 8 hr and 15 hr will provide saturation curves for pulse-labeled DNA against ^{14}C-E. coli DNA (at time point 8 hr) and against ^{14}C-λ DNA (at time point 15 hr), for ^{3}H-λ DNA against ^{14}C-λ DNA, and for ^{3}H-E. coli DNA against ^{14}C-E. coli DNA (the latter two at both time points). From this data, the relative amounts of λ and E. coli DNA present in the pulse-labeled DNA preparations may be calculated. The data reduction protocol given in Table II may be used. The control annealings of ^{3}H-λ DNA against ^{14}C-λ DNA, and of ^{3}H-E. coli DNA against ^{14}C-E. coli DNA permits calculation of the efficiency of self-annealing under these conditions, in step 7.

Figure 4 illustrates a typical set of kinetic curves for pulse-labeled ^{3}H-DNA hybridized against E. coli DNA in the T7 experiment described above in section IV-A. It can be seen that the 2–4 min DNA is about 75% E. coli DNA and the 20–22 min DNA is about 25% E. coli DNA, even though these data are incomplete.

2. Hybridization without Preincubation of Filters. The same DNA substrates are used, and a similar kinetics and saturation experiment is suggested. Details are provided in the flow sheets, Table VII. Data analysis is the same as for the DNA–DNA hybridization with preincubation.

V. CONCLUSIONS

A. Problems Encountered in Hybridization Experiments

Possible problems encountered in hybridization experiments generally are of three types: (1) failure of the DNA to be quantitatively retained by the filter; (2) high RNA or DNA noise; and (3) failure to include the necessary control experiments.

TABLE VI. DNA–DNA Hybridization with Preincubation, Flow Sheet

Preloaded filters containing the following amounts of ^{14}C-DNA will be used:

^{14}C-DNA	0, 5.0, 12.5, 37.5, 100 µg per filter (25 mm diameter)	
	0, 0.4, 1 3 8 µg per minifilter	
^{14}C-E. coli DNA	0, 100, 250, 750, 2000 cpm per minifilter (250 cpm/µg)	
^{14}C-λ DNA	0, 85, 213, 640, 1700 cpm per minifilter (213 cpm/µg)	

^{14}C-DNA filter type: the type of DNA is found between parentheses and semicolons according to the following notation:
(λ DNA; E. coli DNA; salmon sperm DNA)

The amounts of each DNA type, in µg per minifilter, for each time point are presented as the numbers between the parentheses and semicolons. For example, (3; 3; −) means that a 3 µg λ DNA minifilter, a 3 µg E. coli DNA minifilter, and no salmon sperm minifilter would be used at this time point. (3; 0, 0.4, 1, 3, 8; 3) means that a 3 µg λ minifilter, E. coli minifilters containing 0, 0.4, 1, 3, and 8 µg DNA, and a 3 µg salmon sperm minifilter would all be used at this time point.

Added ^{3}H-DNA type

Time of annealing, hr	2 min pulse	^{3}H-DNA types λ	E. coli
0	(3; 3; −)	(3; 3; −)	(3; 3; −)
2	(3; 3; −)	(3; 3; −)	(3; 3; −)
4	(3; 3; −)	(3; 3; −)	(3; 3; −)
8	(3; 0, 0.4, 1, 3, 8; 3)	(0, 0.4, 1, 3, 8; 3; 3)	(3; 0, 0.4, 1, 3, 8; 3)
15	(0, 0.4, 1, 3, 8; 3; 3)	(0, 0.4, 1, 3, 8; 3; 3)	(3; 0, 0.4, 1, 3, 8; 3)
24	(3; 3; −)	(3; 3; −)	(3; 3; −)

Protocol

In brief:
(1) For detailed kinetics, anneal filters in scintillation vials, punch minifilters at times shown, wash, dry, count.
(2) For saturation curves, minifilters are punched at 0 times, annealed in small capped shell vials for 8 or 15 hr, washed, dried, counted.

In detail:
Day 1 Preincubation:

Detailed kinetics of 37.5 μg filters will be done. Six of these filters, three containing λ DNA and three containing E. coli DNA, are placed in six scintillation vials, together with 2.5 ml pm. Incubate these at 65°C for 6 hr.

0 hr DNA saturation curves will be obtained, for example, at the 8 and 15 hr time points. Filters containing the above concentrations of ^{14}C-DNA are obtained, minifilters are punched, placed in small shell vials, covered with 0.2 ml PM, capped with rubber caps, and incubated at 65°C, for 6 hr.

6 hr Punch 2 minifilters from each of the 6 37.5 μg filters; one of these is the 0 hr minifilter, and can be dried and counted. The other is for the 15 hr kinetics point, and is set aside in a small shell vial until about 6 PM day 2. At this time, 0.2 ml ^{3}H-DNA preparation of the appropriate type is added, the vial is capped, and incubated at 65°C overnight.

Day 2 Place the rest of each of these filters in scintillation vials, and add 2.5 ml ^{3}H-DNA prep. There are three ^{3}H-DNA preparations: pulsed, λ, and E. coli; use one of each with each of these six filters. The vials are incubated at 65°C, for a detailed kinetics experiment. At each time point given above, vials are quickly removed from the bath, the filters removed from the vials, a minifilter is punched without drying the filter, the filter is replaced into the vial, and the vial incubated further at 65°C. You will find that the minifilter will stick to the paper punch; remove it with tweezers. Sometimes the filter also adheres to the punch; carefully remove it with the forceps, so as not to tear the filter.

The punched minifilter is washed by immersing and thoroughly shaking in 100 ml 2 × SSC; separate 125 ml erlenmeyer flasks for each filter type are convenient. If so desired, minifilters can be labeled by gently embossing with the point of a forceps or soft pencil. After washing, minifilters are dried under a heat lamp, added to scintillation vials containing 5 ml PPO–toluene, and counted.

For the DNA saturation curves, the 0.2 ml PM is removed with a pasteur pipet, 0.2 ml ^{3}H-DNA preparation is added to the shell vial, the vials are capped, and incubated at 65°C for 8 or 15 hr. The 8 hr minifilters are incubated from 10 AM to about 6 PM day 2. The 15 hr minifilters are set aside after preincubation until about 6 PM day 2; at this time, the ^{3}H-DNA is added, and incubation at 65°C is begun; incubate overnight. After annealing, minifilters are removed from the shell vials, washed as described above, dried, and counted.

TABLE VI. (Continued)

Flow Diagram

Day 1 Other ^{14}C-DNA conc contractors: 0,0.4,1,8; ss 3
Punch mini's, into vials + 0.2 ml PM.
6 hrs, | 65°C
↓
Day 2 15 hr points set aside. ─────────────┐
Remove PM from other shell vials,   │
add 0.2 ml ^{3}H-DNA preparation.   │
↓   │
8 hr   65°C   │
↓   │
Wash, dry, count.   │
                                               ▼
                                        6 PM: add
                                        0.2 ml ^{3}H-DNA
                                        prep

                                        65°C,   15 hr
                                                overnight
                                        Wash, dry, count.

Day 1 6 37.5 µg filters in scintillation vials +
2.5 ml PM.
6 hrs   65°C
Remove filter.

Day 2 Punch 2 mini's from each:
(1) 0 time point: dry, count.
(2) 15 hr point: set aside.
Remove PM from scintillation vials,
add 2.5 ml ^{3}H-DNA preparation to rest
of filter.

2 hr ─────▶ Mini: wash, dry, count.
4 hr ─────▶ Mini: same
8 hr ─────▶ Mini: same
24 hr (overnight) Mini: same

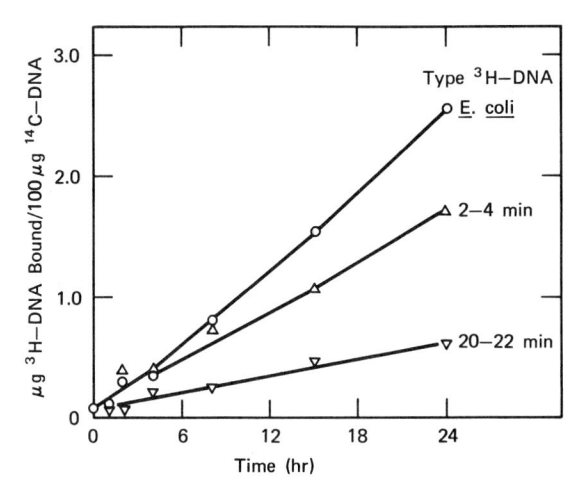

FIGURE 4. DNA-DNA hybridization with preincubation. DNA pulse-labeled with ^{3}H-thymidine for 2 min was isolated from noninfected E. coli cells, and from E. coli cells infected with phage T7 and pulse-labeled at 2–4 min and at 20–22 min after infection. The ^{3}H-DNA was hybridized as described in the text to ^{14}C-E. coli DNA, and the data analyzed as described in Tables I and III. (○———○ , bacterial DNA; △———△ , 2–4 min DNA; ▽———▽ 20–22 min DNA.)

1. **DNA Retention.** The DNA must initially be completely denatured. DNA preparations may be denatured either by heat or by alkali treatment. Alkaline denaturation is less likely to degrade the DNA, and is independent of DNA and salt concentrations. Heat denaturation should be done at low DNA concentration, for example, 100 µg/ml, and in low salt, for example, 0.01 × SSC. The extent of DNA denaturation should be monitored. Denaturation may be monitored using any method that distinguishes single-stranded from double-stranded DNA, for example, the increase in UV light absorbance of 40% upon denaturation (hyperchromic effect), the decrease in viscosity upon denaturation, etc. Some qualitative information can be obtained from the nature of the ethanol precipitate of the DNA. The precipitate of denatured DNA appears snowy (RNA-like); the fibrous quality is completely lost. Partially denatured DNA not only does not stick well to filters, but because of partial self-annealing, it is not completely available for subsequent hybridization.

If the DNA has been excessively fragmented during purification, retention will be incomplete. Raising the salt concentration during loading and during hybridization, for example, to 6 × SSC, and lowering the filtration rate during loading, increases the retention of such preparations.

TABLE VII. DNA–DNA Hybridization: No Preincubation, Flow Sheet

Filters are loaded with the correct amounts of the appropriate ^{14}C-DNA species on day 1 using the procedure given in section II-C using 2 × SSC. Only the four 37.5 μg filters need to be prepared; you have sufficient numbers of the others to provide the needed minifilters.

The same ^{3}H-DNA types will also be used but according to the following table:

		^{3}H-DNA types	
Time of annealing, hr	2 min pulse	λ	E. coli
0	(3; 3; –)	(3; –; –)	(–; 3; –)
2	(3; 3; –)	(3; –; –)	(–; 3; –)
4	(3; 3; –)	(3; –; –)	(–; 3; –)
8	(0,0.4,1,3,8; 3; 3)	(0,0.4,1,3,8; 3; 3)	(3; 0,0.4,1,3,8; 3)
15	(3; 0,0.4,1,3,8; 3)	(3; –; –)	(–; 3; –)
24	(3; 3; –)	(3; –; –)	(–; 3; –)

Protocol

In brief: Very similar to that described in Table VI, with omission of preincubation step, and washing in 0.003 M Tris, pH 9.4 rather than in 2 × SSC.

In detail: Detailed kinetics of 37.5 μg filters will be done. Four of these filters, two containing λ DNA and two containing E. coli DNA will be used. Two minifilters are punched from each of these filters, and the remainder of the filter is placed in a scintillation vial. One of each mini can be washed, dried, and counted immediately; these are the 0 time points. The others are placed in small shell capped vials, and placed aside until about 6 pm day 2. At that time, 0.2 ml ^{3}H-DNA is added and the vials incubated overnight for 15 hr at 65°C for the 15 hr time points. The mini's are then washed, dried, and counted. To each scintillation vial is added 2.5 ml ^{3}H-DNA prep in 2 × SSC, pH 7.0, buffered with 0.01 M Tris Cl, and the vials are then incubated at 65°C. At the times given above, vials are removed from the 65°C baths, the filters removed from the vials, and a minifilter is punched, washed in 0.003 M Tris, pH 9.4. The rest of the filter is replaced into the vial, and the vial incubated further at 65°C.

For the saturation curves, minifilters are punched from appropriate DNA filters, placed in small shell vials, covered with 0.2 ml ^{3}H-DNA preparation, capped with rubber caps, and incubated at 65°C for 8 and 15 hr. After annealing, the vials are chilled, the minifilters removed, washed, dried, and counted.

Minifilters are washed by immersing and thoroughly shaking in 100 ml 0.003 M Tris Cl, pH 9.4. Shaking should be done for some time, and it is suggested that the minifilters be removed and placed in a second 100 ml batch of 0.003 M Tris Cl, pH 9.4; nonspecific binding of ^{3}H-DNA is sometimes a problem with this method.

TABLE VII. (Continued)

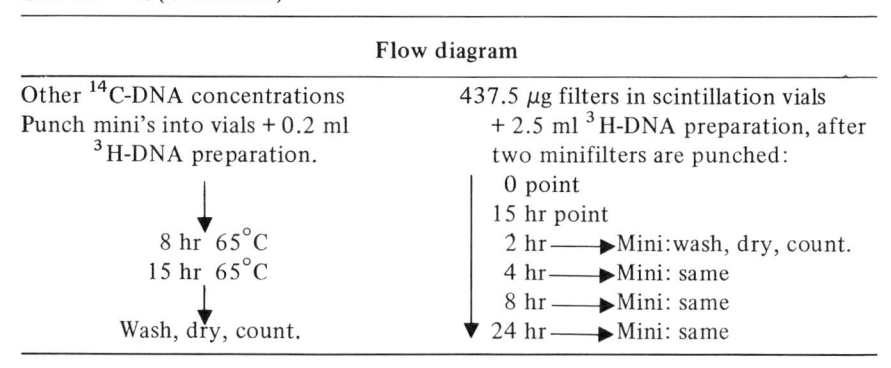

Flow diagram	
Other ^{14}C-DNA concentrations Punch mini's into vials + 0.2 ml ^{3}H-DNA preparation. ↓ 8 hr 65°C 15 hr 65°C ↓ Wash, dry, count.	437.5 μg filters in scintillation vials + 2.5 ml ^{3}H-DNA preparation, after two minifilters are punched: 0 point 15 hr point 2 hr ⟶ Mini: wash, dry, count. 4 hr ⟶ Mini: same 8 hr ⟶ Mini: same 24 hr ⟶ Mini: same

Removal of Mg^{2+} ions from the DNA during purification may reduce the ability of the DNA to bind to the filters [13]. This problem is overcome by including 0.003 M Mg^{2+} in the loading solution. Mg^{2+} is omitted from the wash solution, permitting removal of the excess Mg^{2+}.

2. **RNA Noise.** Any DNA left in the RNA preparation results in a high RNA noise. All RNA preparations should be treated with pancreatic deoxyribonuclease, for example, 10 μg/ml, 15 min, room temperature, in the presence of 0.005 Mg^{2+}. The RNA is then purified from the deoxyribonuclease by phenol extraction of the RNA.

A second source of RNA noise is the presence of basic proteins in the RNA preparation [38]. This noise may be reduced as follows: (1) passage of the RNA preparation two or three times through a nitrocellulose filter; (2) treatment of the RNA preparation with self-digested pronase, for example, 100 μg/ml, 2 hr, 55°C (pronase is self-digested by incubating a 2 mg/ml stock solution in SSC for 1 hr at 37°C); (3) purification of the RNA using MAK column chromatography; or (4) purification of the RNA using Cs_2SO_4 density gradient centrifugation.

3. **Control Experiments.** Hybridization experiments too often lack adequate controls. The most common oversight is failure to include a noise control (blank filter) for each hybridization performed. The noise varies with time and temperature of incubations, RNA or DNA input, washing buffers, and so on; noise controls must be performed when any of these conditions are changed. Such controls include those for both the DNA and the RNA in RNA–DNA hybridization experiments. DNA retention must be determined using a control receiving no RNA in the hybridization mix. DNA retention should be greater than 95% in all experiments. Nonspecific RNA retention must be determined using a blank filter and/or a filter containing completely heterologous DNA,

for example, salmon sperm DNA for an E. coli RNA experiment. The RNA noise should be lower than 0.01% of the input RNA.

The final amount of DNA on the filter after the hybridization and hybrid purification steps must be known with certainty. For this reason, the DNA should be radioactively labeled and its specific activity in counts per minute per microgram of DNA known. Note that this value usually depends on the particular scintillation counter used to assay the counts. The specific activity should be high enough to provide a minimum of about 300 cpm for both the DNA and the RNA in each of the double labels. Most experiments use either ^{14}C or ^{32}P in the DNA and ^{3}H in the RNA, or ^{3}H in the DNA and ^{32}P in the RNA.

B. Comparison of Methods

Advantages and disadvantages of different detection and hybridization methods have been mentioned in appropriate sections above. In summary, the use of filters provides a rapid and inexpensive way to perform a large number of simultaneous hybridization experiments under highly reproducible conditions. However, isolation of the nucleic acid hybrids from the filter is difficult, rendering other methods more useful for preparative experiments. Also, hybrid formation proceeds more slowly on filters. Thus, hybridization in solution is preferred, for example, when $C_0 t$ curves are desired. Recent developments in the use of HA, including the use of urea and low temperatures and the development of batch methods for rapid processing of large numbers of samples, suggest that HA procedures may soon encompass many of the present advantages unique to filter methods [53]. Most workers currently use either filter methods or HA procedures in their experiments.

C. Conclusions

Hybridization experiments have amply proved their versatility and importance as a fundamental research tool for the developmental and molecular biologist, as a glance at the types of recent experiments will show (see section I-A). The physical chemistry of hybridization reactions, using a wide variety of environmental conditions and types of reacting nucleic acids, is under intensive investigation. Technology for hybridization experiments, involving both improvements in current methods and introduction of new techniques, is rapidly developing. There is little doubt that the developmental and molecular biologist will find hybridization techniques indispensable as a research tool in their studies of gene expression at the molecular level.

REFERENCES

[1] Marmur, J., R. Rownd, and C. L. Schildkraut. 1963. Prog. Nucl. Acid Res. 1:231.
[2] Felsenfeld, G., and H. T. Miles. 1967. Ann. Rev. Biochem. 36:407.
[3] McCarthy, B. J., and R. B. Church. 1970. Ann. Rev. Biochem. 39:131.
[4] Kennell, D. E., 1971. Prog. Nucl. Acid Res. Mol. Biol. 11:259.
[5] Wetmur, J. G., and N. Davidson. 1968. J. Mol. Biol. 31:349.
[6] Walker, P. M. B. 1969. Prog. Nucl. Acid Res. Mol. Biol. 9:301.
[7] Crothers, D. M., and B. Zimm. 1964. J. Mol. Biol. 9:1.
[8] Britten, R. J., and D. E. Kohne. 1968. Science 161:529.
[9] Melli, M., C. Whitfield, K. V. Rao, M. Richardson, and J. O. Bishop. 1971. Nature New Biol. 231:8.
[10] Yankofsky, S. A., and S. Spiegelman. 1963. Proc. Nat. Acad. Sci. U.S.49:538.
[11] Bishop, J. O. 1969. Nature 224:600.
[12] Bishop, J. O. 1970. Biochem. J. 116:223.
[13] Gillespie, D. 1968. Methods of Enzymology XIIB:641.
[14] Soeiro, R., and J. E. Darnell. 1969. J. Mol. Biol. 44:551.
[15] Szybalski, W. 1969. Proc. 8th Can. Cancer Congr. 8:183.
[16] Baker, R. F., and C. Yanofsky. 1968. Proc. Nat. Acad. Sci. U.S.60:313.
[17] Imamoto, F. 1968. Proc. Nat. Acad. Sci. U.S.60:305.
[18] Williamson, R., M. Morrison, and J. Paul. 1970. Biochem. Biophys. Res. Comm. 40:740.
[19] Gelderman, A. H., A. V. Rake, and R. J. Britten. 1971. Proc. Nat. Acad. Sci. U.S.68:172.
[20] Brown, I. R., and R. B. Church. 1971. Biochem. Biophys. Res. Comm. 42:850.
[21] Botchan, M., R. Kram, C. W. Schmid, and J. E. Hearst. 1971. Proc. Nat. Acad. Sci. U.S.68:1125.
[22] Taylor, K., Z. Hradecna, and W. Szybalski. 1967. Proc. Nat. Acad. Sci. U.S.57:1618.
[23] Spiegelman, S., and S. A. Yankofsky. 1965. In Bryson and Vogel (ed.), Evolving genes and proteins. Academic Press, New York, p. 537.
[24] Hoyer, B. H., E. T. Bolton, B. J. McCarthy, and R. B. Roberts. 1965. In Bryson and Vogel (ed.), Evolving genes and proteins. Academic Press, New York, p. 581.
[25] Pardue, M. L., S. A. Gerbi, R. A. Eckhardt, and J. G. Gall. 1970. Chromosoma 29:268.
[26] Kuempel, P. L. 1972. J. Bacteriol. 110:917.
[27] Hall, B. D., and S. Spiegelman. 1961. Proc. Nat. Acad. Sci. U.S.47:137.
[28] Hayashi, M., M. N. Hayashi, and S. Spiegelman. 1965. Biophys. J. 5:231.
[29] Bernardi, G. 1965. Nature 206:779.
[30] Walker, P. M. B., and A. McLaren. 1965. Nature 208:1175.
[31] Miyazawa, Y., and C. A. Thomas, Jr. 1965. J. Mol. Biol. 11:223.
[32] Nygaard, A. P., and B. D. Hall. 1963. Biochem. Biophys. Res. Comm. 12:98.

[33] Bautz, E. F. K., and B. D. Hall. 1962. Proc. Nat. Acad. Sci. U.S.48:400.
[34] Bolton, E. T., and B. J. McCarthy. 1962. Proc. Nat. Acad. Sci. U.S.48:1390.
[35] Bolton, E. T., and B. J. McCarthy. 1963. Proc. Nat. Acad. Sci. U.S.50:156.
[36] Britten, R. J. 1963. Science 142:963.
[37] Nygaard, A. P., and B. D. Hall. 1964. J. Mol. Biol. 9:125.
[38] Gillespie, D., and S. Spiegelman. 1965. J. Mol. Biol. 12:829.
[39] McConaughy, B. L., C. D. Laird, and B. J. McCarthy. 1969. Biochemistry 8:3289.
[40] Bonner, J., G. Kung, and I. Bekhor. 1967. Biochemistry 6:3650.
[41] Niyogi, S. K. 1969. J. Biol. Chem. 244:1576.
[42] Kohne, D. E. 1968. Biophys. J. 8:1104.
[43] Bolton, E. T., and B. J. McCarthy. 1964. J. Mol. Biol. 8:201.
[44] Bendich, A. J., and E. T. Bolton. 1968. Methods of Enzymology, XIIB:635.
[45] Mandel, J. D., and A. D. Hershey. 1960. Anal. Biochem. 1:66.
[46] Davidson, E. H., and B. R. Hough. 1969. Proc. Nat. Acad. Sci. U.S.63:342.
[47] Rake, A., A. Gelderman, and R. J. Britten. 1971. Proc. Nat. Acad. Sci. U.S.68:172.
[48] McCarthy, B. J. 1967. Bacteriol. Rev. 31:215.
[49] Denhardt, D. T. 1966. Biochem. Biophys. Res. Comm. 23:641.
[50] Warnaar, S. O., and J. A. Cohen. 1966. Biochem. Biophys. Res. Comm. 24:554.
[51] Weiss, S. B., W. T. Hsu, J. W. Foft, and N. E. Scherberg. 1968. Proc. Nat. Acad. Sci. U.S.61:114.
[52] Kohne, D. E., and R. J. Britten. 1971. Proc. Nucl. Acid Res. II:500.
[53] Kohne, D. E. 1972. Department of Biology, University of California, San Diego, Calif. Personal communication.
[54] Tait, R., and D. Smith. 1972. Department of Biology, University of California, San Diego, Calif. Unpublished observation.

Methods to Study Isoaccepting Transfer RNA Species During Development

LEON S. DURE III

BACKGROUND

The development of specific cells and tissues with unique morphology and functions from undifferentiated progenitors is the result of the acquisition of unique collections of proteins by the various cell types. Thus, to comprehend developmental processes on a molecular basis, we must ultimately comprehend the regulation of the specificity of DNA transcription. However, in unraveling step-by-step the sequence of events that brings new protein into existence in cells, the components of the translation machinery have been suspected of playing a regulatory role; that is, it is possible that the translation machinery may not treat all mRNA the same. Transfer RNA in particular has been singled out as a likely regulatory agent in translation, and perhaps in other cellular processes as well, because of a number of observations that have accumulated over the past ten years. Briefly, these are:

(1) There appear to be more tRNA species than are required to translate the genetic code. In those instances where the total number of species have been determined [1], more than 55 different molecular species per cell have been visualized by chromatographic techniques; yet considering the "wobble" capabilities of tRNA [2] probably less than 40 separate species are needed to recognize the 61 code words and to provide for initiation and termination.

(2) There is a large variation in the levels of the individual tRNA species per

cell [3,4,5]. This may indicate a rather large inequality in the concentration of anticodons in cells.

(3) Suppressor mutations which restore the capability of certain cells to synthesize certain proteins have been shown to involve changes in the code word recognition of certain tRNA species [6].

(4) The methylase enzymes that modify specific bases in tRNA have been found to vary in activity during tissue ontogeny and development [7]. Although the function of the methyl groups on the tRNA molecules has yet to be uncovered, the variation in activity of the enzymes that carry out the methylation suggests that the degree of tRNA methylation changes with development.

(5) Certain tRNA species that read code words beginning with "U" contain substituted adenine nucleotides adjacent to the tRNA anticodon [8]. One of these adenine derivatives is identical to the cytokinin plant growth regulator known to have enormous influence on the development of plant tissues [9].

(6) In certain bacteria a tRNA^{His} species acylated with histidine has been found to participate in the genetic repression of the biosynthesis of the enzymes that synthesize histidine [10], and the repression has been shown to depend upon specific modifications of the tRNA structure that do not influence its adaptor role in translation [11].

(7) The number and levels relative to each other of isoaccepting tRNA species have been found to change during the differentiation of cells, to change in response to hormones and to be different in the cells of different organs of mature organisms. Table I is a resumé of some of the reports that demonstrate changes in the composition of the tRNA pool that accompany developmental changes of various sorts in cells and tissues. This resumé, although not totally complete, indicates the range of developmental situations in which tRNA changes have been found.

None of the observations listed above have directly linked tRNA pool composition with the rate of translation in general or with a differential rate of translation of specific proteins. In fact, the changes in tRNA pool composition may prove ultimately to be the result of developmental changes rather than a causal factor in differentiation or maturation. In fact, it appears more likely that the regulatory functions of tRNA lay outside the translation process itself and involve the control of steady-state processes of the cell as exemplified by the recent findings of Lewis and Ames [10] Singer et al. [11] and Jacobson [12]. Regardless of the level of regulatory influence that tRNA molecules may prove

TABLE I. Resumé of Changes in tRNA Population Associated with Development

---

(1) Sporulation of bacteria
(2) Tissue differentiation
    Animal
      (a) Sea Urchin embryogenesis
      (b) Tadpole metamorphosis
      (c) Liver regeneration, rat
      (d) Erythrocyte maturation, chicken
    Plant
      (a) Seed germination, wheat
      (b) Seedling growth, lupine
      (c) Root growth, soybean
(3) Differences between differentiated tissues
    (a) Liver vs. kidney vs. brain, rat
    (b) Hypocotyl vs. cotyledon, soybean
(4) Specialized population in highly specialized cells
    (a) Recticulocytes, rabbit
    (b) Silk gland, silkworm
    (c) Mammary gland cells, bovine
(5) In response to hormones
    (a) Liver in response to estrogen, rooster
    (b) Liver in response to thyroxine, rat

---

to have, the composition of tRNA pools have been shown to change coevally with developmental changes in ontogeny and in the final maturation of cell types. Thus in mapping the molecular events that characterize a developmental step, a determination of the tRNA population must be considered, even if the meaning of changes in this population is obscure at present.

Since organelles are equipped with their own complement of tRNA species (that are likely transcribed from organelle DNA), identifying organelle species and following their levels relative to cytosol species may prove to be rewarding, since it can provide a tool for following organelle maturation in the developing tissue.

DETERMINATION OF tRNA POOL COMPOSITION DURING DEVELOPMENT

Basically these determinations merely require that (1) tRNA be extracted from the cells, tissues, or organs at several points in development, (2) the tRNA preparation be acylated singly with the individual radioactive amino acids by a homologous enzyme preparation, and (3) the resultant isoaccepting species of acylated tRNA be separated by some form of chromatography. From this the number and relative levels of isoaccepting species existing in the cells at the several developmental stages can be determined. In practice, however, several fundamental things must first be clearly established, if the data collected is to be taken seriously.

Purification of tRNA

The first of these is to establish that all the tRNA of the tissue is extracted and ends up in the final tRNA preparation. This is not particularly important when tRNA is being prepared for purposes other than a comparison of pool sizes during development. But here it is obvious that for our comparisons to be meaningful they cannot be comparisons of just portions of the tRNA pools.

We have found, in our work with plant tissues, that we can extract and purify the total tRNA pool more consistently if we first extract the total nucleic acid fraction from the tissue. Of course, a large portion of the tRNA pool can be separated from the ribosomal RNA by centrifuging a tissue homogenate at 100,000 × g for several hours and using the supernatant as the starting material. Yet we have found that this procedure rarely yields more than 70% of the tissue's tRNA. We prefer to homogenize the tissue in buffer, pH 7.5–8.0, containing 0.01 M $MgCl_2$, 0.001 M EDTA, 0.01 M KCl, 0.001 M mercaptoethanol, and a detergent; followed by a low-speed centrifugation (8000–12,000 × g) for about 15 min; and then to extract the total nucleic from this supernatant by routine phenol procedures. (Naturally, we reextract the low-speed pellet with the same buffer in order to solubilize occluded material.) As for the detergent, we have found that 1% SDS insures a complete solubilization of all RNA, but that all too frequently much of the tRNA recovered contains nicks in the polynucleotide chains. Using 1% NaDOC (sodium deoxycholate) on the other hand solubilizes all the RNA and yields tRNA that for the most part is structurally undamaged. We believe that SDS solubilizes too many deleterious enzymes that manage to hydrolyze tRNA molecules at some point in the tRNA purification. Consequently, we prefer NaDOC as the detergent. Routinely we extract the low-speed supernatant first with 80% phenol in the cold followed by a reextraction of the phenol and interface layer with pH 8.5 buffer at room temperature. All succeeding manipulations are performed as close to 0°C as possible. The combined aqueous phases are then made 2% in acidic potassium acetate, pH 5.0, to lower the charge density of the nucleic acids and precipitated with 2.5 vol of very cold ethanol. We allow this precipitation to proceed overnight in a freezer (−20°C) and then resuspend the precipitate in buffer, pH 7.5, 0.01 M $MgCl_2$, 0.001 M EDTA, and 0.001 M mercaptoethanol.

This resuspension should contain all the tRNA and rRNA of the tissue and usually most of the DNA. If an insufficient volume is used to resuspend this precipitate, the Mg salt of the rRNA will remain insoluble. We prefer not to centrifuge this material out, but rather to dilute the nucleic acid further to solubilize the rRNA. Any material remaining insoluble upon dilution is denatured protein and can be centrifuged out at this time. We keep the preparation 0.01 M $MgCl_2$ at all times to maintain the tRNA in its proper secondary and tertiary configuration so as to render it less susceptible to nuclease hydrolysis and to prevent its renaturation into an inactive configuration.

The redissolved nucleic acid is next made 2% in acidic potassium acetate and reprecipitated with 2.5 vol of very cold ethanol. This second precipitation should rid the preparation of all the phenol that up to now would mask any spectral measurement of nucleic acid content. The precipitate is again dissolved in buffer, pH 7.5, 0.01 M $MgCl_2$, 0.001 M EDTA, and 0.001 M mercaptoethanol. Here again it should be dilute enough to allow the rRNA to solubilize in the presence of 0.01 M $MgCl_2$. The nucleic acid content of the preparation can now be determined spectrally by assuming that 1 mg/ml of a rRNA, tRNA, and DNA mixture in 0.01 mg $MgCl_2$ at pH 7.5 at room temperature should give about 22 A_{260} units (in a 1 cm lightpath). Preferably, this measurement should be made with a scanning spectrophotometer so that the purity of the preparation can be estimated using as a criterion for pure nucleic acid the following: $A_{320} = 0$; $A_{280} < 1/2\ A_{260}$; A_{231} = bottom of the spectral trough and $A_{220} < A_{260}$. EDTA absorbs in the lower wave length region of this spectrum and its absorption varies with the concentration of other ions. Thus the reference cells should contain all the constituents of the buffer solution.

The virtue of maintaining all the rRNA in with the tRNA now becomes apparent since the total amount of rRNA and tRNA, the degree of rRNA breakdown (if any), and the ratio of tRNA to rRNA can all be measured by subjecting about 1 A_{260} unit of the preparation to SDS gel electrophoresis as described by Loening [13]. This is very valuable information since contamination of the tRNA with small fragments of degraded rRNA must be ruled out.

Figure 1 (upper portion) shows a gel of such a nucleic acid preparation from green cotton cotyledons at this stage of purification. Here, both cytosol and chloroplastic rRNA species are present, and although the cytosol rRNA spe-

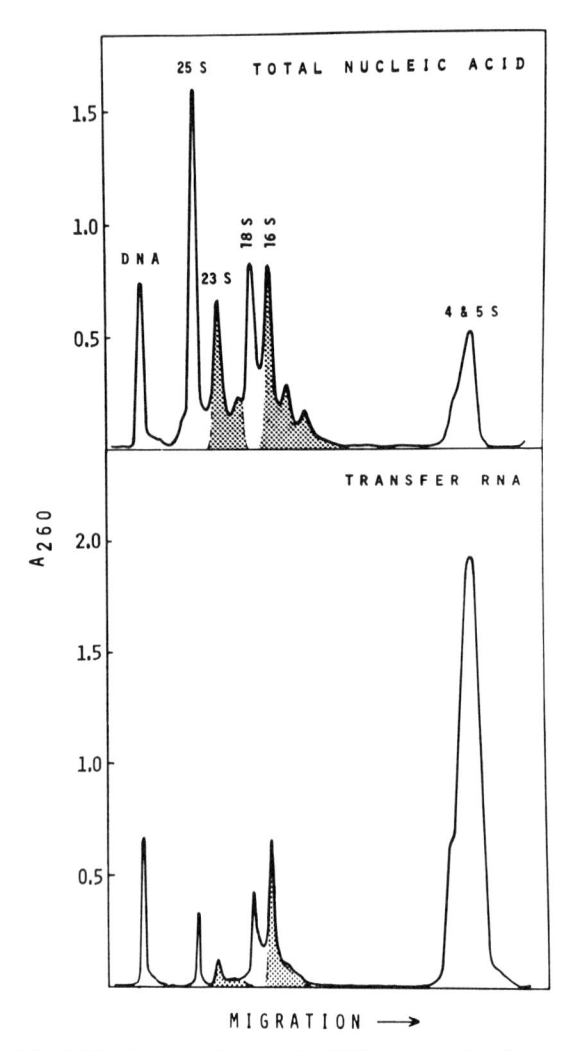

FIGURE 1. The SDS–gel electrophoresis of a tRNA preparation from green cotyledons before (upper gel) and after (lower gel) the DEAE–cellulose column separation of tRNA and low molecular weight RNA from DNA and rRNA. Nucleic acids were extracted, purified, and electrophoresed on SDS–polyacrylamide gels. The positions of the various nucleic acid species on the gels were determined by scanning the gels for absorbancy at 260 nm and are identified by the $S_{20,w}$ value commonly ascribed to them. Shaded portions of the profile represent chloroplastic rRNA.

cies are present in the proper proportions, one to the other, the heavy chloroplastic rRNA species is largely degraded (a universal problem regardless of the investigator or source of chloroplasts). However, none of the breakdown fragments appear to overlap into the 4 and 5 Svedberg units (S) species on the gel. It is possible with gels such as this to estimate the amount of DNA, cytosol rRNA, chloroplastic rRNA, and tRNA present in the preparation by cutting out the areas of the recorder chart paper they occupy and calculating what portion of the 1 A_{260} unit loaded on the gel they comprise. The molecular weights of all these species are known [14], and since one molecule of 5 S and 5.8 S RNA is present for each cytosol ribosome and one molecule of 5 S RNA for each chloroplast ribosome, the amount of 5 S and 5.8 S RNA that should be present in the preparation can be calculated. These calculations predict that about 3% of the 25 + 18 S cytosol rRNA should be present as 5 S and 5.8 S RNA and that about 1.8% of the chloroplastic rRNA should be present as 5 S RNA. Thus by calculating the amounts of the two classes of rRNA in the preparation, the amount of 5 S and 5.85 RNA that contaminates the tRNA in the 4 and 5 S peak on the gel can be determined, and from this the amount of tRNA in the preparation can be determined.

In the case of cotton tissue, regardless of the state of plastid maturation, we always get an amount of tRNA that calculates back to 13–15 tRNA molecules per ribosome in the cell. This is the same value others have obtained for E. coli cells [15] and for sea urchin cells [16], and it may prove to be a nearly universal relationship between ribosomes and tRNA. Thus from this gel, the amount of tRNA in the preparation can be determined and from this the amount extracted per unit of tissue. Should this gel profile show a great deal of rRNA degradation that produces fragments that overlap into the 4 and 5 S region of the gel, start over, because the estimation of tRNA in the preparation is obliged to be shaky.

The next step in preparing tRNA involves getting rid of most of the rRNA and DNA. This can be done by precipitating the rRNA from the nucleic acid preparation by making it 1.5–2 M in NaCl. If kept close to 0°C for several hours, the rRNA will precipitate as the sodium salt leaving DNA and tRNA in solution. Unfortunately, a small amount of tRNA usually precipitates also (as revealed by a gel profile of the precipitate). For this reason we separate tRNA from the bulk of the other nucleic acid by DEAE–cellulose column chromatography. This column separation utilizes DEAE in a routine fashion; the column is equilibrated, washed, and loaded in 0.3 M NaCl, which allows any residual protein to wash through, and tRNA is eluted batchwise with 1 M NaCl. The pH is buffered at 7.5 throughout and all the solutions are again 0.01 M in $MgCl_2$. If this column is loaded and eluted cold, more rRNA elutes in the 1 M NaCl fraction; if it is loaded and eluted at room temperature, less rRNA elutes. This simply means that the more secondary structure rRNA is allowed to have (by cold temperatures), the less binding sites interact with the column and more of this RNA is displaced by the 1 M NaCl. Yet performing this step at room temperature may result in nuclease damage to the tRNA. These parameters have to be determined empirically for each tissue. Figure 1 (lower portion) is a SDS gel electrophoresis profile of the 1 M NaCl eluate of the same preparation shown in the upper portion of Figure 1. The amount of tRNA in the 1 M NaCl elution fraction can be calculated from this gel profile by cutting and weighing, and the 5 S and 5.8 S contamination that is based on the amount of rRNA found in the earlier gel can be taken into account in determining the actual amount of tRNA present.

In the case of the preparation from green cotton cotyledons shown in Figure 1, about 12% of the material in the 4 and 5 S region of the gel is 5 S and 5.8 S RNA. (Another way of determining the low molecular weight ribosomal RNA contamination of tRNA is to run an SDS polyacrylamide gel that is much less porous, that is, a 5 or 7.5% gel, which will effect a separation of these types.) Using the procedures outlined above we calculated that tRNA comprised 65% of the A_{260} absorbing material in the preparation. The other 35% was comprised of 5 S and 5.8 S RNA and the rRNA and DNA that eluted in 1 M NaCl and is easily identified on the lower profile of Figure 1.

Next, the 1 M NaCl eluate is diluted 1:3 with buffer that is 0.01 M $MgCl_2$ and precipitated with 2.5 vol of very cold ethanol. The dilution prevents the precipitation of the NaCl. This precipitate overlaid with the ethanol:buffer solution is a good way to store the tRNA, since very little can happen to it in this state.

Now that we have calculated the amount of tRNA extracted and purified per unit tissue, the question is "how do we know we have it all?" First, we know that we have already made a good estimate of the amount of tRNA in the preparation by demonstrating that it apparently is not contaminated with rRNA degradation fragments. Second, we have shown that there appear to be between 13 and 15 tRNA molecules per ribosome in the tissue. However, the only way to be convinced that all the tRNA of the tissue is now in the 1 M NaCl eluate is to repeat the extraction several times using 1% SDS and omitting the $MgCl_2$ throughout. It is also a good idea to use other published methods for extracting tRNA for comparison. If in all these extractions no greater yield of tRNA is ever encountered, then complete extraction can be assumed with some conviction.

Charging of tRNA

Once a total extraction and purification of the tRNA has been established, the next obligation is to prove that all the tRNA species have survived these procedures undamaged. This, of course, can only be established by the acylation reaction, and by the demonstration that each species functions in translation. This latter requirement is generally ignored because of the time and effort required to test each species in this fashion, and thus the acylation reaction has become the sole criterion for the intactness of the individual tRNA species in most studies of this kind.

If the proper controls are run, the acylation reaction can provide us with a fairly accurate estimate of the percentage of the tRNA preparation that will accept each of the 20 amino acids and, from this, the total percentage of the preparation that can be charged. Unfortunately, very few studies have bothered to make this latter determination. We feel that it is important since it is an indication of the degree of damage done to the tRNA during purification, or of the degree of contamination of the preparation with non-tRNA nucleic acid heretofore not realized. It must be kept in mind that if we intend to attach any significance to any changes in the tRNA pool we find during development, we cannot base any conclusions on tRNA preparations that can only be partially charged, that is, that accept much less amino acid than theoretically possible. The preparation of tRNA from green cotton cotyledons shown in Figure 1 could be 92.9% charged. Had it been, say, 65% chargeable, little importance could be given any chromatographic measurement of the number and levels of isoaccepting tRNA species, because there is no way of demonstrating that the damage to the 35% of the molecules that rendered them functionless (for example, loss of the terminal 3 nucleotide sequence cytidylic–cytidylic–adenylic acid [CpCpA terminus]) is random for all species.

Setting up the acylation reaction to determine the amount of tRNA in the preparation that will accept each amino acid is relatively simple, since we are interested here only in the extent of charging rather than in optimizing the rate of charging or in studying the enzymology of the reaction itself. A homologous enzyme preparation must be prepared that should include synthetase activity for all the tRNA species, but need not contain the total amount of each synthetase present in the tissue, since we are calculating tRNA levels per unit of tissue and not enzyme units per unit of tissue. The enzyme preparation should not contain any small molecules such as free amino acids or nucleotides, nor any endogenous tRNA. Finally, it should be prepared in solutions that tend to maximize the stability of the enzymes. We have found with the tissues of cotton seedlings that the following procedure satisfies most of the above listed requirements. The tissue is homogenized in buffer, pH 8.0 that contains 0.01 M $MgCl_2$, 0.001 M EDTA, 0.005 M mercaptoethanol, and that is 20% in glycerol. After the homogenate has been centrifuged at 17,000 × g for 30 min the supernatant is applied to a DEAE-23–cellulose column equilibrated with the same homogenizing solution including the glycerol. The enzyme preparation is eluted batchwise from the column with the buffer solution made 0.4 M in NaCl. This eluate fraction is then dialyzed against the same buffer that is 50% in glycerol for 36 hr with several changes of the buffer-glycerol solution. This final step reduces the volume of the eluate and makes it 50% in glycerol, in addition to lowering the NaCl concentration. A preparation such as this from green cotton cotyledons acylates over 90% of cotton tRNA from any cotton tissue, more slowly with some amino acids than others, but unfortunately has no activity for tyrosine whatsoever. (We have yet to stabilize the tyrosine synthetase(s) from cotton tissues.) We store the synthetase preparation at $-20°C$ or in liquid nitrogen.

The reaction mixture we use contains from 0.5 to 2.0 A_{260} units of tRNA, from 0.3 to 1.0 mg protein of the synthetase preparation, and a ^{3}H- or ^{14}C-amino acid, ATP, and 0.01 M buffer, pH 7.5, 0.01 M $MgCl_2$ and 0.01 M NH_4Cl all in 0.25 ml. Since the nucleotide triphosphates at neutral pH are strong chelators of Mg, the ratio of ATP to Mg is crucial to tRNA structural integrity. Consequently, the optimal concentration of ATP should be determined for the acylation of each amino acid. In our system this concentration ranges between 0.001 M and 0.005 M. The amino acid concentration should be high enough to allow for complete charging within 20–40 min. The reaction is followed by removing 50 μliter aliquots at intervals and determining the tRNA dependent radioactivity incorporated into acid insoluble material by the paper disk method of Bollum [17]. It is important that the reaction time be long enough to reveal the true plateau level of charging. That is, the last two or three time points should show no further increase in incorporation. This will also show if there is any decay in the aminoacyl–tRNA formed, which becomes evident after the rate of acylation becomes negligible. Since unknown reactions that are deleterious to charging apparently take place when crude enzyme preparations are used, it is wise to use enough enzyme to insure that the acylation reaction is complete within about 30 min. It is not usually necessary to determine the pH value that will give the maximum rate of charging for each amino acid, unless the rate of charging with a specific amino acid is extremely slow at pH 7.5. Naturally, it is a good idea to perform some reactions at high tRNA levels and at low enzyme levels to show that rate is initially linear with enzyme concentration. Such a demonstration is presented in Figure 2 (upper portion).

There are a number of controls that should be performed with each amino acid that are essential. First, there are a number of amino acids (or radioactive contaminents) that bind to the paper disk and give high radioactivity backgrounds.

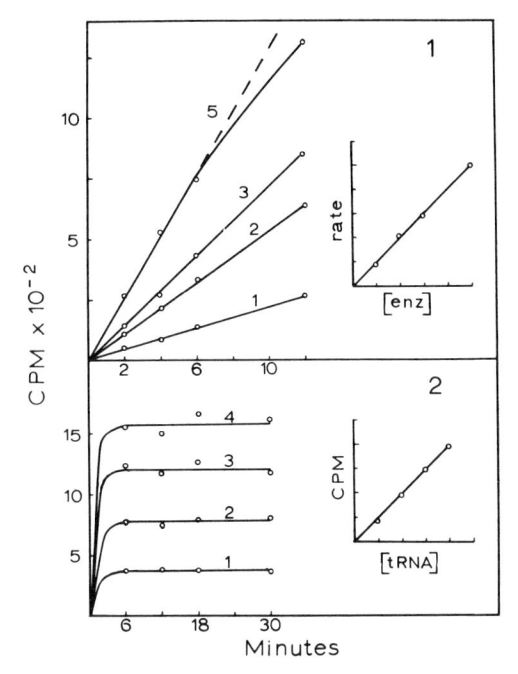

FIGURE 2. Characteristics of tRNA aminoacylation reaction. (1) The effect of enzyme concentration on the rate of acylation of tRNA from green cotton cotyledons with ^{14}C leucine. Multiples of a very low level of the enzyme preparation (3×10^{-3} A_{280} units) and 0.75 A_{260} units of tRNA in 0.25 ml were used and short time points assayed. Insert: Initial rate with the several concentrations of enzyme plotted against enzyme concentration. (2) The effect of tRNA concentration on the extent of acylation of tRNA from green cotton cotyledons with ^{14}C leucine. Multiples of 0.15 A_{260} units of tRNA and 0.145 A_{280} units of the enzyme preparation in 0.25 ml were used. Insert: Plateau level of tRNA-acylated plotted against tRNA concentration.

These can be determined by omitting tRNA or ATP from the reaction mixture. Next, to demonstrate that all the radioactivity has been incorporated into aminoacyl—tRNA linkage, disks from a duplicate reaction mixture should be treated with hot trichloroacetic acid (80°C) for 30 min. This procedure will discharge the amino acid rendering it acid soluble. To insure that there are no unknown complications to acylation occurring in the reaction, several levels of tRNA should be used to demonstrate a linear relationship between tRNA concentration and the amount of tRNA charged. Figure 2 (lower portion) gives a typical demonstration of this sort. Finally, and of great importance, the integrity of the tRNA chains should be demonstrated by charging tRNA that has been melted and allowed to reform its tertiary structure. This can easily be accomplished by heating the aliquot of tRNA in the buffer, Mg and NH_4Cl reaction mixture to 80°C for 10 min and cooling before adding the ATP, amino acid, and enzyme. Transfer RNA molecules that have sustained breaks in the polynucleotide chain can still be acylated by its cognate synthetase in many cases. If the tRNA is first heated, the individual fragments dissociate and do not reassociate upon quick cooling. By comparing the percent charged with the individual amino acids between heated and nonheated tRNA, the amount of nicked tRNA can be estimated. This factor becomes very important when the number and levels of isoaccepting species are to be determined by the chromatographic separation of the isoaccepting species, since, in some chromatographic procedures, the nicked molecules will separate from their intact counterparts and be mistaken for unique isoaccepting species.

There are several other controls that should be performed also. There is a possibility that some tRNA survives the purification protocol still in the acylated state, and hence is not acylated in the reaction mixture. This can be checked by incubating an aliquot of the tRNA preparation in 1.8 M Tris buffer, pH 8.0, for 15 min to deacylate any charged tRNA, and then charging the tRNA after dialyzing it back to its original buffer and ionic environment. The possibility that some of the synthetases may acylate the wrong tRNA in the in vitro reaction can be ruled out by carrying out an acylation reaction with each amino acid in the presence of the other 19 nonradioactive amino acids. Presumably the nonradioactive amino acids and their synthetases will outcompete the misacylation reaction. Finally, there is the possibility that Asn and Gln can be enzymatically deamidated during the course of the acylation reaction, and that the resulting radioactive Asp and Glu react with their cognate synthetases and tRNA species producing spuriously high values for the amount of $tRNA^{Asn}$ and $tRNA^{Gln}$ in the tRNA preparation. Consequently, $tRNA^{Asn}$ and $tRNA^{Gln}$ should always be assayed in the presence of nonradioactive Asp and Glu. Conversely, since ATP and ammonium ion can lead to the formation of Asn and Gln from Asp and Glu, KCl should replace NH_4Cl in the acylation of Asp and Glu.

Now that a total extraction of the tissue tRNA has been demonstrated and the total tRNA acceptance of each tRNA preparation has been determined, we are in position to determine the number and relative levels of isoaccepting species in each of the tRNA preparations for some of the amino acids. Any changes we observe between the tRNA preparations from the tissue at different developmental stages should be real in vivo differences because of the pains we have already taken in characterizing the tRNA preparations.

Separation of Isoaccepting Species

In choosing what amino acids should be used for examining isoaccepting species we can compare the percent of the total tRNA-acylated values for each amino acid for the several tRNA preparation. These values may be significantly different between the tRNA preparations for certain amino acids, in which case they would obviously be the amino acids to choose, since either the numbers or relative levels of isoaccepting species change relative to each other or relative to the rest of the tRNA pool.

The most popular method for separating isoaccepting tRNA species has been the reverse phase column first introduced by Weiss and Kelmers [3]. There are several types of these columns [18,19], but all of them utilize the same principle for the separation of tRNA molecules. This involves loading a solution of tRNA-acylated with a single radioactive amino acid onto a column comprised of an inert matrix that is coated with an essentially hydrophobic layer that contains positively charged amine groups. The tRNA molecules interact with the column in two ways: the negatively charged phosphate groups of the tRNA bind with the positively charged amines, and the nucleotide bases of the tRNA interact with the hydrophobic coating of the matrix. The bound tRNA molecules are eluted with a salt gradient, and frequently very nice separations of isoaccepting species are achieved. The tRNA molecules that differ only by a single nucleotide have been separated with one type of these columns [20].

However, there are several aspects of this method that can cause problems in a developmental study of tRNA. First, the recovery of radioactivity from these columns is not always equal to that loaded. In fact, occasionally it is far too low (less than 70%) to give meaningful data for a developmental study. That is, one does not know if the uneluted radioactivity represents a random loss from each of the isoaccepting species or a preferential loss from specific species. Since we are interested in comparing the levels of individual species between the tRNA preparations, incomplete elution of radioactivity from the column is a serious problem. Second, these reversed phase columns will often separate nicked tRNA molecules from unnicked but otherwise identical molecules. This gives rise to elution peaks that represent spurious species, and the levels of these spurious species depend on the amount of the tRNA that gets nicked during purification or during the acylation reaction. As we have pointed out, it is possible to detect nicked tRNA for a given amino acid in the tRNA preparation by comparing the amount of tRNA acylated before and after melting and quick-cooling of an aliquot of the preparation. Those amino acids that show a decrease in acylation with tRNA that has been so treated should <u>not</u> be used to measure levels of isoaccepting species with these columns. Moreover, there is the possibility that some tRNA gets nicked during the acylation reaction itself and thus may generate spurious species in the column elution profile. This possibility can be assayed for by pooling separately the elution fractions that contain each peak of radioactivity, adding carrier rRNA, and precipitating the tRNA and rRNA with 95% ethanol. This precipitate is redissolved in a small volume of buffer, MgCl$_2$ solution, and heated to 80°C for 10 min to discharge the amino acids and melt the tRNA, and then quick-cooled. The solution is then subjected to reacylation by the enzyme preparation, ATP, radioactive amino acid, etc., and if the elution peak contained undamaged tRNA it will be reacylated; if it contained nicked tRNA (a spurious species) there will be no reacylation whatsoever. In order to verify that each elution peak from the reverse phase column is a valid species, the above procedure should be carried out routinely.

With the cotton system we encountered numerous instances of spurious species and incomplete elution yield of radioactivity. For these reasons, we have utilized another means for determining the number and levels of isoaccepting tRNA species for most of the amino acids.

In this procedure the reaction mixture that gives complete acylation with a given amino acid within 30–40 min is scaled up so as to produce 40,000–60,000 cpm of ^{14}C-aminoacyl–tRNA (α1–1.5 ml reaction mixture). The reaction mixture is immediately applied to a small column of DEAE-23-cellulose (0.9 × 10 cm) that has been equilibrated with 0.01 M sodium acetate, pH 4.5, 0.01 M MgCl$_2$, 0.01 M mercaptoethanol and 0.3 M NaCl. The column is washed with this buffer until all free ^{14}C-amino acid and protein has washed through. The ^{14}C-aminoacyl–tRNA is then eluted batchwise with the same buffer made 1.0 M in NaCl. This eluate (5–10 ml) is diluted with 1 vol of distilled water to reduce the NaCl concentration, and carrier rRNA is added to assist in precipitating the tRNA (7 A$_{260}$ units/ml of diluted eluate). The nucleic acids are then precipitated with 2.5 vol of very cold ethanol. The recovery of ^{14}C-aminoacyl–tRNA should be that predicted from the 0.25 ml reaction mixture used to establish the amount of tRNA in the tRNA preparation that will accept the given amino acid. (This precipitate can be dissolved in a small volume and applied to a reverse phase column if that procedure is to be used.)

We dissolve this precipitate in 1 ml of 0.01 M sodium acetate, pH 5.5, 0.001 M EDTA, and add to this solution Takadiastase ribonuclease T1 (150 enzyme units/A$_{260}$ unit of nucleic acid). This is incubated for 30 min at 37°C after which additional ribonuclese T1 is added (60 enzyme units/A$_{260}$ unit) and the incubation continued for an additional 60 min.

The purpose of this incubation is to digest the ^{14}C-aminoacyl–tRNA into specific fragments. Ribonuclease T1 specifically cleaves polynucleotides at the site of guanine residues producing guanosyl-3′-phosphate at the 3′ termini. Thus, digesting ^{14}C-aminoacyl–tRNA with this enzyme produces only one radioactive oligonucleotide fragment from each aminoacyl–tRNA molecule—the fragment containing the amino acid. The nucleotide length and composition of this fragment depends on the position of the guanine residue nearest the CpCpA–amino acid terminus of the molecule. Isoaccepting tRNA species that produce different aminoacyl oligonucleotides in the digestion can be distinguished and their relative concentrations measured if the different aminoacyl oligonucleotides are separated by column chromatography. A pH of 5.5 is not the optimum pH for the ribonuclease T1 digestion, but it is used so as to prevent discharge of the amino acid which is promoted by pHs above neutrality. We have observed very little discharge during this digestion incubation with cotton tRNA except in the cases of arginyl–tRNA and prolyl–tRNA. The action of ribonuclease T1 on aminoacyl–tRNA is diagrammatically presented in Figure 3.

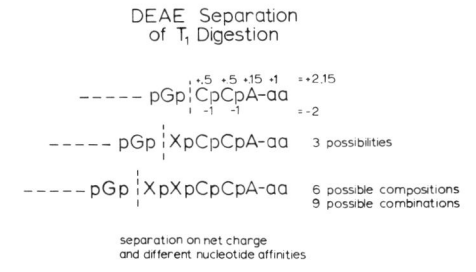

```
                    DEAE Separation
                      of T₁ Digestion

                      +.5  +.5  +.15  +.1   ≈ +2.15
        - - - - - pGp │ CpCpA-aa
                      │  -1  -1   -1         ≈ -2

        - - - - - pGp │ XpCpCpA-aa       3 possibilities

        - - - - - pGp │ XpXpCpCpA-aa     6 possible compositions
                      │                  9 possible combinations

                    separation on net charge
                    and different nucleotide affinities
```

FIGURE 3. Diagram of the action of ribonuclease T1 on ^{14}C aminoacyl–tRNA. Vertical dashed line indicates position of cleavage. Approximate electrostatic charge on the ionized groups of the ^{14}C aminoacyl oligonucleotides at pH 4.5 are shown.

This digestion mixture is applied directly to a DEAE-32–cellulose column (1 X 24 cm) that has been equilibrated with 0.01 M sodium acetate, pH 4.5. This pH is used to produce about one half of a net positive charge on cytosine residues and a slight positive charge on adenine residues. Urea, which is often used in the chromatography of oligonucleotides, is omitted in this procedure to allow maximum interaction between the nucleoside residues and the column matrix. This allows the separation of aminoacyl oligonucleotides that differ in nucleotide composition but not in nucleotide number. Radioactivity that is not retained by this column (positivity charged ^{14}C-aminoacyl oligonucleotides) is applied to a carboxymethyl-cellulose (CM-32) column of similar size equilibrated with the same buffer. The radioactive aminoacyl oligonucleotides are eluted from the DEAE column with a linear gradient (300 ml–300 ml) of 0.0–0.4 M NaCl that is 0.01 M sodium acetate, pH 4.5, and the CM column is eluted with a linear gradient (100 ml–100 ml) of 0.0–0.2 M NaCl also buffered at pH 4.5 with 0.01 M sodium acetate. There are very few aminoacyl oligonucleotides that are positively charged at this pH and the maximum net positive charge will be rather small, hence 0.2 M NaCl is sufficient to elute all of them. Elution is carried out at 30 ml/hr and 1 ml fractions are collected. This column may be run at room temperature, since most aminoacyl oligonucleotides are stable at pH 4.5. Each 1 ml fraction is mixed with 10 ml of a scintillation mixture designed for counting aqueous samples and its radioactivity determined.

If possible, the elution profiles of these columns should be monitored at 260 nm with a flow-through cell and recorder in order to verify the completeness of the ribonuclease T1 digestion by visualizing the A_{260} elution profile of the digested carrier nucleic acid that is the source of the bulk of the eluting oligonucleotides. This profile should always be the same, provided the same carrier nucleic acid is used in all experiments.

There is obviously a serious limitation to this technique in ascertaining the number and relative levels of isoaccepting tRNA species. Isoaccepting species that differ in nucleotide composition only in other parts of the polynucleotide chain, including the anticodon region, will generate the same aminoacyl oligonucleotide fragment upon digestion with ribonuclease T1, and thus not be distinguished by this technique. However, the different species demonstrated by this technique are unequivocally unique species, since differences in the CpCpA–amino acid containing fragments indicate a difference in the primary structure of isoaccepting species. Modification of the primary structure of tRNA species by methylation, alkylation, or other processes is also not manifested by this technique, since these modifications are not found on the C-C-A stem of tRNA molecules. It is conceivable that tRNA molecules having initially the same primary structure become more or less modified during development. These modifications would not be revealed by the chromatography of the ^{14}C-aminoacyl oligonucleotides. However, such modifications are not thought to influence directly the cells' capacity for translating specific code words and thereby to influence the rate of translation. These modifications may directly influence the regulation by tRNA of other steady state processes [11].

Some Results Obtained from Cotton Seed Development. Utilizing the procedures outlined above, we determined the amount of tRNA in cotton cotyledons from several developmental stages that would accept all 20 amino acids, and compared these values with those obtained with tRNA from cotton roots and from partially purified chloroplasts [21,22,23]. We also determined the number and relative levels of isoaccepting species for many of the amino acids in all these tRNA preparations.

Table II shows the percent of the total tRNA of each of these preparations that can be charged with 5 amino acids. This table at the bottom also shows the total percent of the tRNA that can be charged with the 20 amino acids, which is over 90% in each case. Notice that there is essentially no difference in the percent of the tRNA that will accept these 5 amino acids in the tRNA from cotyledons of young embryos or dry seeds and from roots. Some differences in these values are noted in tRNA from germinated cotyledons (both greened and etiolated) and distinct differences are noted when the tRNA from chloroplasts is compared with the other tRNA preparations.

About 80% more tRNA per cotyledon is present in germinated cotyledons, and the chromatographic separations of the isoaccepting species for these five amino acids (Figures 4 and 5) show that this increase is due to an increase in chloroplast tRNA per cotyledon. A detailed examination of elution profiles shown in Figures 4 and 5 will show how this fact is established.

Figure 4 shows the elution profile of isoleucyl, valyl, and methionyl oligonucleotides produced by the ribonuclese T1 digestion. This figure shows that with every tRNA preparation three different isoleucyl oligonucleotides are produced from isoleucyl–tRNA. These isoleucyl oligonucleotides indicate that at least three tRNA^{Ile} species exist in these tissues and that their relative levels are the same in the tRNA from the young embryo and dry seed cotyledons and from roots. Further, two of these species have increased relative to the third during germination, in etiolated cotyledons as well as in green cotyledons, to the extent that they comprise about 50% of the tRNA^{Ile} after 5 days of germination. The same two species are seen to be the predominant species in chloroplastic tRNA. Our interpretation of these changes in isoleucine isoacceptor levels is that the species which increase in cotyledons during germination and which predominate in the tRNA from partially purified chloroplasts are chloroplastic tRNA species. The alleged chloroplast species are shaded in this and other figures. It may be argued that the isoleucyl oligonucleotides that are seen here to increase in relative amount are not the result of an increase in the levels of existing species, but represent the de novo appearance of two new tRNA^{Ile} species that happen to yield the same isoleucyl oligonucleotide on ribonuclease T1 digestion as existing species. However, the chromatography of isoleucyl–tRNA on a reverse phase column [23] showed that the

TABLE II. Percent of Cotton tRNA Charged with Several Amino Acids[a]

Amino acid	Source of tRNA					
	Young embryo cotyledons	Dryseed cotyledons	Roots	Green cotyledons	Etiolated cotyledons	Chloroplasts
Ile	3.2	3.2	3.3	3.3	3.4	4.4
Leu	10.0	9.8	10.2	11.2	11.0	11.1
Lys	5.2	5.3	5.5	3.6	3.7	4.0
Met	3.5	3.3	3.5	4.7	4.7	5.8
Val	9.0	8.9	9.0	8.8	8.6	6.6
Total tRNA charged (sum of 20 amino acids), %	92.6	92.3	91.9	92.9	92.7	93.1

[a] Transfer RNA was prepared from the tissues indicated and charged to completion with each amino acid. The percent of the tRNA charged was calculated from assumptions given in reference 23.

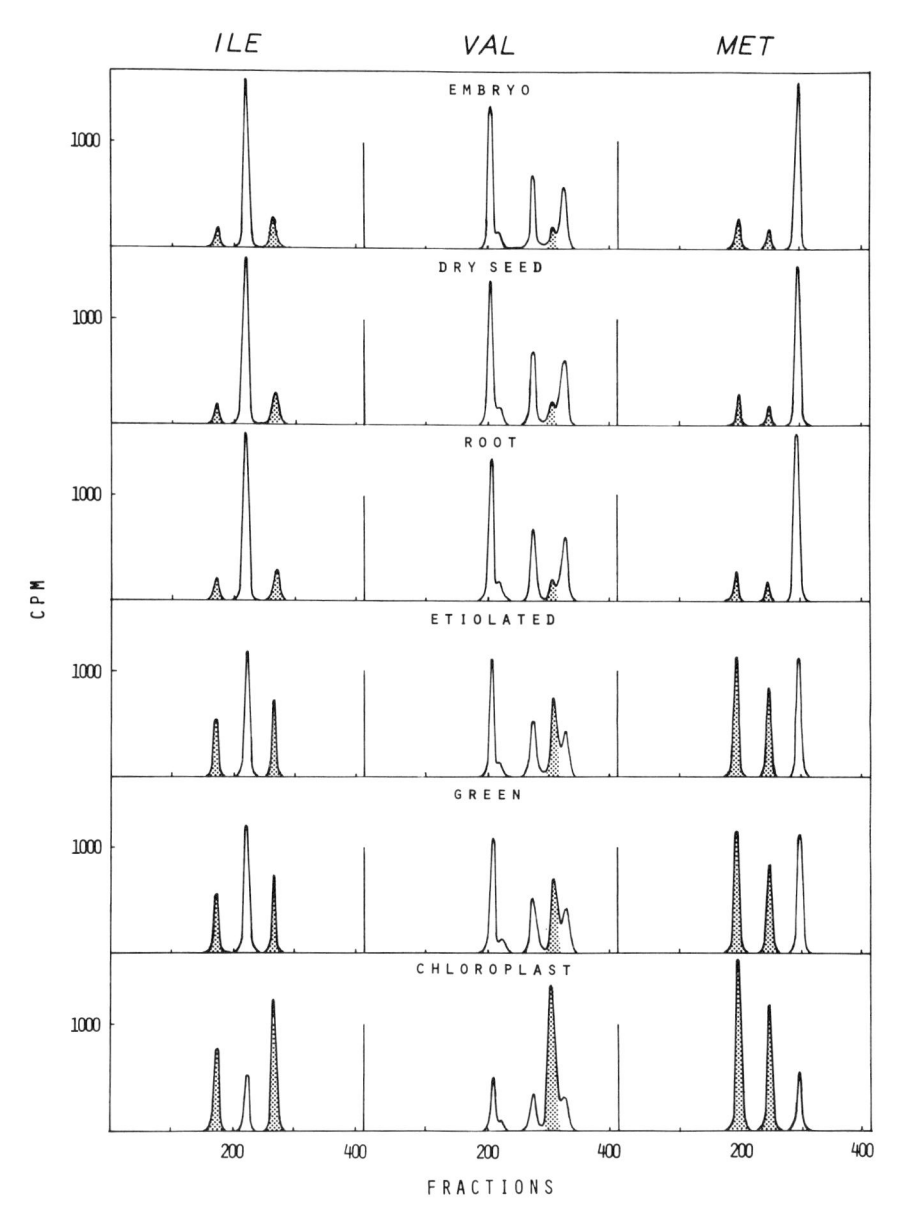

FIGURE 4. Radioactivity elution profiles of ^{14}C isoleucyl-, ^{14}C valyl, and ^{14}C methionyl oligonucleotides from DEAE-32 columns. Transfer RNA from the tissues indicated in the figure were charged with the indicated ^{14}C amino acid by a cotton cotyledon enzyme preparation and ^{14}C aminoacyl oligonucleotides were prepared from the charged tRNA by RNA T1 digestion and chromatographed as described in the text. Shaded elution peaks represent aminoacyl oligonucleotides from chloroplastic aminoacyl–tRNA. [From Merrick and Dure, 1972.]

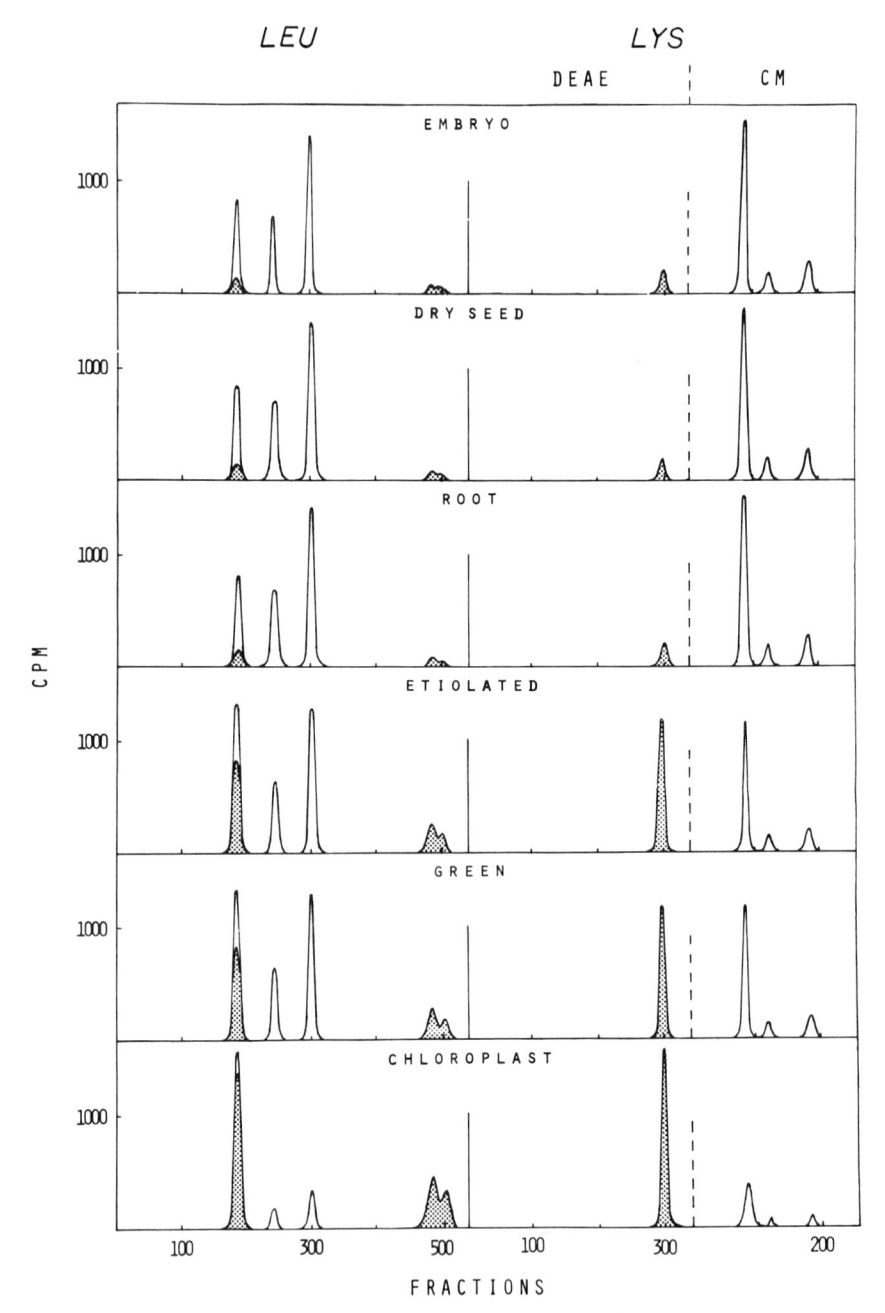

FIGURE 5. Radioactivity elution profiles of ^{14}C leucyl and ^{14}C lysyl oligonucleotides from DEAE-32 and CM-32 columns. Experimental details are presented in the legend to Figure 4 and in the text. [From Merrick and Dure, 1972.]

two minor species existing in the dry seed cotyledons are the species that increase in amount during germination and that are concentrated in chloroplasts. The elution profiles of isoleucyl—tRNA from the reverse phase column also showed that two cytoplasmic tRNA^{Ile} rather than one exist in these tRNA preparations. These two cytoplasmic species apparently produce identical isoleucyl oligonucleotides on ribonuclease T1 digestion, and thus appear as one species on the DEAE—cellulose column elution profile.

The information from the DEAE and reverse phase column taken together shows that two chloroplastic and two cytoplasmic tRNA^{Ile} species exist in all the tissues examined (including the young embryo cotyledons and roots) and that the chloroplastic species increase markedly during germination. Further, the increase in the chloroplastic species is shown not to be light dependent. The quantitative identity of the DEAE column profiles obtained with young embryo and dry seed cotyledon tRNA and root tRNA shows that not only do these tissues have the same levels of total tRNA^{Ile} relative to the total tRNA (Table II), but that they have the same levels of isoaccepting tRNA^{Ile} species.

The same pattern observed for tRNA^{Ile} species is reiterated in the case of tRNA^{Val} and tRNA^{Met} in Figure 4. There are five valyl oligonucleotides evident in this figure, one of which appears to be derived from chloroplastic tRNA by the criteria given above. Four code words exist for valine and, if chloroplastic and cytoplasmic protein synthesis are mutually exclusive in their use of tRNA, and if chloroplast protein synthesis uses the entire genetic code, there should exist at least one other chloroplastic tRNA^{Val}. Unfortunately, the reverse phase column did not resolve valyl—tRNA well enough to determine if the chloroplastic valyl oligonucleotide seen in the DEAE—cellulose column elution profile was produced by two chloroplastic tRNA^{Val} species. Notice here that the levels of the cytoplasmic tRNA^{Val} species are found not to change relative to one another during cotyledon development nor to differ from that found in root tRNA.

The DEAE column chromatography of methionyl oligonucleotides show two chloroplastic species and one cytoplasmic species. We have previously shown that the methionyl—tRNA that produces the middle methionyl oligonucleotide in the elution profile can be formylated for form N-formylmethionyl—tRNA by an endogenous cotton enzyme and by E. coli transformylase [22]. This fact further substantiates our assumption that species that increase during germination and that are concentrated in the chloroplast tRNA preparation are chloroplastic species, since formyl methionyl—tRNA has been shown to initiate chloroplastic but not cytoplasmic protein synthesis in plants. There should be at least two cytoplasmic tRNA^{Met} species also, one for polypeptide chain initiation and another for the internal positioning of methionine in translation, but we were not able to demonstrate more than one by other types of chromatography.

In Figure 5, the elution profiles of leucyl oligonucleotides from the DEAE—cellulose column and lysyl oligonucleotides from the DEAE— and CM—cellulose columns are presented. Five leucyl oligonucleotides were resolved indicating the existence of at least five tRNA^{Leu} species. However, when these preparations of tRNA were charged with an E. coli synthetase preparation and then digested with ribonuclease T1, only a portion of the leucyl oligonucleotide eluting first from the DEAE column was formed. This portion was larger in tRNA from germinated cotyledons than from younger cotyledons and roots and was almost equivalent to that formed with the cotton synthetase preparation in the chloroplast tRNA. This we interpret as indicating that the first eluting leucyl oligonucleotide is produced from two tRNA^{Leu} species—one cytoplasmic and one chloroplastic—and that the E. coli synthetase preparation charges only the chloroplastic species. (Further evidence for this interpretation is presented in reference 24.) Thus the amount that the chloroplastic tRNA^{Leu} species contributes to the first eluting leucyl oligonucleotide (shaded portion of the first peak in Figure 5) was obtained with the E. coli synthetase preparation. From this there appear to be six tRNA^{Leu} species in cotton—three cytoplasmic and three chloroplastic. Assuming that these species contain a wobble capability in their anticodons, three species are sufficient to recognize the six leucine code words. Notice again that, although the chloroplast species increase in amount per cell during germination, there is no change in the levels of the cytoplasmic species relative to each other nor in the levels of the chloroplastic species relative to each other during cotyledon development nor between young cotyledon and root tRNA.

Only one of the lysyl oligonucleotides was retained by the DEAE—cellulose column, whereas three others were retained by the CM—cellulose column, indicating that they bear a net positive charge at pH 4.5. Only a limited number of lysyl oligonucleotides would be positively charged at this pH, and consequently it is possible to assume the nucleotide composition of these three lysyl oligonucleotides as being, in order of elution, ApCpCpA—lysine, CpCpCpA—lysine and CpCpA—lysine, with positive charges of about 0.4, 0.7, and 1.2 electrostatic units (ESU), respectively. (Free lysine is also retained by the CM—cellulose column at pH 4.5, but it elutes from this column earlier in the salt gradient than any of these three lysyl oligonucleotides.)

Our original purpose for investigating the number and levels of iso-accepting tRNA species in developing cotton cotyledons was to see if any of the developmental transitions that this tissue goes through are reflected in a coincident change in its tRNA pool. Our total findings on this subject and their possible meaning are given in reference 23. Briefly, as can be surmized from the data presented here for the five amino acids illustrating our techniques, we found no changes in the number and levels of cytoplasmic tRNA species during cotyledon development. We did find a large increase in the total amount of chloroplast species that takes place during germination in the dark as well as in the light. Furthermore, we observed that chloroplast tRNA species are present in cotton roots (which surprised us but few others). However, as shown in Figures 4 and 5, the levels of the chloroplast species do not change relative to one another, but only relative to the cytosol tRNA.

In summary, these types of experiments on tRNA pools illustrate the obligation for extremely critical quantitation that must be employed in studying the molecular bases of tissue development and maturation.

REFERENCES

[1] Gallo, R. C., and S. Pestka. 1970. J. Mol. Biol. 52:195.
[2] Crick, F. H. C. 1966. J. Mol. Biol. 19:548.
[3] Weiss, J. F., and A. D. Kelmers. 1967. Biochemistry 6:2507.
[4] Yang, W. K., and G. D. Novelli. 1968. Proc. Nat. Acad. Sci. U.S. 95:208.
[5] Muench, K. H., and P. A. Safille. 1968. Biochemistry 7:2799.
[6] Garen, A. 1968. Science 160:149.
[7] Borek, E. (Ed.) 1971. Symposium on transfer RNA and transfer RNA modification in differentiation and neoplasia. In Cancer Res. 31:591.
[8] Söll, D. 1971. Science 173:293.
[9] Armstrong, D. J., W. J. Burrows, F. Skoog, K. L. Roy, and D. Söll. 1969. Proc. Nat. Acad. Sci. U.S. 63:834.
[10] Lewis, J. A., and B. N. Ames. 1972. J. Mol. Biol. 66:131.
[11] Singer, C. E., G. R. Smith, R. Cortese, and B. N. Ames. 1972. Nature New Biol. 283:72.
[12] Jacobson, R. B. 1971. Nature New Biol. 231:17.
[13] Loening, U. 1967. Biochem. J. 102:251.
[14] Leaver, C. J., and J. Ingle. 1971. Biochem. J. 123:235.
[15] Watson, J. D. 1970. Molecular biology of the gene (2nd ed.). W. A. Benjamin, New York. p. 85.
[16] Brown, D. D., and E. Littna. 1966. J. Mol. Biol. 20:95.
[17] Bollum, F. J. 1966. In G. L. Cantoni and D. R. Davies (Ed.), Procedures in nucleic acid research. Harper and Row, New York. 296p.
[18] Weiss, J. F., R. L. Pearson, and A. D. Kelmers. 1968. Biochemistry 7:3479.

[19] Pearson, R. L., J. F. Weiss, and A. D. Kelmers. 1971. Biochem. Biophys. Acta 228:770.
[20] Gefter, M. L., and R. L. Russell. 1969. J. Mol. Biol. 39:145.
[21] Dure, L. S., III and W. C. Merrick. 1971. In N. K. Boardman, A. W. Linnane, and R. M. Smillie (Ed.), Autonomy and biogenesis of mitochondria and chloroplasts. North-Holland, London. 413 p.
[22] Merrick, W. C., and L. S. Dure, III. 1971. Proc. Nat. Acad. Sci. U.S. 68:641.
[23] Merrick, W. C., and L. S. Dure, III. 1972. J. Biol. Chem. 247:7988.
[24] Merrick, W. C., and L. S. Dure, III. 1973. Biochem. 12:629.

Methods for the Study of Hybridization and Reassociation of Nucleic Acids Extracted from Cells of Higher Animals

R.B. CHURCH

SECTION I INTRODUCTION

The double-helix structure of native DNA depends on the complementary relationships between nucleotide pairs. In 1959 Marmur and Doty showed that, when aqueous solutions of native DNA were heated, the two strands of the duplex molecule could be dissociated. They also showed that, during slow cooling of the heat-denatured bacterial DNA, the separated complementary strands recognized each other in a reassociation reaction which reestablished the original duplex molecule. The reassociation of single-stranded DNA from different bacterial species to form hybrid molecules was described by Schildkraut, Marmur, and Doty [1961]. Their observations led to the development of various hybridization techniques to examine DNA/DNA and DNA/RNA duplexes. Due to the size of the genome of higher animals it was then anticipated that the enormous dilution of individual nucleotide sequences would make reassociation of these nucleic acids impractical. However, Bolton's group at the Carnegie Institution observed reassociation of vertebrate DNA in 1964 which was followed by a hypothesis formulated by Waring and Britten [1966] that some nucleotide sequences were repeated to varying degrees in the DNA of vertebrates. The general occurrence of repeated sequences in DNA and techniques for the characterization of the various classes of nucleotide sequence reiteration has been elegantly described by Britten and Kohne [1968]. Recently, Laird [1971], Flamm [1971], and Bostock [1971] have provided detailed examinations of the possible biological relationships of the nonreiterated and reiterated DNA sequences in the genomes of complex organisms, respectively.

Influence of Reiterated DNA Base Sequences on Hybridization.

Almost all of the evidence for the existence of reiterated sequences has been obtained from reassociation experiments. DNA reassociation involves two processes. The first is an initial nucleation reaction in which various lengths of complementary sequences form a stable duplex. The criteria of the reaction conditions will set the length and specificity of nucleotide sequence required for this nucleation reaction to occur [McCarthy and McConaughy, 1968]. After the initial nucleation reaction stabilizes the two strands, a zipper reaction completes the nucleotide base-pairing along the rest of the duplex molecule. The first part of the hybridization reaction is usually the rate-limiting process unless the reaction involves very highly reiterated sequences such as the adenylic-thymidylic (AT)-rich sequences in the mouse. The rate of renaturation of fully denatured DNA is kinetically a second-order reaction with a maximum rate of reaction some 20–25°C below the mean thermal denaturation temperature (T_m) of native DNA [Wetmur and Davidson, 1968] for viral and bacterial nucleic acids. Nuclear DNA extracted from eukaryotic organisms contains base sequences which do not follow the expected second-order kinetics of reassociation, but reassociate very much faster than would be expected if each sequence were present once per genome, as well as sequences which follow the expected second-order reassociation kinetics. If nucleotide sequences are repeated within a haploid genome their effective concentration is increased by that relative amount, hence, reassociation of the reiterated sequences is faster than would be expected for the genome size. The sequences which reassociate at a rate consistent with the genome size are present once, or are single copy, base sequences. In the terminology introduced by Britten and Kohne [1968] the rate of reassociation may be expressed by $C_0 t$, which is defined as the product of the nucleic acid concentration expressed as moles of nucleotides per liter (C_0) times the incubation time in seconds (t). Therefore, $C_0 t\ 1/2$ is the product of the initial concentration of denatured DNA expressed as molarity of nucleotides and time in seconds at 50% reassociation. The data must be corrected for fragment size and the effect of base composition [Wetmur and Davidson, 1968] and for standard phosphate buffer [Britten, 1970]. An easy approximation in practice is to express $C_0 t$ in terms of absorbancy, as

$$C_0 t = (A_{260/2}) \times \text{incubation time (hr)}$$

A $C_0 t$ of 1 (mole × sec/liter) results if 83 μg of DNA (400 nucleotide fragment size) is incubated in 0.12 M sodium phosphate buffer (PB) for 1 hr at 60°C.

When the haploid genome contains only unique or nonrepeated nucleotide sequences, the size of the genome can be estimated directly from the $C_0 t$ 1/2 value. The reassociation of double-stranded DNA from various sources is shown in Figure 1. The proportionality between the $C_0 t$ 1/2 that is required, for completion of one half of the reassociation reaction of DNA, and the genome size is only true in the absence of repeated DNA sequences, that is, T4, E. coli, and unique mouse DNA. The reassociation curve for total mouse DNA reveals the presence of three general categories of DNA base sequences within the haploid genome. The reassociation profile suggests that the mouse genome contains a very rapidly reassociating fraction which contains the AT-rich satellite and has

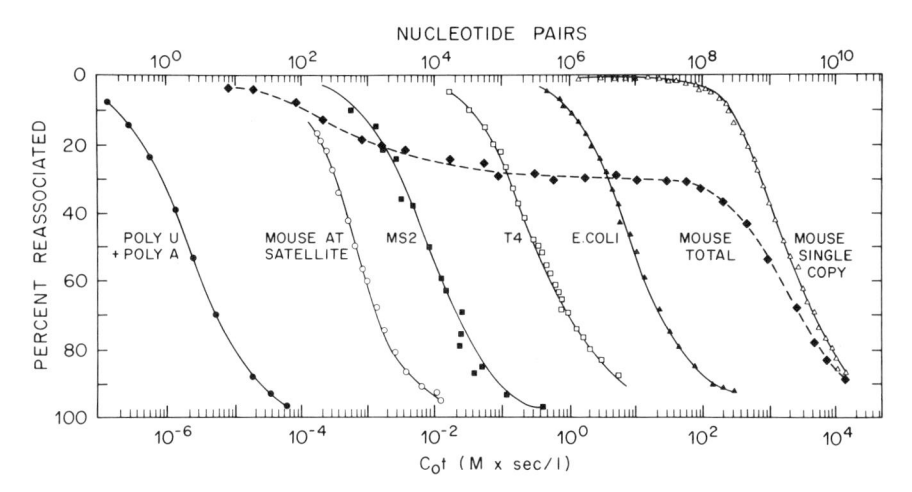

FIGURE 1. Reassociation of DNA from various sources. The reassociation kinetics of DNA, from various sources, in 0.12 M PB at 60°C. Unlabeled total mouse DNA (2 mg/ml) was mixed with ^{3}H-labeled single copy mouse DNA (1 μg/ml $C_0 t$ 220), both 400–500 nucleotides, and ^{14}C-labeled E. coli DNA (10 μg/ml) 550–600 nucleotides in 0.12 M PB. The mixture was heat-denatured, quickly cooled to 60°C and 50 μliter aliquots removed at the appropriate time ($C_0 t$) intervals for analysis on hydroxyapatite. The ^{3}H-labeled DNA (230,000 cpm/μg) isolated from mouse L-cells was heat-denatured and incubated at 60°C in 0.12 M PB to $C_0 t_{220}$. The single-stranded DNA was eluted from hydroxyapatite with 0.14 M PB, concentrated by vacuum dialysis, heat-denatured and reassociation allowed to proceed to $C_0 t_{220}$ in 0.12 M PB at 60°C. The nonrenatured sequences which were eluted from the hydroxyapatite in 0.12 M PB were used for the renaturation kinetics presented. The MS2, Poly U + Poly A and T4 renaturation profiles are those presented by Britten and Kohne [1968]. The mouse satellite reassociation kinetics were carried out in 0.05 M PB at 60°C with 0.1 μg ^{3}H-satellite DNA per ml. The AT-rich satellite was isolated, from the same ^{3}H-labeled cell DNA used for the isolation of single copy DNA for the reassociation experiment presented after fractionation on a CsCl gradient.

a reiteration of about 10^6. Sequence analysis of this AT-rich fraction which comprises about 10% of the genome suggests that the repeating units have a corrected complexity of 140 base pairs [Sutton and McCallum, 1971].

The second rapidly reassociating fraction, sometimes called intermediate, makes up approximately 20–25% of the mouse genome and reassociates at an average rate of from a few to 10^5 times faster than is expected for nucleotide sequences present only once per haploid genome. In view of the low RNA and DNA concentrations and the relatively short reaction times used for most molecular hybridization studies, these must be the DNA base sequences involved in the duplex reaction. Therefore, the design of hybridization experiments utilizing nucleic acids isolated from higher organisms must consider the criteria of reassociation as having prime importance.

Reaction Criteria

Criteria can be defined by the stringency of base-pairing required by the incubation conditions (see below). The rapidly reassociating or reiterated sequences found in the genomes of higher organisms reassociate as families of similar but not identical nucleotide sequences [Britten and Kohne, 1968]. As a consequence, molecular hybridization with the reiterated nucleotide sequences will rarely display absolute base sequence complementarity since the chance of the two DNA strands originally paired in native DNA of reacting with other sequences of the reiterated family is much greater [McCarthy and McConaughy, 1968].

Similarly, the presence of reiterated DNA base sequences in the RNA/DNA hybridization reaction means that RNA sequences will seldom have the chance of reacting with their original transcriptional site within a family of reiterated DNA sequences [Church and McCarthy, 1968]. The reassociation criteria which include salt concentration, concentration of organic solvents, temperature, nucleic acid fragment size and concentration in combination with time of incubation will govern the base sequence mismatching tolerated in duplex formation. The degree of base sequence mismatching can be estimated by determination of the Tm of the duplexes formed. Laird, McConaughy, and McCarthy [1969] established that a 1.5% change in base-pairing is reflected in a 1°C change in the mean thermal denaturation temperature (T_m). The particular choice of reassociation criteria for an experimental system will depend on the practical aspects of labeling in the biological system and some compromise between the extent of reaction and the specificity chosen by the investigator. Theoretically, with ultimate criteria, all sequences could conceivably behave as unique sequences. Under the conditions used in Figure 1, approximately 65% of the mouse DNA sequences reassociate at a rate constant which is consis-

REASSOCIATION OF NUCLEIC ACIDS

tent with the expected second order kinetics predicted for the mouse genome if each sequence were present once. The degree of specificity of base-pairing is dependent on the conditions of reassociation, hence the distinction between reiterated and unique sequences is an arbitrary one [McCarthy and Church, 1970].

Reassociation Reaction Conditions

The optimal reaction conditions for the reassociation of bacterial and viral DNA's have been investigated by Marmur, Round, and Schildkraut [1963] and more recently by Wetmur and Davidson [1968]. In general, we note: (1) The rate of reaction increases with sodium ion concentration above 0.01 M. (2) The incubation temperature has a flat maximum 15–30°C below the T_m of the native DNA. (3) The incubation time and concentration of nucleic acids must be high enough to permit sufficient random nucleation collisions between complementary strands. (4) The size and homogeneity of the DNA fragments affects the rate of reassociation hence to allow the unit genome concept to have meaning most workers use DNA fragments of about 400 nucleotides.

Therefore, to achieve reproducible results within any experimental reassociation system, the cation concentration, the temperature of incubation, the DNA and RNA concentration, and the DNA and RNA fragment size must be controlled. The investigator can achieve the desired degree of base pair matching in the duplex formed by manipulation of any or all of these factors. Complete denaturation of the native DNA duplex is required to enable an accurate estimation of the 0 time point.

SECTION II ISOLATION AND CHARACTERIZATION OF MAMMALIAN NUCLEIC ACIDS

Preparation of Mammalian RNA

Mammalian RNA can be fractionated in a number of ways; at the nuclear cytoplasmic level; by isolation of polysomes from which 28 S and 18 S ribosomal RNA and presumptive messenger RNA can be obtained; by extraction of the chromatin gel; or by differential extraction with a combination of phenol and temperature. The following procedure is applicable to the isolation of heterogenous nuclear RNA from purified nuclei or for total cellular RNA [Church and McCarthy, 1968]. All steps are carried out at 4°C unless noted.

(1) Freshly excised tissue is homogenized vigorously in 0.25 M sucrose, 0.03 M $CaCl_2$, 0.01 M Tris (pH 7.4) (10/1 v/w). Alternatively for nuclear

RNA, nuclei, purified as described for the isolation of DNA, are homogenized to obtain complete nuclei suspension.

(2) An equal volume of 0.28 M LiCl, 0.02 M sodium acetate, 0.003 M $MgCl_2$, and 1% SDS (pH 6.1) is added, and the mixture homogenized further in a glass-Teflon homogenizer.

(3) The viscous white suspension is then sonicated in a BRANSON Sonifier (LS) for 1 min at peak output to disrupt the chromatin gel and increase hybridization efficiency [Church and McCarthy, 1968].

(4) An equal volume of freshly redistilled water-saturated phenol (pH 7–7.5) at 70°C is added and the mixture is then shaken for 10 min before being cooled to 4°C.

(5) The white cloudy mixture is centrifuged for 10 min at 5000 X g at 4°C and the aqueous supernatant removed. The supernatant will be slightly cloudy for nuclear RNA and quite cloudy for cellular homogenates.

(6) The interphase is then reextracted with an equal volume of 85°C phenol for 10 min while shaking, then cooled and spun as before, and the supernatant pooled with the first supernatant.

(7) The RNA can then be precipitated from the aqueous supernatant by the addition of 2 vol of ice cold ethanol for greater than 4 hr at −20°C or if the supernatant is very cloudy, further deproteinized by the addition of an equal volume of room temperature phenol before ethanol precipitation.

(8) The flocculent white precipitate is collected by centrifugation at 2000 X g for 10 min and taken up in 0.01 M $MgCl_2$, 0.01 M Tris, pH 7.4 and digested with 10 μg/ml of electrophoretically pure deoxyribonuclease (Worthington) for 1 hr at 37°C.

(9) The mixture is further treated with phenol as in step 7 before precipitation with ethanol once more. After draining off the ethanol, the deoxyribonuclease digestion step is repeated, followed by two further deproteinizations with phenol as before.

(10) After precipitation, the RNA is dissolved in 1/10 X SSC or 0.03 M PB and eluted from G-50 Sephadex to remove oligonucleotides, protein, and glycogen.

(11) The eluted fraction from G-50 Sephadex is then passed over a Chelex 100 (200–400 mesh, Biorad) resin column in the sodium form to remove traces of heavy metals.

(12) The major fraction is then precipitated by the addition of 2 vol of ice cold ethanol and stored at −20°C.

(13) The precipitate is collected by centrifugation at 10,000 X g for 20 min

at 4°C and suspended in 1/10 × SSC or 0.03 M PB at a concentration of 10–15 mg/ml for storage at −20°C.

These procedures were designed to maintain low cation concentrations in order to preclude accumulation of salt during the preparation of RNA. In the case of brain RNA isolation, it was found that further purification by the cetyltriethyl ammonium (CTA) bromide method of Bellamy and Ralph [1968] was advantageous.

In reassociation studies utilizing mammalian RNA [Church and McCarthy, 1968], increased hybridization efficiency occurred when the labeled RNA was degraded to a relatively homogenous population of molecules sedimenting at about 4–6 S. These authors also noted that RNA used in reassociation reactions was a more effective reactant if the RNA solution was heated before use.

The considerable secondary structure contained in mammalian RNA is, presumably, destroyed by the heating step.

The binding of the poly (A) 3' terminal end sequences of at least some messenger RNA species to "Millipore" filters under conditions which might be used in DNA/RNA hybridization reactions must be considered [Kates, 1970]. The unique properties of Poly (A) allow this polymer to bind to denatured proteins and Millipore filters in the presence of 0.5 M KCl. This characteristic of poly (A) has been used to isolate potential messenger RNA species [Lee, Mendecki, and Brawerman, 1971]. Many laboratories have succeeded in isolating presumptive mRNA's coding for a number of proteins. The ultimate in RNA preparations for reassociation studies would be a "pure" mRNA population.

Some characteristics of RNA which must be considered in the design of hybridization reactions are:

(1) RNA which has a large amount of secondary structure, that is, "hairpins," must be hybridized at temperatures above the T_m of the RNA to melt out secondary structure.
(2) For unique sequence reassociation reactions which are for extended periods of time, the RNA must be ultrapure and preferably passed over Chelex or SE-Sephadex columns to remove heavy metals and prevent degradation.
(3) For the same type of reactions, high temperatures without formamide will result in excessive RNA degradation. RNA may be sheared to 4–6 S before hybridization to minimize the effects of molecular weight.

in vitro Labeling of RNA

Although several methods of in vitro labeling of RNA have been tried in the past none has proven to be ideal for molecular hybridization reactions. Often the greatest limitation to mammalian in vivo gene activity studies is the lack of sufficiently high specific activity RNA.

The random in vitro methylation of RNA in the presence of labeled dimethyl sulfate has been used extensively since described by Smith, Armstrong, and McCarthy, [1967]. The success of this technique lies with the purity of the dimethyl sulfate, RNA free from detectable contamination of degraded DNA, basic proteins, and polysaccharides.

Recently, Commerford [1971] described a technique for the iodination of cytosine and DNA with ^{125}I. This method has been modified and used for ^{125}I in vitro labeling of RNA for hybridization studies by Getz, Altenburg, and Saunders, [1972]. They have succeeded in obtaining specific activities of greater than 200,000 cpm/μg of human lymphocyte RNA.

The dimethyl sulfate in vitro labeling of RNA involves:

(1) 0.5–1.0 mg of RNA dissolved in 0.1–0.2 ml of 0.1 M PB, pH 7.4 is prepared in a silicone-coated vial. The uniformity of labeling is increased when the RNA to be labeled is sheared to 4–6 S. Reproducible results require RNA purified by elution from SE-50 Sephadex or Chelex 100. The volume and RNA concentrations are maximums for efficient labeling because of the two phase system of methylation.

(2) The RNA mixture is heated to 85°C and quickly cooled to 25°C for the methylation incubation.

(3) Labeled ^{14}C or ^{3}H dimethyl sulfate in benzene with the highest specific activity available (greater than 150 millicuries (mC)/mmole) is made up to the desired stock solution by addition of 0–20 mg of analytical grade nonlabeled dimethyl sulfate to give a 0.07–0.27 M solution in 0.5 ml of diethyl ether. The molarity of the solution and the specific activity will depend on the extent of labeling required. For example, dimethyl sulfate with a specific activity of 150 mC/mmole made to 0.27 M with 20 mg of unlabeled dimethyl sulfate in 0.5 ml of ether will result in a stock solution with a specific activity of approximately 300 microcuries (μC)/mg. For higher specific activities no nonlabeled carrier dimethyl sulfate is added.

(4) Add 10–20 μliter of the dimethyl sulfate stock solution to the RNA mixture. The reaction is incubated in a tightly stoppered silicone-glass vial with vigorous shaking for 10–60 min at 25°C.

(5) The time of incubation is determined by the extent of in vitro methylation desired in the RNA. If in vitro methylation exceeds 7% of the RNA bases, the specificity of base-pairing of such labeled RNA is reduced.

There is a direct correlation, during the initial stages of the reaction, between the time and concentration of dimethyl sulfate reagent and the extent of RNA bases methylated.

(6) After the reaction the RNA is precipitated with 2 vol of ice cold ethanol and left for 4 hr at $-20°C$.

(7) The RNA precipitate is spun out of the solution, the pellet dissolved in 1/10 × SSC and reprecipitated with ethanol.

(8) Finally, the RNA is eluted from a G25 Sephadex column in 0.1 M NaCl, 0.01 M sodium acetate. The eluted fractions are precipitated with 2 vol of ethanol overnight at $-20°C$.

(9) The location of the radioactivity can be checked by its stability in alkali. Complete digestion is observed by treatment of the methylated RNA with 0.3 M KOH for 3 hr at $50°C$.

(10) Lawley and Brookes [1963] have shown that methyl groups were attached to 65% guanine, 24% adenine, and 11% cytosine residues.

(11) Specific activities of 2440 cpm $^3H/\mu g$ of mouse RNA have been obtained when 1 mg of RNA/ml in 0.15 ml 0.1 M PB was reacted with 500 μC of dimethyl sulfate. Smith, Armstrong, and McCarthy [1967] and Morrison, Paul, and Williamson [1972] have shown that when RNA labeled in vivo with ^{14}C and ^{32}P is methylated in vitro with ^3H-dimethyl sulfate that the hybridization and thermal dissociation properties of the two labels in the RNA/DNA duplex are fairly similar.

The best way of labeling RNA in vitro would appear to be the iodination, with ^{125}I, a technique perfected by Getz, Altenburg and Saunders [1972]. The procedure involves:

(1) Making a stock solution of carrier free ^{125}I by diluting NaI (100 mC/ml) with distilled water to give a final concentration of 5 mC/ml. The stock solution is stored in the dark at $-20°C$.

(2) 1 mg of purified RNA is dissolved in 0.1 M sodium acetate, 0.04 M acetic acid, pH 5.0, at $0°C$. The solution is made 6.25×10^{-5} M KI, 0.5 mC ^{125}I and 2.3×10^{-3} M thallium chloride ($TlCl_3$) in that order to a total volume of 2.0 ml.

(3) The reaction mixture is heated to $60°C$ for 10–30 min and then chilled in an ice bath.

(4) 0.1 ml of a freshly prepared 0.1 M Na_2SO_3 solution is added and the pH raised to 8.7 by addition of 0.15 ml of 1 M ammonium acetate, 0.5 M NH_4OH.

(5) The mixture is reheated to $60°C$ for 20 min and chilled in an ice bath.

(6) The mixture is then eluted from a G-25 Sephadex column (0.6 × 75 cm) with H_2O followed by elution from HA with 0.2 M PB.
(7) The fractions comprising 1 void vol are pooled and lyophilized to dryness.
(8) The RNA is dissolved in 2.0 ml of 0.01 M Tris HCl pH 8.0. The reaction mixture is made 50 μg/ml Pronase (self-digested nuclease-free, Calbiochem) and incubated for 30 min at 25°C. The labeled ^{125}I solution has an unidentified, phenol-soluble, Pronase-digestible contaminant.
(9) Radioactive ^{125}I can be counted in a standard toluene-based liquid scintillation system with discriminators set at 20-1000 with 20% gain (Packard 3375). Since there is considerable spillover into the ^3H and ^{14}C channels, RNA labeled with ^{125}I can only be used conveniently with ^{32}P-DNA for reassociation.
(10) The mixture is then extracted three times with chloroform:isoamyl alcohol (24:1), twice with ether, and purged with dry N_2.
(11) The RNA is precipitated by addition of 1/10 vol 20% potassium acetate, pH 5, followed by 2.5 vol ice cold ethanol for 16 hr at −20°C.

Preparation of Mammalian Nuclear DNA

Nuclei are prepared by a procedure originally described by Chauveau, Moule, and Rouiller, [1956] as modified by Church and McCarthy [1968].

(1) Freshly excised tissue, preferably spleen or testes, is rinsed with ice cold distilled water and plunged into ice cold 0.32 M sucrose, 0.01 M Tris HCl (pH 7.6), 0.03 M $MgCl_2$ in approximately a 1:10 ratio (w/v).
(2) The tissue is quickly minced with scissors and rapidly homogenized by 2-10 passages through a motor-driven Teflon-glass homogenizer at 4°C.
(3) The homogenate is filtered through washed cheesecloth (four layers) and once through miracloth (Chicopee Mills, N.Y.) to remove connective tissue and cell debris.
(4) The filtrate is centrifuged at 1200-1500 × g for 10-15 min at 4°C.
(5) After centrifugation, the cloudy supernatant is discarded and the whitish nuclear pellet suspended in approximately 5 vol of ice cold 0.01 M Tris HCl (pH 7.6) before adding an equal volume of ice cold 0.075 M NaCl, 0.01 M Tris HCl, 0.025 M EDTA.
(6) The mixture is shaken and spun for 5 min at 3000 × g at 4°C. The white nuclear pellet is then suspended in 5-10 vol of the same buffer.
(7) The mixture is then placed on 2 vol (to the total) of ice cold 2.2 M sucrose, 0.01 M Tris HCl, 0.005 M $MgCl_2$, and spun at 35,000 × g for 20 min at 4°C.

(8) The clear white nuclear pellet is then fully suspended in 10 vol (w/v) ice cold distilled H_2O. The homogenous suspension is made 0.05 M EDTA, 0.075 M NaCl and 1% SDS at 4°C. The nearly clear viscous mixture can be adjusted to obtain a manageable viscosity with 1/10 × SSC.

(9) The mixture is made 1 M with respect to sodium perchlorate ($NaClO_4$) for deproteinization or made 200 μg/ml with self-digested Pronase (Calbiochem) and incubated for 2 hr at 37°C. All clumps should have disappeared by this time.

(10) An equal volume of chloroform/octanol (10/1) is added, and the white cloudy mixture shaken for 5–10 min at room temperature, cooled to 4°C and spun at 4°C until a tightly packed interphase is obtained.

(11) The chloroform/octanol extraction of the viscous aqueous phase is repeated until a minimum interphase is detected. Finally, the viscous aqueous phase is removed and precipitated with 2 vol of ice cold ethanol.

(12) The precipitated DNA should spool out readily as a crystal clear gel on a glass rod.

(13) The gel-like precipitate is blotted dry and taken into solution in 0.03 M PB or 1/10 × SSC. Solubilization should be rapid and complete. We prefer to start again if the sample is cloudy at this stage.

(14) RNA contamination can be removed by dialysis against 0.25 N NaOH for 15 hr followed by dialysis against 0.03 M PB or 1/10 × SSC for 10 hr at 15°C or the mixture can be made 1 × SSC and incubated with electrophoretically pure boiled ribonuclease (Worthington) (5 min at 10 mg/ml) at 10–20 μg/ml for 30–45 min at 37°C. A mixture of 4:1 units of pancreatic : T1 ribonuclease activities has given good results.

(15) The ribonuclease can be removed by making the solution 50 μg/ml with respect to self-digested Pronase and incubation continued for 30 min at 37°C.

(16) The residual protein is then removed by repeated phenol and chloroform/octanol extractions until no visible interphase is evident (usually 2–3 times).

(17) The DNA is then precipitated with ice cold ethanol until the precipitation mixture is clear after spooling.

(18) The DNA is then checked for nuclease activity by incubating an aliquot with labeled RNA and DNA to test any loss in acid-precipitable radioactivity of each sample.

(19) The final sample in 1/10 × SSC or 0.03 M PB is then centrifuged for 1 hr at 10,000 × g in the presence of homogenously dispersed, acid-washed

Norite. After precipitation with ethanol again, the final product should be crystal clear.
(20) DNA can be stored under ethanol or in an appropriate buffer in the presence of a drop of chloroform.
(21) Purity is determined by a spectral scan from 230 to 300 mμ and by melting an aliquot in a recording spectrophotometer. There should be very little increase in optical density below 65°C and a normal hyperchronicity of greater than 33 and 20% is required for native and sheared DNA, respectively.

Denaturation of DNA is such a common procedure and the parameters have been known for so long [Marmur and Doty, 1959] that it may appear trite to emphasize the matter. However, for successful reassociation experiments, it is absolutely essential that nucleic acid preparations be not only as pure as possible but that the denaturation of all double-stranded molecules be complete before the reassociation reaction commences. The reassociation reaction consists of a two step process, nucleation and zippering. If renatured DNA is examined at intervals throughout the reaction, the initial reaction products are much richer in GC pairs than the final duplexes. Therefore, the nucleation sites appear to involve nuclei rich in GC regions [Thrower and Peacock, 1968], with a reassociation rate which is slightly faster than the lower G + C regions of the genome [Wetmur and Davidson, 1968]. Incomplete denaturation will be reflected in low hypochromatic shifts in optical melting studies and by incorrect estimates of the percentage of reiterated sequences in a genome. The apparent rapid reassociation at 0 time is discussed under DNA reassociation.

Denaturation can be accomplished by holding the high concentration of sheared DNA (1–8 mg/ml) required for some studies in 0.03 M PB in boiling water for 10 min after the buffer has reached 95°C.

The solution is then plunged into an acetone dry ice bath to cool but is not frozen. For denaturation of high molecular weight DNA which is to be loaded onto membrane filters, we prefer to hold DNA concentrations of less than 100 μg/ml in 1/10 × SSC for 10 min in a boiling water bath. The mixture is immediately poured into sufficient ice cold 4 × SSC to give a final DNA concentration of less than 10 μg/ml. By cooling all denaturation solutions as quickly as possible to 4°C the "snap-back" and rapid "apparent" reassociation is minimized. Laird [1971] has suggested 5–7% of the initial optical reassociation is due to base-stacking while the strand cross-linking of Alberts and Doty [1968] may be responsible for some DNA structure.

The addition of an organic solvent, such as formamide, may be required to lower the T_m to a convenient working temperature if an investigator is primarily interested in the very rapidly reassociating DNA sequences.

If the specially built air-operated shear press developed by Britten and Kohne [1968] is used to shear DNA by passage through a needle valve with a pressure drop of 3.4 kilobar (50,000 psi) the DNA is denatured unless a salt concentration of above 0.6 M PB is used to increase the T_m.

A successful combination of shearing technique, removal of all cations (particularly heavy metals) and denaturation will provide reproducible rates of reassociation with a minimum of aggregate formation.

Preparation of DNA Fragments

All DNA sequence fragments used for reassociation should be analyzed for length distribution in alkaline sucrose gradients or by sedimentation velocity analysis by moving boundary sedimentation in an alkaline high-salt solution (that is, 0.9 M NaCl, 0.1 M NaOH) where molecular weights can be calculated from the relationship of Studier [1965]:

$$S_{20,w} = 0.0528 \, M^{0.4}$$

In alkaline sucrose gradients caution must be exercised in the estimation of the molecular weights of fragments sedimenting slower than about 5 S. Fragments sedimenting at 4.5 S have been estimated to have a single-strand molecular weight of 66,000 dalton corresponding to a single-strand fragment length of 200 nucleotides [Saunders et al., 1972] after shearing by extensive sonication. Laird [1971] has used one passage through a pressure cell at 12,000 psi to shear mouse DNA of a molecular weight of 11.5×10^6 dalton, down to a homogenous single-strand molecular weight of 1.2×10^5 dalton. This corresponds to a fragment length of about 400 nucleotides. Laird [1971] estimated molecular weights by band velocity sedimentation, using the coefficients of Studier [1965], during sedimentation at 42,040 rpm at 25°C in a Spinco AnD rotor using a band forming centerpiece 331346.

In our laboratory we have used sonication and passage of native DNA through French Pressure Cells to shear macromolecules to a homogeneous fragment population. In our hands, a Branson Sonifier model W-185C (up to 4 min of total sonication time at 4°C) results in more heterogeneity and fragment end denaturation than does fragmentation by shearing through a Pressure Cell.

The Pressure Cell used must be carefully calibrated as to its shearing efficiency since the size and angle of the orifice and the velocity, as measured by pressure drop, effect the fragment size and homogeneity. Therefore a standard curve of the empirical relationship between pressure and molecular weights of the fragments produced is essential. Flow rates for shearing of high molecular weight DNA, at 4°C, through a pressure cell should be less than a uniform 1 ml/min at as steady a pressure as possible.

The effect of fragment size on the apparent reassociation as distinguished on HA columns compared to optical reassociation is illustrated in Figure 2 for mouse DNA. Reproducible distributions of DNA fragment lengths, suggested by a uniform sedimentation peak in alkaline sucrose gradients, have been reported by Saunders et al. [1972]. They purged 250 μg/ml of purified DNA in 2 × SSC with N_2 for 10 min in a plastic beaker. Ultrasonic fragmentation

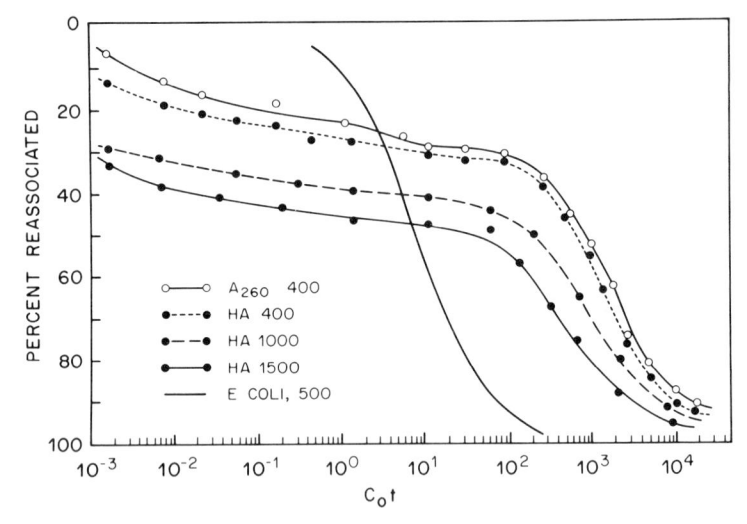

FIGURE 2. Effect of fragment size on HA reassociation analysis. The effect of fragment size on the apparent rate of reassociation assayed by hyperchromicity at 260 nm and by elution from HA. Labeled ^{3}H mouse DNA (42,000 cpm/μg) was sheared at various pressures to produce DNA fragments of 400 (2 × 12,000 psi), 1000 (1 × 5500 psi) and 1500 (1 × 4000 psi) nucleotide size respectively. The DNA samples were heat-denatured and reassociated in 0.12 M PB at 60°C to the indicated $C_o t$ values in the presence of 10 μg ^{14}C-E. coli DNA. Duplicate samples were removed at each time interval and subjected to: (1) elution from HA with 0.12 M PB and 0.4 M PB as described in the text; (2) or denatured in 0.12 M PB in a Gilford 2400 recording spectrophotometer in a temperature program with a 1°C rise per 2 min. The optical reassociation was calculated from the relative hyperchromicity of the reassociation duplex relative to analogous sheared native DNA. The optical analysis of renaturation for the longer fragments is not shown since considerable variation was observed. The close correspondence between hyperchromicity and HA analysis of DNA fragments 400 nucleotides in length depends on the DNA being passed over Chelex-100. The calibration of the French Pressure Cell for use in shearing DNA to known fragment size was carried out by Bell [1971]. (See also Laird, 1971 and Grouse, Chilton, and McCarthy, 1972.)

is then accomplished in 5 ml samples in an ice bath with a Branson Sonifier, equipped with a microtip, using 10 sec pulses at 1 min intervals for a total sonication time of 3 min. This pulse-cool procedure seems to minimize the "tail" denaturation and provide uniform fragments. The sonicated DNA fragments are then dialyzed for 6–12 hr against 10^2–10^3 vol of 0.03 M PB, concentrated by lyophization and stored at 4°C.

Procedure for the Estimation of the Molecular Weight of DNA Fragments

(1) Sheared labeled DNA (15 µg/ml) is denatured at pH 12.5 by addition of 0.5 to 1.0 M NaOH and left for 10 min at room temperature.
(2) The solution is cooled to 4°C and neutralized by the addition of 0.1 vol of 1 M PB (pH at room temperature approximately 6.4–6.6).
(3) Aliquots of 0.25 ml are back-layered onto 4.75 ml 5–20% sucrose gradients (in 0.12 M NaCl, 0.001 M Tris HCl, pH 7.6) and spun at 37,000 rpm for 6 hr at 4°C.
(4) A marker DNA (E. coli or E. coli rDNA) with a different label is added to the original sample at a concentration of 5 µg/ml.
(5) After centrifugation, 1 drop fractions are collected directly on GF/C (Whatmann) filter discs (22 mm).
(6) Each disc is then placed in a filter holder and rinsed twice with 5 ml of 5% TCA followed by 2 ml of ethanol.
(7) The filter discs are dried and assayed for radioactivity in a scintillation system programmed for dual label counting.
(8) The molecular weight estimation is calculated from the midpoint of gradient distribution using the relationship between molecular weight and sedimentation coefficient developed by Studier [1965].

Since this relationship is not convincing at low molecular weights, sedimentation analysis should be carried out as well in control experiments [Laird, 1971].

SECTION III IMMOBILIZATION OF SINGLE STRANDED DNA

The analysis of genetic transcription was first examined by RNA/DNA molecular hybridization by Hall and Spiegelman [1961]. The RNA/DNA duplex was formed in buffer solution and analyzed by equilibrium density-gradient centrifugation. The extensive time required to reach equilibrium restricted the use of hybridization until single-stranded DNA was found to absorb to nitrocellulose by Bautz and Hall [1962]; to be mechanically immobilized as a single-stranded molecule in agar [Bolton and McCarthy, 1962]; to form cross-linked gels by exposure to UV irradiation [Britten, 1963]; and to be adsorbed to nitrocellulose filters by Gillespie and Spiegelman [1965]. Each of these procedures allows molecular hybridization to be carried out rapidly and easily. The purpose of fixing the single-stranded DNA to filters or other solid matrix is to reduce as far as possible the complications of DNA/DNA self-reannealing during the hybridization reaction. Molecular hybridization specificity considerations has been the subject of two recent reviews [McCarthy and Church, 1970, and Kennell, 1971].

Nitrocellulose Absorption of RNA/DNA Hybrids

The discovery by Nygaard and Hall [1964] that nitrocellulose strongly absorbed single-stranded DNA along with any hybridized RNA allowed RNA/DNA duplexes formed in solution to be trapped for assay on nitrocellulose filters. Although this technique is of more use in viral and bacterial studies, it is of value in special reassociation experiments with fractionated mammalian DNA or separated strands. A typical in solution hybridization experiment might involve:

(1) Hybridization can take place in any suitable conditions with high specific activity labeled DNA in RNA excess reactions or high specific activity labeled RNA in reaction with separated single-strand or fractionated DNA.
    The corresponding macromolecule in the duplex usually has a different low specific activity label.
(2) The reassociation reaction is stopped by chilling to 4°C by a 30-fold dilution with ice cold 0.1 × SSC.
(3) In DNA/DNA reassociation reactions the hybridization mixture is treated with Sutton [1971] S1 exonuclease which digests all single-stranded nucleic acids. The S1 nuclease shows deoxribonuclease activity in 0.25 M K^+ and deoxyribonuclease and ribonuclease activity in 0.5 M K^+. The reaction is stopped by rapid cooling to 4°C, diluted 5-fold, and the salt concentration increased to 0.25 or 0.5 M K^+ depending on whether the reaction is DNA/DNA or RNA/DNA reassociation. For efficient enzyme activity, 50 μg of E. coli DNA (sheared) and 20 μg/ml of Sutton [1971] S1 nuclease is added, and the mixture is incubated at 50°C for 1/2 hr.
(4) The reassociation mixture is filtered through presoaked (6 × SSC) Bac-T-Flex type B6 (Schliecher and Schuell, U.S.); Millipore HA (Millipore Corp, U.S.), or MF50 (Sartorius, Germany) nitrocellulose filters adjusted to 0.5 M Na^+. High vacuum should be avoided since retention is reduced by vacuum suction washing.

(5) Nonspecific RNA/DNA interactions can be reduced by addition of highly purified 0.1 mg/ml 4 S E. coli RNA during dilution of the reaction mixture. An aliquot is precipitated by the standard method with 5% TCA as an input control.

(6) The filters are then washed twice with 20 ml of ice cold 2 × SSC, dried, and counted in a liquid scintillation system.
Percent hybridization is calculated from:

$$\frac{^3\text{H-DNA}/^{14}\text{C-DNA in hybrid fraction}}{^3\text{H-DNA}/^{14}\text{C-DNA in the TCA-precipitable fraction}} \times 100$$

A similar equation for RNA/DNA reassociation is used.

The filter-trapping method is a fast convenient method for assay of reassociation reaction $C_0 t$ aliquots provided proper optical and HA controls are included.

Immobilization of Single-Stranded DNA in Agar

Single-stranded DNA was first immobilized in an agar gel by Bolton and McCarthy [1962] for DNA/DNA homology studies. The technique has been used for both RNA/DNA and DNA/DNA hybridization studies since as reviewed by Bendich and Bolton [1968].

The preparation of DNA–agar involves:

(1) Making a 4% agar suspension of 8 g of Ionager 2 (Oxoid) per 100 ml distilled water and sterilizing for 10 min at 10 psi.

(2) High molecular weight DNA, 100 μg/ml, in 1/10 × SSC is denatured for 10 min at 98°C while the sterilizer is cooling.

(3) The denatured DNA is poured into the 90°C agar solution and the mixture shaken vigorously to disperse the single-stranded DNA through the viscous agar solution.

(4) The hot viscous mixture is poured into a beaker in an ice bath. The agar gels in about 1 min if the depth of agar solution is kept to a minimum.

(5) The agar is cut into pieces and forced through a 35-mesh stainless steel screen with a syringe.

(6) The DNA–agar particles are washed in a tea-bag with 25 ml of 2 × SSC at 60°C for 12 hr. The 2 × SSC should be changed two or three times. This wash procedure removes the free DNA from the gel and prevents self-reassociation.

(7) The DNA-agar suspension is then washed in a Buchner funnel with low suction for storage in a tightly stoppered container over a drop of chloroform.

(8) Assay of the amount of DNA immobilized in the agar can be determined by the difference (A_{260}) between the DNA extracted from the DNA agar by treatment with 5 ml of 0.5 M $NaClO_4$ at 100°C for 5 min and the absorbing materials extracted from agar after the same treatment.

(9) 1 g of 4% agar has the capacity to trap approximately 100 μg of DNA but agar batches differ in capacity.

(10) Reassociation with DNA–agar is considered in section IV. The leaching of 10–30% of the immobilized DNA from the DNA agar and the susceptibility of agar to degradation with increased temperature limit the procedure somewhat.

Immobilization of Single-Stranded DNA in UV-Treated Gels

When single-stranded DNA molecules are treated with UV irradiation, cross-linkage occurs between the DNA strands of the solution. The UV-DNA gel immobilization technique was developed by Britten [1963]. The most extensive use of the technique has been by Georgiev and coworkers [1967] for RNA/DNA hybridization studies. The immobilization of single-stranded DNA is accomplished by the formation of insoluble gels after exposure to UV radiation in the following manner:

(1) For the best gels very high molecular weight native DNA (mol wt is greater than 8×10^6) is dissolved in H_2O to a concentration of 2–2.5 mg/ml. It may be necessary to stir gently at 4°C for some time to get the necessary concentration, however very pure DNA should not present problems.

(2) The solution is denatured for 20 min in a boiling water bath.

(3) The water may be evaporated off by prolonged exposure to 80°C temperatures in a petri dish. The dry film left on the very clean siliconed petri dish is nearly all single-stranded DNA. Alternatively the solution can be rapidly cooled by plunging the mixture into an acetone dry ice bath. The cold DNA solution is then poured (a thin film of liquid) into a smooth, ultraclean, siliconed petri dish (60 μg/cm^2). The film is air dried at 0°C. The former high temperature drying of small fragments of reiterated DNA is required to prevent reassociation.

(4) The dry denatured DNA film is then radiated by an UV lamp (600–800 erg/mm^2). The amount of irradiation required to cause sufficient cross-linkage will depend on the molecular weight of the DNA. More energy is required for gel formation of low molecular weight DNA films.

(5) It is important to <u>immediately</u> wash the film from the petri dish with 6–8 ml of 2 × SSC and spin the gel from the buffer at 1000 rpm for 5 min.

The success achieved for DNA gel stability depends on the rapidity with which the washing of free DNA from the gel is accomplished. Reiterated free DNA will reassociate and leach during the subsequent hybridization reactions.

(6) The gel is washed gently with three more 10 ml washes of 2 × SSC and spun out as before.

(7) The "loosely cross-linked DNA" is then eluted from the gel by incubating the gel in 10 ml of 2 × SSC at 65°C for 36 hr. The gel is spun out of solution and washed once more with 10 ml of 1/10 × SSC at 65°C. After centrifugation, the gel is ready for hybridization reaction experiments.

Although this technique for the immobilization of single-stranded DNA has been of most use where membrane filters have not been available, it offers a great deal of promise for studies of reiterated DNA sequences. The major contribution to molecular hybridization attributable to the gel method is in the very high concentrations of DNA which are possible. As is noted elsewhere, small fragments of DNA are difficult to immobilize on membrane filters, especially prefractionated reiterated DNA sequences. Gels do suffer from the same leaching problems as are common with the agar technique. However, with the proper controls and with sufficient care in the preparation and washing of the gel, I believe much more use will be made of reiterated DNA fraction gels in the future.

Immobilization of Single-Stranded DNA on Membrane Filters

The membrane filter hybridization technique was developed by Gillespie and Spiegelman [1965] and described in detail by Gillespie [1968]. Denatured DNA is immobilized on a nitrocellulose filter before the reassociation reaction commences. The Bac-T-Flex B6 or MF50 (Schleicher and Schuell and Sartorius, respectfully) and HA type of Millipore nitrocellulose filters are suitable. Each batch of filters should be checked for oily surfaces. These filters are clogged and will not retain DNA efficiently. We prefer to load 145 mm filters and cut suitable small filters (1–24 mm diam) with appropriate paper punches as opposed to loading many independent 24 mm filters. The uniformity of loading of the large filter is checked by analysis of a number of randomly selected filters for DNA content by the diphenylamine reaction or preferably by monitoring labeled DNA. Variation in retention by acceptable filters is less than 3%. The single-stranded DNA retention capacity of B6 filters is usually about 100 μg/24 mm filter. We have had batches of filters which had loading capacities of as high as 150 μg/filter and as low as 50 μg/filter. Therefore, retention properties of each batch must be monitored at least once with radioactive DNA. The procedure is as follows:

(1) A carefully selected 145 mm filter is placed in the filter apparatus and washed with 1000 ml of 4 × SSC at 90°C under low vacuum. This hot prewash with 4 × SSC helps to remove excess wetting and softening agents. These substances may have considerable absorption at 260 mµ. Other sizes of filters are loaded with relative volumes of buffer.

(2) The purified DNA dissolved in 1/10 × SSC at 100 µg/ml is heat-denatured at 95°C for 15 min. The denaturation solution is quickly cooled in a dry ice acetone bath with dilution to 1000 ml with cold 4 × SSC. DNA concentration is then less than 10 µg/ml of buffer.

(3) To retain isolated repetitive DNA which has been sheared, reassociated and fractionated on HA, the filter wash and DNA dilution should be with 6 × SSC, 0.05 M KOH, 0.001 M $MgCl_2$ to increase the retention of single-stranded DNA.

(4) To load the filter, the ice cold single-stranded DNA (<10 µg/ml) is slowly passed through the filter by normal gravity in 4 × SSC. If the flow rate is too high, the retention of single-stranded DNA will be greatly retarded.

(5) A rough indication of the retention of single-stranded DNA by the membrane filter can be estimated from the A_{260} of the input solution versus that of the filtrate. A note of caution, however; it is essential that in each set of experiments the filter retention properties be determined with radioactive DNA, since A_{260} absorbing material can be eluted from the filter.

(6) In some cases the impurities or filter batch will show reduced retention of single-stranded high molecular weight DNA below the expected 70–90% levels. With fractionated low molecular weight repetitive DNA, 50% retention is average. Retention can be improved by increasing the salt concentration to 6 × SSC, in the presence of 0.05 M KOH and 0.001 M $MgCl_2$ and loading at 4°C.

(7) When the sample has passed through the filter, it may be desirable to recycle the filtrate to increase the recovery of single-stranded DNA by the filter.

(8) The 145 mm filter is then washed with 1000 ml of 4 or 6 × SSC at the loading temperature with low vacuum followed by 200 ml of 4 or 6 × SSC at medium vacuum.

(9) The area of effective loading is then marked with a soft pencil, the filter removed from the filtration apparatus, blotted on clean washed filter paper, and left to dry for a few minutes at room temperature.

(10) The filter is then treated for 1 hr at room temperature in the Denhardt

[1966] mixture to eliminate background noise. The Denhardt [1966] preincubation mixture consists of 0.02% each of Ficoll (Pharmacia, mol wt 400,000), polyvinylpyrrolidone (Sigma. mol wt 360,000), and bovine albumin (Armour, fraction V) in 4 × SSC.

(11) At the end of the preincubation the filter is blotted on a clean filter paper to remove excess moisture and dried for a few minutes.

(12) The 145 mm filter is then cut into small filters of the desired size (that is, diameter 2, 5, 7, 22 mm) and the DNA content assayed by the diphenylamine reaction after treatment with deoxyribonuclease, or preferably by radioactivity, of a random selection of the small filters.

(13) The small filters are air dried at room temperature in partly open petri dishes for 2 hr at room temperature before being baked at 60°C for 16 hr or 4 hr at 80°C.

(14) The baked filters are stored dry in covered containers at 4°C. Control filters contain equal amounts of bacterial DNA and are treated in a similar fashion.

(15) A 145 mm diameter B6 filter has an effective diameter of 110 mm. A typical loading input would be from 7–8 mg of single-stranded DNA. Retention of 5.5–6 mg is to be expected. When the 110 mm effective diameter filter is cut into small filters with a diameter of 5 mm each filter will contain approximately 12 μg of single-stranded DNA. Satisfactory results have been obtained from 1 mm diameter filters containing 0.1 μg of radioactive DNA.

Immobilization of Density-Fractionated DNA

To determine whether a particular density of DNA is complementary to the RNA species under study it is possible to fractionate DNA on preparative CsCl density gradients before hybridization.

(1) For the preparative ultracentrifuge, 10 ml of CsCl containing 200 μg of sheared DNA at a refractive index of 1.4000 is added to a 12 ml centrifuge tube, the tube is layered with parafin oil and spun for 72 hr at 37,000 rpm to reach equilibrium.

(2) Gradients are monitored with a micro-flow cell (0.125 ml, 1 cm light path) at 260 mμ and the fractions collected. The refractive index is determined on alternate fractions (36 fractions).

(3) Each fraction is diluted to 5 ml with 4 × SSC and the DNA denatured at pH 12.5 by addition of NaOH. After 15 min at 30°C the fractions were cooled to 4°C and neutralized with HCl.

(4) Each fraction is adsorbed to a 24 mm B6 nitrocellulose filter as described above.
(5) After treatment with the Denhardt [1966] preincubation mixture the filters can be cut to appropriate sizes for controls, dried, and baked overnight at 60°C.
(6) Hybridization is carried out under appropriate conditions using duplicate filters, cut from 22 mm original, for each CsCl density fraction. This technique has been used extensively for analysis of G + C rich ribosomal cistrons [Brown and Weber, 1968].

Estimation of Single Stranded DNA Concentration During Reassociation Reactions

The accurate estimation of the concentration and complexity of single-stranded DNA in reassociation reactions utilizing either DNA or RNA is subject to considerable error. The leaching of single-stranded DNA from gels and agar is well known. However, the benefit of <u>accurate</u> monitoring of the retention of single-stranded DNA by membrane filters and the subsequent elution of some immobilized DNA during the hybridization reaction cannot be over emphasized. In-solution reactions must include the proper controls to estimate the rate of the homologous DNA/DNA reassociation.

In reactions where the single-stranded DNA is immobilized any DNA eluted from the matrix not only reduces the effective concentration of DNA available for reaction in the immobilized state but complicates the kinetics of the formation of homologous and heterologous duplexes. The kinetics by elution of labeled single-stranded DNA from membrane filters during an incubation reaction indicates that 95% of the elutable DNA is free of the filter by 4 hr at 67°C in 2 × SSC [Schultz, 1969]. There is a very rapid elution of this imperfectly immobilized DNA during the first 2 hr of incubation followed by a very slow elution of DNA during the remaining incubation reaction to 72 hr. Something like 20–30% of the adsorbed DNA can be eluted during incubation.

Therefore, the following procedure was developed for immobilization of low molecular weight DNA on membrane filters.

(1) The loading of <u>completely</u> denatured DNA is carried out in 6 × SSC with or without 0.01 M $MgCl_2$ at 0–4°C to prevent renaturation of reiterated sequences.
(2) The concentration of DNA in solution is <5 μg/ml for loading by gravity on prewashed filters (6 × SSC).
(3) The filtrate is recycled since very seldom is more than 50% of the DNA retained on the first passage.

(4) The filter is washed as before, air dried at room temperature for 2 hr and baked for 4 hr at 80°C.
(5) The filter is then placed in the appropriate reassociation reaction buffer (25 ml) and incubated for 4–6 hr at the reaction temperature chosen.
(6) The filter is removed from the incubation mixture, blotted dry and incubated with the preincubation mixture of Denhardt [1966] for 1 hr at room temperature. This mixture presumably blocks all reactive sites which have become exposed on the membrane filter during incubation.
(7) The filter is blotted, cut into small filters, dried, and baked overnight at 60°C.
(8) The incubation mixture is made 5% with respect to TCA after addition of 500 μg of carrier RNA and the precipitate collected for assay of the eluted DNA.
(9) The DNA concentration on a random selection of filters is determined by the diphenylamine reaction or preferably by radioactivity. Our experience has been that very little of the remaining DNA is eluted during either the reassociation reaction or thermal melting procedure. It is assumed, but has not been studied, that the proportion of DNA which elutes represents a random not a specific set of base sequences. Elution of less than 10% of the retained DNA is found during incubation and thermal dissociation. The retention of DNA by nitrocellulose membrane filters can be measured by:
   (a) The decrease in optical density at 260 mμ of the DNA solution before and after passage through the filter.
   (b) The use of low specific activity (^{14}C-DNA 100 cpm/μg, is our preference) DNA for retention assay is the preferred method.
   (c) Elution of the filter-bound DNA by treatment with 0.5 N HClO$_4$ at 75°C for 15 min. The OD read at 260 mμ of the extracted versus that of a control filter is used to estimate filter-bound DNA concentration.

SECTION IV REASSOCIATION OF HYBRIDIZATION REACTIONS WITH IMMOBILIZED (REITERATED) SINGLE-STRANDED DNA

Molecular RNA/DNA hybridization has been used extensively in the last ten years to obtain estimates of genetic activity. The method is a powerful tool for base sequence analysis but presents problems of interpretation for DNA isolated from the complex genomes of higher organisms. This section will deal with methods of low $C_0 t$ reassociation, which due to low nucleic acid concentrations and short reaction times, involve primarily only reiterated DNA base sequences. These sequences may be isolated $C_0 t$ fractions representing a given fraction of the genome or the 5–80% reiterated sequences found in various DNA's. The agar, UV gel and membrane filter RNA/DNA and DNA/DNA hybridization or reassociation reactions provide specificity of reaction for bacterial and viral nucleic acid studies. They seldom provide cistron specificity for mammalian systems under these low $C_0 t$ conditions [McCarthy and Church, 1970]. Exceptions to this may be the high criteria ribosomal or transfer RNA hybridization reactions, although some heterogeneity may exist there as well. The criteria or specificity of the reaction must be ascertained for each biological system examined hence the conditions given are to be used as guide lines only.

DNA-Agar Hybridization

The amount of agar–DNA required for an experiment will depend on the specific activity of the labeled DNA or RNA. The procedures for incubation of RNA/DNA and DNA/DNA reactions are similar. All labeled DNA is sheared prior to the hybridization reaction.

(1) 0.5–1.0 g of DNA–agar is incubated with 0.5–1.0 ml 2 × SSC of the radioactive nucleic acid solution for 15–18 hr at 60°C. The conditions of salt, time, and temperature will depend on the criteria designated. DNA is eluted from the agar at accelerated rates at temperatures over 60°C.

(2) Incubation is carried out in a screw-capped silicone-treated glass container (that is, scintillation or smaller similar vial) for a given time.

(3) At the predetermined incubation time the incubation mixture is transferred quantitatively to a 10 mm tea bag tube. The tea bag tube is constructed from a silicone-treated glass tube (18 cm × 10 mm) which has one end capped with Saran screen (MS 904, National Filter Corp.) held in place by a Neoprene-O-ring 9 mm inside diameter. The tube is placed in a standard test tube (18 × 150 mm) on a wire support such that the Saran screen is at least 3 cm from the bottom of the test tube.

(4) The incubation vial is washed with 10 ml of 2 × SSC at 60°C, and the solution is subsequently transferred to the tea bag tube with the agar–DNA.

(5) The tea bag tube is then transferred through a series of five or more washes, each consisting of 15 ml of 2 × SSC at 60°C. The tea bag tube is moved up and down frequently for 15 min in each wash fraction. The tea bag tube is carefully drained at the end of each step before proceeding to the next wash fraction.

(6) The efficiency of washing unassociated nucleic acid from the DNA–agar can be assayed by monitoring acid-precipitable labeled nucleic acid in each wash fraction.

(7) The RNA or DNA in double-stranded duplexes with DNA–agar can be recovered in one step by washing the tea bag tube with 15 ml of 0.01 × SSC at 65°C. Usually three 15 min wash fractions are sufficient to quantitatively remove all labeled nucleic acid.

(8) Alternatively the RNA/DNA or DNA/DNA duplex can be thermally dissociated by washing the tea bag tube with 15 ml fractions of 0.01 × SSC commencing at 40°C. Each successive 15 min step comprises a 15 ml 0.01 × SSC wash and a 5°C increase in temperature until the RNA/DNA is all melted (about 75°C).

(9) The eluted labeled nucleic acid in each fraction is assayed by addition of 50 µg of rRNA carrier and 5% TCA precipitation in the cold, followed by collection of the precipitate on membrane or glass fiber filters. DNA leached from the agar which is duplexed to RNA will lower the observed thermal stability.

(10) Controls include incubation of the labeled nucleic acid with a bacterial DNA–agar, incubation of a labeled bacterial nucleic acid with the mammalian DNA–agar under study, etc. The former provides an estimate of the specificity of reaction, the latter, an estimate of DNA–agar background noise or nonspecific binding.

(11) Competition and saturation experiments with DNA–agar are described at the end of this section.

(12) A typical DNA/DNA reaction contains 1 µg ^{14}C-labeled DNA fragments (2500 cpm/µg) and 4 µg ^{3}H-labeled DNA fragments (220 cpm/µg from mouse incubated with 0.5 g of agar containing 60 µg of high molecular weight single-stranded mouse DNA in the presence of increasing (to 1200 µg) amounts of bacterial and unlabeled mouse DNA.

A typical RNA/DNA reaction contains 5 µg ^{3}H kidney RNA (230 cpm/µg) and 5 µg ^{32}P liver RNA (100 cpm/µg) incubated with 0.5 g of agar containing 36 µg of single-stranded mouse DNA in the presence of increasing amounts of unlabeled mouse and bacterial RNA (to 900 µg) [McCarthy and Hoyer, 1964].

DNA-gel Hybridization

The UV radiation cross-linked DNA gel/RNA hybridization has been exploited by Georgiev and coworkers [1967]. The technique is similar to the DNA–agar method for RNA/DNA duplex analysis.

(1) Cross-linked DNA gels containing 1–10 mg of DNA are incubated with the labeled RNA preparation to be examined in 0.5–2 ml of 2 × SSC at 65°C in a tightly sealed glass centrifuge tube.
(2) At the predetermined incubation time the gel is carefully removed from the incubation media with forceps or spun down at 1500 × $\underline{g}$ for 5 min at 4°C.
(3) The gel is washed 2–5 times with 10 ml aliquots of 2 × SSC at 65°C. The DNA gel/RNA duplex is recovered by centrifugation after each wash.
(4) The wash fractions can be assayed for the unassociated labeled RNA by precipitation with TCA.
(5) The extent of RNA/DNA duplex formation can be assayed directly by drying the gel to a film and direct counting in a liquid scintillation system or by increasing the temperature of the last 10 ml wash to 85°C in 1/10 × SSC. The melted labeled RNA can be collected by acid precipitation.
(6) The DNA gel/RNA duplex can be thermally dissociated with increasing temperature by subsequent stepwise (15 min per step) increases in temperature from 50°C in 1/10 × SSC. Each fraction is then assayed for the labeled RNA melted from the duplex at each temperature.
(7) If ribonuclease is to be used in the assay conditions the RNA/DNA gel incubation mixture is treated with 50 μg/ribonuclease/ml of 2 × SSC (10 ml) for 30 min at 37°C. The ribonuclease-resistant RNA/DNA duplex is then assayed in the standard manner.

Although the DNA gel technique has the disadvantage of DNA leaching from the gel yielding apparently lower thermal stability than other techniques, the method does allow a convenient and fast method of assaying RNA/DNA duplexes formed under conditions of <u>vast single-stranded DNA excess</u>.

DNA Filter Hybridization

The reassociation of radioactive DNA fragments with unlabeled high molecular weight DNA adsorbed to nitrocellulose filters has been used to study the complementarity between DNA oligonucleotides, fractionated DNA, and total DNA. The normal low $C_0 t$ reassociation reactions are primarily reflections of the kinetics of the reiterated base sequence reactions of mammalian genomes. The ratio of filter-bound DNA to that in solution is usually about 10:1 to minimize in-solution reassociation of the labeled DNA fragments. The specificity of DNA/DNA base-pair matching can be determined more precisely than for RNA/DNA reactions since the kinetics of denaturation of native DNA allow definitive controls. In vitro synthesized complementary RNA (cRNA) is the only comparable cRNA/DNA control reaction [Melli and Bishop, 1970]. In most cases the reiteration and complexity of RNA sequences is not a measurable parameter.

The DNA/DNA duplex formation and the incidence and effect of partially related base sequences in DNA has been studied by McCarthy and McConaughy [1968, 1970a, 1970b]. The success of filter hybridization and the confidence of the interpretation depends in large measure on sufficient and proper control reactions. Some of the general considerations to bear in mind in the design of filter hybridization reactions are:

(1) RNA impurities and secondary structure, etc., which influence the temperature chosen for the reaction (see section I).
(2) Complete denaturation of DNA is required for proper retention of DNA by membrane filters (see section I).
(3) The specificity of the base-pair reaction as defined by the criteria chosen for the reaction (see section I).
(4) The preparation of DNA filters with low RNA background adsorption by the preincubation treatment.

Controls for filter hybridization should include:

(1) The presence of a filter-bound DNA from a completely heterologous source (E. coli, B. subtilis) in each reaction vessel. The nonspecific base-pairing of the labeled RNA with this heterologous DNA is a function of the criteria of the reassociation conditions. The nonspecific hybrid serves as a "zero" control. RNA background noise includes nonspecifically bound ribonuclease-resistant radioactivity adsorbed to these filters [see (5)].
(2) The use of radioactive DNA to monitor retention of DNA by the filter during the incubation and particularly during thermal dissociation. This control provides a quantitative check on DNA concentration.
(3) The use of a parallel series of reactions without the presence of the homologous DNA filters to ascertain the degradation of labeled RNA during the incubation. The TCA-precipitable radioactivity after the incubation is considered the input value for labeled RNA in calculations.
(4) The same RNA control in saturation or competition experiments is a requirement for determining the actual concentration of surviving labeled RNA (input). Cold competitor RNA at high concentrations often shows ribonuclease activity which "mimics" homologous dilution curves during competition experiments.

(5) An aliquot of the same control as in (4) treated with ribonuclease provides a direct estimate of RNA noise. The ribonuclease-resistant product may be due to secondary structure or contamination with basic protein or degraded DNA. The contamination of labeled RNA with degraded DNA can be detected by monitoring the alkali stable (0.3 M KOH 30°C for 16 hr), acid-precipitable radioactivity in the labeled RNA preparation.

(6) The contamination of basic proteins is more serious since they bind to membrane filters and RNA. These proteins can be removed by HA chromatography, passing RNA through membrane filters or by treatment with Pronase for 30 min at 37°C. The procedure involves the use of single-stranded DNA immobilized to filters as described in section II (filter-bound DNA). The conditions will vary with the biological system under study and the compromise made between the extent of reaction which can be measured accurately by the specific activity of the labeled nucleic acid available and the amount of base-pair mismatching which can be tolerated in the hybrid [McCarthy and Church, 1970] (Figure 3).

The hybridization parameters are:

(1) Salt concentration can vary from 1/10 × SSC to 6 × SSC with increasing base-pair mismatching at a given temperature. Usually 2–4 × SSC are selected as a compromise between the higher rate of reaction obtained at higher salt concentration and a greater demand for base-pair matching in low salt conditions [Church and McCarthy, 1968].

(2) Volume of reaction and concentration of labeled nucleic acid in solution depends on the amount of nucleic acid available. We have used filters with 0.1 µg of DNA in 100 µliter of buffer. Very small volumes introduce a handling problem, since in order to introduce a number of 5 mm diameter filters into a 10 × 40 mm specimen vial at least 0.2 ml is required. The mass of labeled nucleic acid required for incubation volumes of greater than 2 ml becomes quite large for high concentrations of nucleic acid.

(3) Temperature of incubation is chosen in combination with salt concentration to obtain the desired stringency of base-pairing. The higher the temperature the higher the stringency on base-pairing and the lower is the rate and extent of reaction. Thermal degradation and DNA elution from filters are practical limitations to high temperatures. The optimal temperature of the RNA/DNA hybridization reaction is influenced by the homogeneity of the RNA population isolated from mammalian cells, the G + C content of the sequences, the secondary structure of

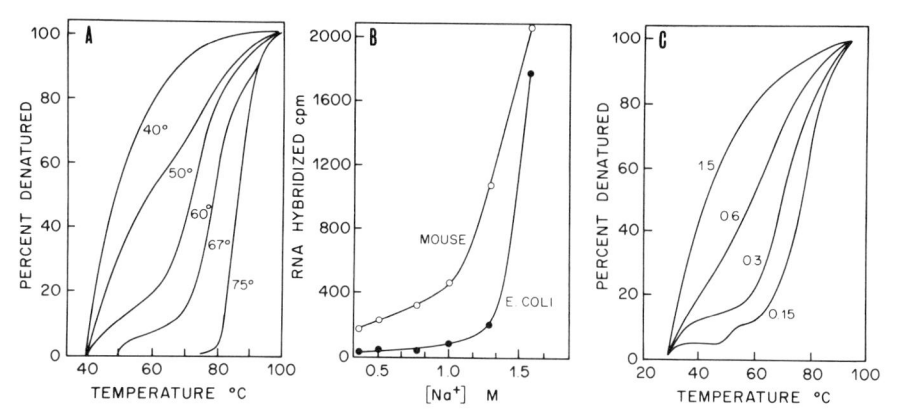

FIGURE 3. Effect of reaction conditions or criteria on the RNA/reiterated DNA hybridization reaction. The effect of hybridization conditions or criteria on the extent and quality of the RNA (labeled in vivo)/mouse reiterated filter-bound DNA (low $C_o t$) reaction. (a) Dependence of the thermal denaturation of RNA-DNA hybrids formed by incubating 100 µg ^{3}H mouse spleen RNA with 10 µg ^{14}C filter-bound DNA in 0.2 ml of 4 × SSC, 10^{-2} M TES, for 20 hr at the indicated temperatures. The filters were removed from the incubation mixture, washed three times with 4 × SSC at the reaction temperature and finally thermally dissociated in 2 ml aliquots of 1 × SSC. Triplicate filters were assayed for each point. The pulse labeled ^{3}H-RNA melted from the RNA/DNA duplex and that remaining in the duplex was monitored. The ^{14}C-DNA remaining on the filter during the thermal dissociation was assayed for filter retention. (b) The effect of Na$^+$ concentration on the hybridization of 5 µg ^{3}H-RNA isolated from spleen with 10 µg homologous ^{14}C-DNA and heterologous ^{32}P-E. coli DNA adsorbed to nitrocellulose membrane filters. The reaction mixtures, set up in duplicate, were incubated in 0.2 ml of the buffers indicated (SSC) for 20 hr at 68°C. The significance of nonspecific binding of labeled RNA to heterologous DNA in high salt concentrations is easily recognized in these low $C_o t$ reactions. (c) The effect of salt concentration (SSC) on the thermal stability of pulse labeled tritiated L-cell RNA (100 µg)/filter-bound mouse DNA (10 µg) hybrids formed under low $C_o t$ conditions at the indicated Na$^+$ concentration in 0.2 ml of buffer (SSC, 10^{-2} M TES) for 20 hr at 68°C. The filter-bound duplexes were thermally dissociated in 2 ml aliquots of SSC held for 10 min at each 5°C temperature increment. The treatments 1, 2, 4, and 10 × SSC are represented in the ionic concentration series. For a complete analysis see Church and McCarthy [1968] and Shearer and McCarthy [1970].

the RNA which must be melted (that is, hairpins), the specificity of base-pairing desired, and the fragment size of the RNA. Church and McCarthy [1968] noted that efficiency of hybridization increased when the large heterogeneous RNA of mammals is degraded to 6 S fragments, however much smaller fragments show a decreased rate of reaction and thermal stability [McConaughy and McCarthy, 1970, Birnstiel, Sells, and Purdom, 1972]. The presence of hairpin loops will drastically reduce the rate of reaction and influence the stability and apparent ribonuclease resistance of the RNA/DNA hybrid. Therefore, it is essential to choose and standardize the incubation temperature with care [McCarthy and Church, 1970]. For rapidly labeled nuclear RNA from mammals, for mammalian rRNA and for "pure" messenger the optimal reaction temperatures are approximately 20°C below, equal to, and 10°C below the T_m of DNA/DNA duplexes from the same organism, respectively.

(4) The time of incubation is determined by the reassociation $C_0 t$ desired. The incubation should be as short as possible to reduce RNA degradation. The final incubation time will depend on the nucleic acid concentrations available.

These hybridization parameters have been investigated in a mammalian and comparable bacterial RNA/DNA reassociation system by Church and McCarthy [1968].

Basic RNA/filter-bound DNA reassociation experiments are as follows.

(1) Filters appropriately prepared with immobilized DNA as described in section III are marked, soaked in 1 × SSC—with or without formamide, and mounted in series on nonreactive straight pins. Up to 10–5 mm filters can be incubated in 0.2 ml of buffer in a 10 × 44 mm specimen vial. At least two of the filters contain immobilized heterologous DNA to act as noise controls.

(2) The purified labeled RNA to be hybridized is dissolved in the buffer to be used in the reaction (that is, 2 × SSC, 10^{-2} M TES or 2 × SSC, 30% formamide, 0.4% SDS) and heated to 85°C to reduce secondary structure and quickly cooled to the incubation temperature.

(3) For saturation experiments the concentration of labeled RNA in the buffer should coincide with the highest concentration to be used in the experiment. Other less concentrated points are obtained by dilution with the same buffer.

(4) For competition experiments the labeled RNA concentration should be as high as possible in the incubation buffer. Each reaction vial receives a standard volume and concentration. The unlabeled competitor RNA is taken up in the incubation buffer at the highest concentration to be used in the experiment (that is, 5–10 µg/ml). The appropriate aliquot series of unlabeled RNA samples are removed and placed in the incubation vials. The reaction mixtures are then made up to a uniform volume with the same buffer (that is, 0.2 ml) before heating and cooling to the incubation temperature selected.

(5) The filter-bound DNA is added at the incubation temperature and the reaction vessel capped tightly or sealed with paraffin oil.

(6) TES buffer is particularly useful in maintaining pH 7.2 in the citrate buffer at incubation temperatures above 70°C. The reassociation reaction is concentration dependent hence the volume of the incubation reaction should be kept to a minimum which can effectively wet the filter. The effect of volume concentration has been investigated by Church and McCarthy [1968].

(7) The choice of buffer, temperature, and formamide is arbitrary (see below). Conditions of incubation have been studied by McCarthy and McConaughy [1968] McCarthy and Church [1970] and Schmeckpeper and Smith [1972].

(8) The reaction time for low $C_0 t$ reassociation reactions is usually between 16–72 hr at the chosen temperature (that is, 2 × SSC at 67°C or 2 × SSC 30% formamide, 0.4% SDS at 45°C for 24 hr). Reaction scatter is reduced by constant shaking during the incubation period while RNA reduced to 4–6 S increases the efficiency of hybridization [Church and McCarthy, 1968].

(9) The proper controls include labeled RNA alone, labeled RNA with competitor RNA, and no RNA in reaction vials with and without heterologous filter-bound DNA. Input of labeled RNA is estimated from the acid-precipitable labeled RNA remaining at the end of the reaction.

(10) At the end of the incubation reaction without formamide (that is, 2 × SSC 10^{-2} M TES at 65°C) the filters are carefully removed from the incubation vials, drained, and washed three times for 10 min in 15 ml of the incubation buffer at the incubation temperature.

(11) The portion of filters to be counted are washed once more with 15 ml of 1 × SSC, 10°C below the reaction temperature, blotted dry, dried, and counted in a scintillation system. The last wash in 1 × SSC is to reduce the salt quenching during counting.

(12) For incubation reactions with formamide (2 × SSC, 30% formamide, 0.4% SDS at 45°C) a portion of the filters are carefully removed from the incubation vials, drained of remaining buffer, and washed twice with 15 ml of 2 × SSC with 30% formamide for 10 min. The final two washings are with 15 ml of 2 × SSC and 1 × SSC for 10 min each, respectively.

(13) The washed and dried RNA/filter-bound DNA hybrids assayed in (11) and (12) are sometimes referred to as "raw" hybrids since it is speculated that "tails" of ribonuclease-sensitive sequences are assayed.

Church and McCarthy [1968,1970] have shown that the proportion of labeled RNA in RNA/DNA duplexes sensitive to ribonuclease decreases with increasing criteria. These results were interpreted as evidence for increased base-pair matching in the duplex formed at high reassociation criteria. However, since the extent of reaction is so drastically reduced the high criteria incubation conditions are not often practical. Tails and "loops" may be eliminated by ribonuclease treatment, but RNA secondary structure may add to the apparent RNA/DNA nuclease-resistant product [McCarthy and Church, 1970]. If RNA which can be hybridized is to be eluted from low $C_0 t$ RNA/DNA duplexes for other studies, the treatment of the hybrid with ribonuclease will result in the elution of degraded molecules.

After removal of the filter from the reaction vial, it is washed with the same buffer at the same temperature. However, RNA/DNA duplexes formed early in the hybridization reaction are relatively unstable and have a measurable dissociation constant [Church, 1971 unpublished] which influences the results of ribonuclease treatment [Church and McCarthy, 1968]. A relationship exists between the washing volume and the extent of dissociation of imperfectly paired DNA/DNA duplexes [McCarthy and McConaughy, 1970a and 1970b]. The reader is referred to the series of papers by McCarthy and coworkers outlining their studies of related base sequences in the DNA of simple and complex organisms [1968, 1970] and to the review on specificity of hybridization by McCarthy and Church [1970]. The effect of volume, salt concentration, and temperature on the specificity of reaction is shown in Figure 3.

(14) In studies which warrant ribonuclease treatment a portion of the filters from (11) and (12) are treated as follows:
  (a) The filters are incubated in 5 ml of 2 × SSC for 30 min at 37°C in the presence of a mixture of 5 µg/ml pancreatic ribonuclease and 10 units/ml of T1 ribonuclease.
  (b) At the end of the reaction the filters are washed twice with 15 ml of 2 × SSC at 37°C, once with 5 ml of 1 × SSC at room temperature, blotted, dried, and counted in a scintillation system.
(15) Each filter is rinsed with two washes of chloroform (5 ml) to remove the toluene and fluor after counting and placed in 2 ml of 1/10 × SSC at 40°C for the thermal characterization of the RNA/DNA duplex (see thermal analysis below).

The Use of Formamide in Nucleic Acid Reassociation

Renaturation of DNA and hybridization of RNA with filter-bound DNA or DNA in solution are normally studied under reaction conditions involving elevated temperatures. The optimal rate of reassociation occurs some 20°C below the T_m or mean thermal denaturation temperature of the native DNA. The size of eukaryotic genomes necessitates long incubation times for unique sequence reassociation which may be accompanied by extensive thermal degradation. Some experiments utilizing amino acyl–tRNA require low temperatures since the ester linkage is unstable at high temperatures [Nass and Buck, 1970]. In hybridization experiments in which sheared, fractionated DNA is immobilized on membrane filters, elution of the immobilized DNA is enhanced at high temperatures. For these and other reasons techniques have been examined which allow the use of low temperatures, 25–50°C, with the reassociation criteria expected for higher reaction temperatures.

The use of organic solvents as denaturants was originally explored by Helmkamp and Ts'o [1961]. The principle was exploited by Bonner, Kung, and Bekhor [1967] for RNA/DNA hybridization at 25°C in formamide. Formaldehyde hydroxymethylates free amino groups [Grossman, 1968] and thereby prevents hydrogen bonding in nucleic acids. This hydroxymethylation can be reversed as Schmeckpeper and Smith [1972] have shown that the formaldehyde reaction has no irreversible effects on DNA reassociation.

Conditions for DNA renaturation and RNA/DNA hybridization in formamide solutions at low temperatures which retain high specificity and reaction rates were described by McConaughy, Laird, and McCarthy [1969]. They found that for the range 45–90°C, every 1% formamide in the reassociation reaction reduced the T_m of double-stranded DNA 0.72°C.

The extent of nonspecific hybridization among related base sequences is dependent on temperature and ionic strength [Church and McCarthy, 1968]. These authors showed that at conditions of high criteria the rate and extent of reaction was drastically reduced. Specificity of conditions is, therefore, easily adjusted by manipulation of ionic strength and formamide concentration using the relationship of 1% formamide to 0.72°C change in T_m. Many authors have used this relationship on the assumption that the effect of formamide on helix disruption is the same as its effect on reassociation.

Very recently Schmeckpeper and Smith [1972] examined the effect of formamide on RNA/DNA reassociation by a comparison of the thermal stabilities of the duplexes formed at a given criteria. It is significant to note that, although increasing formamide concentrations in reassociation buffers increased the T_m of duplexes formed there was no simple linear relationship between T_m of the RNA/DNA duplexes formed and formamide concentrations. In the systematic survey carried out by Schmeckpeper and Smith [1972] it was reported that under some conditions (2 × SSC, 50% formamide (F), 33°C) the rate of reaction was greatly retarded. The presence of unstable hybrids in the duplexes formed at very specific reaction conditions (2 × SSC, 70% F, 33°C) was also suggested by the presence of a duplex RNA/DNA component which melted with a low T_m. Schmeckpeper and Smith [1972] have suggested two guidelines for calculating equivalent reassociation conditions.

(1) For reactions above 45°C, 1% formamide reduces the T_m 0.72°C [McConaughy et al., 1969].
(2) For experiments equivalent to 2 × SSC at 68°C the nonlinear relationship shown in Figure 4 is applicable.

The data presented in Figure 4 shows the relationship between thermal stability of RNA/DNA hybrids and formamide concentration. In order to com-

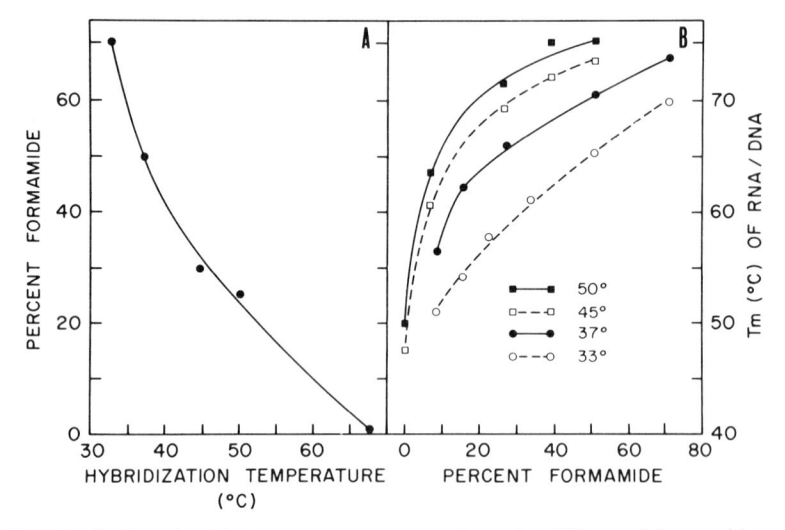

FIGURE 4. Relationship between temperature, thermal stability, and formamide concentration. (A) The relationship between temperature of hybridization and formamide concentration in the incubation buffer necessary to produce a criterion equivalent to 68°C, 2 × SSC. The hybridization reaction contained approximately 60 μg complementary in vitro synthesized cRNA in reaction with 4.5 μg of filter-bound mouse satellite depleted DNA in 0.1 ml 2 × SSC, 10^{-3} M EDTA in various concentrations of formamide [Schmeckpeper and Smith, 1972]. (B) The relationship between the thermal stability of mouse satellite-depleted DNA/cRNA hybrids and the formamide concentration in the incubation mixture. Temperatures of hybridization were 33, 37, 45 or 50°C. All thermal stabilities were determined, after hybridization in 0.1 ml 2 × SSC, 10^{-3} M EDTA at the concentrations of formamide noted, in 0.5 × SSC. The data after Schmeckpeper and Smith [1972] with additions from our laboratory [J. Crozier, unpublished] for thermal stabilities at 33 and 37°C for pulse labeled L-cell RNA and satellite-depleted mouse DNA hybrids formed in 2 × SSC and melted in 0.5 × SSC.

pare equivalent systems (that is, 2 × SSC at 68°C vs 2 × SSC, 50% formamide at 33°C) one must have a measure of base mismatching. In fact, as shown by Schmeckpeper and Smith [1972], the increased reassociation may be incorrectly interpreted as a rate effect when in fact the reassociation criteria in the apparently equivalent formamide incubation is lower. Therefore, for any investigation in which formamide is utilized, the control reactions must ascertain the equvalent base-pair matching by careful analysis of reaction rate, extent, and thermal stability of the product. This is especially relevant if the reaction is to be carried out at temperatures below 45°C where some variance from the relationship of 1% formamide to 0.72°C established by McConaughy et al. [1969] may be evident.

The formamide used in our laboratory is obtained from Eastman Kodak Company and passed over a Chelex-100 resin column (BioRad, 100–200 mesh) to remove UV absorbing materials. The criterion used for solvent purity includes optical density readings of less than 0.12 when 100% formamide is observed at 270 mμ in 1 cm path-length cuvettes. Most optical measurements on nucleic acids are made at 260 mμ. However, since formamide absorbs strongly at 260 mμ, all optical measurements with formamide present are monitored at 270 mμ where DNA absorption is still 80% of that of 260 mμ and absorption by the formamide is less than 0.12 [McConaughy et al., 1969].

Secondly, for analysis of reassociation reactions, carried out in formamide, on HA it is necessary to dilute the formamide concentration to _below_ 1% with 0.03 or 0.12 M PB before application to the HA column. Reassociation reactions to be analyzed on HA should be carried out _without_ sodium citrate since SSC adversely affects the ability of HA to separate structural differences.

For the above reasons, our laboratory tries to avoid the use of formamide whenever possible for reassociation reactions with filter-bound DNA and in-solution DNA. When formamide is necessary, the minimum incubation temperature used is 45°C. High criteria conditions such as 30% formamide, 2 × SSC at 45°C is convenient for mammalian RNA/DNA reassociation studies.

Saturation Hybridization Experiments

Saturation experiments are designed to estimate the number of DNA sequences complementary to a given population of RNA molecules. This is theoretically accomplished by holding the DNA input constant while increasing the RNA input in a series of incubations. The amount of RNA which will form a duplex with DNA sequences decreases as a percentage of the RNA input. The percentage of DNA involved in the reaction can be calculated from the plateau value of the incubation reactions. The plateau value is a function of the complexity of the

RNA and concentration of each species of RNA in the spectrum. Saturation experiments with filter-bound DNA have been very useful in the estimation of the number of cistrons coding for ribosomal RNA. Saturation experiments with total mammalian cellular RNA are uninterpretable because of reiterated sequences and the complexity of RNA populations which react in low $C_0 t$ reactions.

The saturation plateau of cell RNA will not level off completely but continue to rise as RNA complementary to unique DNA sequences form RNA/DNA duplexes. The rate of the RNA/unique DNA filter reaction is too low to be easily observed. The extended incubations lead to thermal degradation and a decrease in the proportion of unstable intermediate RNA/DNA duplexes. These intermediate RNA/DNA hybrids are responsible for nucleation at an accelerated rate but are characterized by low thermal stability. These duplexes have been shown to be the reversible component in the RNA/DNA hybridization reaction [Church, unpublished]. Numerous studies have noted a <u>decline</u> in apparent saturation values at incubation times of greater 20 hr. This is primarily a reflection of RNA degradation.

The use of ribonuclease treatment to remove nonspecifically paired regions of the raw hybrid has been the subject of controversy. Preference is given to stringent reaction conditions and thermal stability analysis [Church and McCarthy, 1968]. The saturation plateau of raw RNA/DNA hybrid continues to increase more rapidly than does the ribonuclease-resistant duplex under standard conditions. An example of the effect of stringency on ribonuclease resistance is shown in Figure 5.

Saturation Experiments for RNA Complexity Studies

The kinetic complexity of RNA molecules can be calculated using RNA/DNA hybridization on membrane filters [Birnstiel et al., 1972]. The object of these experiments is to assay base sequence complexity of RNA and establish the complexity of RNA species in animal cells. Since the reassociation of DNA follows second order kinetics (see section I) the half period of reassociation is inversely proportional to the molar concentrations of the DNA complements. Britten and Kohne [1968] have established that $C_0 t_{1/2}$ is a measure of the base sequence complexity of DNA. In RNA/DNA hybridization experiments where RNA is in 100-fold excess (RNA-driven) of complementary DNA sequences, the reaction can be expressed by the linear curve of the double reciprocal plot, 1/hybridization vs 1/time [Bishop, 1969]. Bishop [1969] has proposed that at a given RNA input the rate of hybridization is directly proportional to the concentration of RNA and inversely proportional to the sequence complexity of the RNA. If this relationship is true, the reaction is

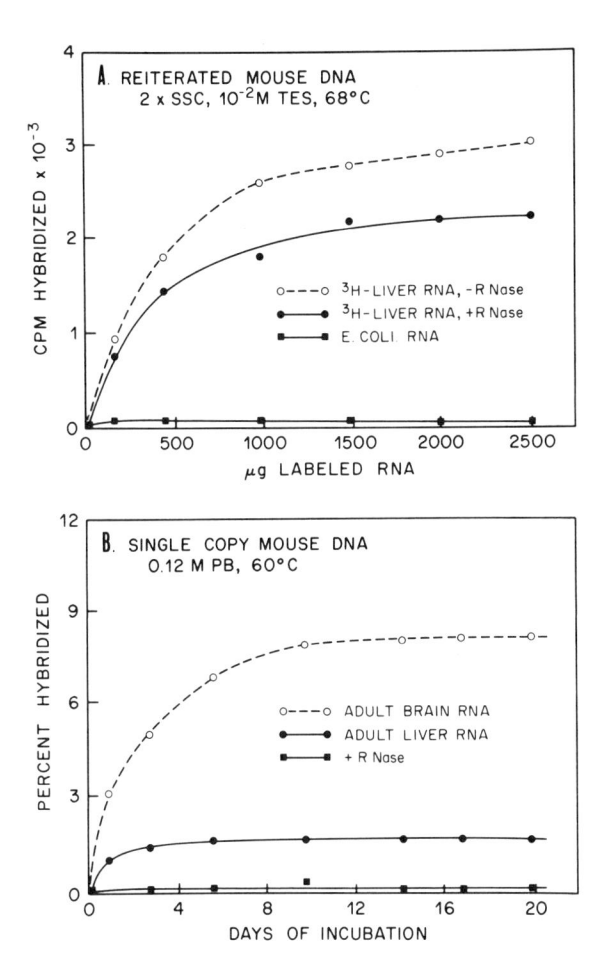

FIGURE 5. Saturation experiments with reiterated and single copy DNA. The saturation of complementary reiterated and single copy mouse DNA by mouse RNA preparations. (a) The effect of ribonuclease treatment on the RNA/reiterated DNA duplex in the saturation of 10 μg mouse DNA (bound to a filter) with increasing amounts of 30 min pulse-labeled mouse liver RNA. The reaction was incubated in 0.3 ml of 2 × SSC, 10^{-2} M TES for 18 hr at 68°C. The raw hybrid was assayed after three 15 ml washes of 2 × SSC at 68°C, dried, and counted. The filters were washed in chloroform and buffer to remove the toluene and fluor before being incubated with 10 μg ribonuclease/ml for 20 min at 37°C. The ribonuclease-resistant RNA/DNA duplex was then dried and counted. No true saturation such as found in ribosomal RNA is evident [Church and McCarthy, 1968]. (b) The saturation hybridization reaction of vast excesses of unlabeled mouse RNA with labeled mouse ^{3}H-DNA fractioned at C_ot 220 (single copy). Samples of 0.5 μg ^{3}H-DNA and 600 μg liver RNA and 600 μg brain RNA in 50 μliter of 0.12 M PB were incubated 60°C for the time indicated. The proportion of single-stranded vs double-stranded molecules was determined by HA chromatography elution at 0.12 M and 0.4 M PB. The RNA transcriptional complexity of mouse brain and mouse liver (adult) is measured by the extent to which the labeled DNA forms an RNA/DNA duplex [Brown and Church, 1971; Hahn and Laird, 1971].

governed by the molar concentration of nucleotide sequences in solution. For filter hybridization Birnstiel et al. [1972] have suggested that RNA/DNA hybridization with homogeneous RNA species present in excess (100 fold) can be characterized by $C_r t_{1/2}$; where C_r is the molar concentration of RNA nucleotides in solution and $t_{1/2}$ is the time taken to reach 50% of the apparent saturation value. Within limits, $C_r t_{1/2}$ is independent of the filter DNA content and the degree of RNA fragmentation. For homogeneous RNA populations $C_r t_{1/2}$ increases linearly with base sequence complexity of the RNA molecules. In these studies Birnstiel et al. [1972] established the optimal rate temperature (T_{opt}) in 6 × SSC (pH 7.2), 50% formamide, and in 0.15 M sodium acetate (pH 5), 60% formamide for bacterial and Xenopus RNA species.

The slope of the straight standard curve which links $C_r t_{1/2}$ to the ϕ X bacteriophage–cRNA sequence complexity is 9.3×10^{-9} mole sec/dalton in 6 × SSC.50% formamide.

Therefore, the simpler the complexity of a population of RNA molecules the faster the initial rate of reaction will be. The values presented in Table I from Birnstiel et al. [1972] reflect the relative complexities of a number of RNA species. At present only mammalian rRNA and a few fairly homogeneous presumptive messenger RNA (that is, hemoglobin) molecules have been isolated with sufficient purity for reliable complexity analysis. Complimentary in vitro synthesized RNA is not a good source of mammalian RNA for complexity analysis unless pure DNA cistrons for a given sequence(s) are used as template since transcription is not random.

The Use of Saturation RNA/DNA Hybridization to Assay Presumptive Messenger RNA Purity

When a presumptive messenger RNA has been isolated for a particular protein, its purity can be rapidly assayed by RNA/DNA hybridization. From the molecular weight of the RNA the analytical complexity ($C_r t_{1/2}$) can be calculated [Birnstiel et al., 1972]. From a comparison of the analytical and kinetic complexity one can estimate the RNA sequence complexity.

The procedure for kinetic complexity analysis was originally defined by Birnstiel et al. [1972]. A typical procedure may include:

(1) DNA is immobilized on nitrocellulose filters as described in section II.
(2) Before the incubation reaction the DNA filters are soaked for 4 hr in 6 × SSC·50% formamide at room temperature.
(3) The labeled RNA in 6 × SSC·50% formamide is heated to 85°C and

TABLE I. Analytical and Kinetic Complexity of RNA in 6 × SSC · 50% Formamide[a]

Source of RNA	Complexity, dalton × 10^{-6}	Complementary DNA, %	Genomic redundancy	$C_r t_{1/2} \times 10^3$, mole sec/l	Kinetic complexity, dalton × 10^{-6}
φX 174 cRNA	1.6	95	1	15	Std.
4 S E. coli tRNA	0.025	0.06	60	6.7	0.78
23 X 16 S B. subtilis rRNA	1.6	0.64	8	12	1.4
4 S Xenopus tRNA	0.025	0.009	6.5×10^3	7.8	0.90
28 S Xenopus rRNA	1.5	0.051	6.1×10^2	11	1.3
28 + 18 S rabbit rRNA	2.5	0.03	2.5×10^2	17	2.0

[a] After Birnstiel et al. [1972].

cooled to the incubation temperature. The amount of RNA should be in 100-fold excess over the DNA filter concentration.
(4) The DNA filters are added to the reaction mixture, the vial tightly sealed, and the reaction gently shaken at the chosen incubation temperature. Incubation temperatures for rabbit and HeLa cell ribosomal RNA are 62 and 65°C, respectively [Birnstiel et al., 1972].
(5) The filters are removed at the chosen times and plunged into ice cold 6 × SSC before being washed in three aliquots of 50 ml of each of 2 × SSC at room temperature.
(6) The filters are then removed and incubated for 30 min with 10 μg/ml ribonuclease in 10 ml of SSC at room temperature.
(7) The filters are washed, dried, and counted as described above. For thermal elution studies the RNA/filter DNA hybrid is handled as outlined in the next section.

Saturation Hybridization of rRNA Molecules

The hybridization of ribosomal RNA molecules with total cellular DNA is a unique system since the family of ribosomal DNA sequences is discrete and the ribosomal RNA molecules can be obtained in large quantities in pure form. Gene linkage studies in Xenopus by RNA/DNA hybridization have been carried out by Brown and Weber [1968]. The kinetic complexity of similar Xenopus RNA populations has been examined by Birnstiel et al. [1972].

The following modification of the Brown and Weber [1968] procedure can be used for examination of the G + C rich ribosomal DNA sequences (Figure 6).

(1) Filter-bound DNA is prepared in the manner described above from CsCl gradients. The 22 mm B6 filters are marked as to CsCl fraction and then transferred to a scintillation vial after the filters from one or more gradients are mounted on a pin.
(2) The incubation mixture must be shaken carefully to remove all trapped air bubbles.
(3) Filters containing heterologous DNA are interspersed with the homologous DNA filters.
(4) 1.5–3.0 μg ^{3}H-rRNA is added to the 1 ml of 4 × SSC incubation solution for 1–10 filters and additional ml for each subsequent 10 filters.
(5) The incubation mixture is incubated in a tightly closed vial, with gentle shaking, for 18 hr at 70°C.
(6) At the end of the reaction period the stock of filters suspended on a pin are removed from the reaction, drained carefully and washed with two 20 ml aliquots of 2 × SSC at 70°C.

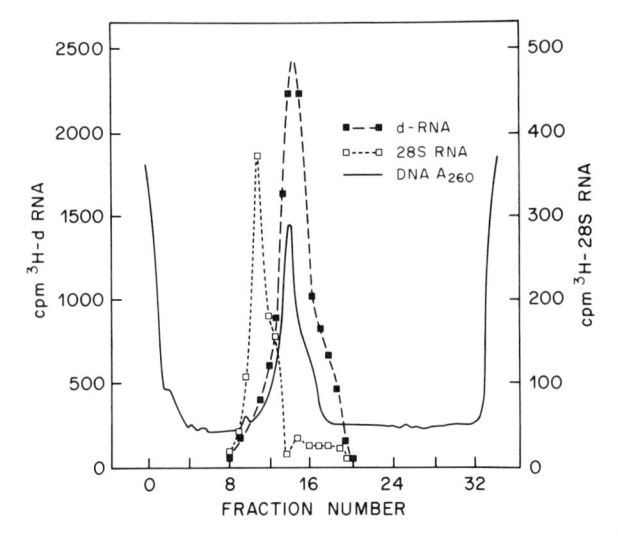

FIGURE 6. RNA/DNA hybridization with CsCl fractionated DNA. The hybridization of 28 S RNA and rapidly labeled RNA (d-RNA) with CsCl fractionated Gallus domesticus DNA. 200 μg of DNA was fractionated on a CsCl gradient, monitored at 260 mμ, alkaline-denatured, and fixed to nitrocellulose filters. Each aliquot was divided into six parts. Two were hybridized with ^{3}H-28 S RNA, two with ^{3}H-18 S RNA (not shown) and two with rapidly labeled ^{3}H-d-RNA. All filters were suspended on stainless steel dissecting pins in order of fraction number and hybridized with ^{3}H-labeled RNA in 1.0 ml of 1 × SSC, 10^{-2} M TES for 15 hr at 66°C. The hybridized filters were washed, dried, and counted. Each point is the mean of duplicate determinations and results are plotted in relation to the absorbance profile of the DNA [after Schultz, 1969].

(7) The filters are incubated with 50 μg/ml of ribonuclease in 5 ml of 2 × SSC at room temperature with gentle shaking.

(8) The batch of filters are washed with three 10 ml aliquots of 2 × SSC to remove the ribonuclease.

(9) Finally each filter is placed in 10 ml of 2 × SSC for 30 min before being washed in a filter holder with 10 ml of 2 × SSC at room temperature.

(10) The filters are blotted dry, dried, and counted in a toluene-based scintillation system.

(11) DNA remaining on the filter is assayed by washing the filter twice with 5 ml of chloroform to remove the fluor and hydrolyzing the DNA at 100°C in the presence of 1.0 N HCl for 15 mm. Brown and Weber [1968] report the optical density of 1 mg hydrolyzed DNA/ml in 1.0 N HCl to be 27.8 at 260 mμ.

Competition Hybridization

The only method currently available for proving differences in base sequence among heterogenous populations of cellular RNA is RNA/DNA hybridization competition. The interpretation of such experiments rests on the assumption that two RNA molecules which have sufficiently similar base sequences will compete with each other for any complementary sequence in the DNA. The definition of <u>sufficiently</u> <u>similar</u> varies with the conditions under which the nucleic acid sequences are allowed to react. The extent of reaction obtained using a given amount of RNA, DNA, and competitor RNA varies with the volume, time of incubation, temperature, and ionic strength [Church and McCarthy, 1968; Bishop, 1969]. Therefore, in species where reiterated sequences exist, the use of hybridization conditions of low stringency will result in the RNA transcribed from one DNA sequence of a sequence family reacting with all members of the sequence family. Under conditions of high stringency, cross-reaction among sequences of a gene family will be restricted to the most closely related members, resulting in a lower extent of hybridization. The RNA/DNA duplex is characterized by a higher thermal stability containing fewer mismatched base-pairs.

Competition reactions as usually carried out with the hybridization of labeled RNA to filter-bound DNA in the presence of excess unlabeled RNA under low $C_0 t$ conditions assays those molecules transcribed from reiterated DNA sequences. Therefore, only differences between families of related genes, defined by the criteria of the reaction conditions, will be detected. The method is not very sensitive to differences between gene products within the same sequence family, therefore, the differences observed between two RNA molecule populations is always an underestimate. The RNA/DNA filter hybridization technique cannot be used to prove identity of two RNA molecule populations, but only to indicate differences. Therefore great care must be taken in the interpretation of low $C_0 t$ competition results. DNA/DNA hybridization under low $C_0 t$ conditions using a similar procedure have been reported [Schultz and Church, 1972].

Competition Hybridization by Presaturation

In 1969, Soeiro and Darnell described competition experiments with HeLa cell RNA in which the filter DNA was exposed to saturating amounts of unlabeled RNA before exposure to labeled RNA. The procedure for presaturation competition experiments is as follows:

(1) Filter-immobilized DNA is prepared as described in section II.
(2) The unlabeled RNA (100–2000 µg depending on the filter DNA concen-

tration and specific activity of the labeled RNA) is taken up in 2 × SSC, 0.4 % SDS or 10^{-2} M TES is heated to 85° and cooled to the incubation temperature (67°C) before the filters are added to 0.2 ml aliquots for incubation.
(3) The incubation with unlabeled RNA is continued for 16–20 hr after which the filters are removed and washed three times with 20 ml of 2 × SSC for 15 min at 67°C.
(4) The filters are then returned to 0.2 ml of 2 × SSC at 67°C for reaction with labeled RNA.
(5) After a further 16–20 hr of incubation the mixture is washed as described in (3).
(6) The ribonuclease sensitive sequences are digested with ribonuclease (5 µg/ml pancreatic, 5 units/ml T1) for 30 min at 37°C in 10 ml of 2 × SSC.
(7) The ribonuclease is removed by two washes in 2 × SSC (10 ml) and the filters blotted, dried, and counted in a liquid scintillation system.
(8) Control experiments include the use of heterologous DNA filters in the reaction vials with the homologous DNA filters. The presence of at least two reactions with only the heterologous DNA present to assay background nonspecific binding noise and the acid-precipitable labeled RNA remaining at the end of the incubation (input). Lastly, the inclusion of labeled RNA during the first but not the second incubation as an assay for degradation during incubation.

The presaturation experimental method may be useful in the selective hybridization of a small proportion of RNA molecules in a cellular preparation. For example, to assay for hormonal induction of RNA sequences, one would presaturate a hybridization system with normal cytoplasmic polysomal RNA (free from rRNA) followed by hybridization with labeled hormonally induced polysomal RNA (free from rRNA). The greatly enriched labeled hormonally induced RNA can then be eluted and characterized even though unlabeled normal RNA is present. The interpretation is severely handicapped by the presence of unstable RNA/DNA components formed during incubation.

Analysis of the Thermal Stability of DNA/DNA and RNA/DNA Duplexes

The extent to which two polynucleotide strands will associate is a function of the complementarity between base sequences. The thermal stability of such duplex molecules therefore is a function of the length of the molecules, the base composition, and the relative proportion of matched and mismatched basepairs. The thermal stability of a duplex molecule is directly related to the proportion of mismatched base pairs such that a 1°C difference in T_m of the duplex is an indication of 1.5% mismatched bases [Laird et al., 1969]. McConaughy and McCarthy [1970a, b] have presented evidence for an increase in base sequence specificity in pairing with increases in chain length, salt concentration, and temperature. McCarthy's group has also shown that species-specific interactions occur with oligonucleotides with an increase in specificity and thermal stability as fragment chain length increases. The thermal stability of mouse oligonucleotide/mouse DNA duplexes was always lower than the corresponding bacterial duplex of similar fragment size, presumably due to reiterated sequences.

Thermal Melting of RNA or DNA/Filter-Bound DNA Duplexes

The DNA filter technique [Gillespie and Spiegelman, 1965] provides a convenient way of analyzing the thermal stability of RNA/DNA or DNA/DNA molecules. There are two ways of analyzing the thermal stability of filter-bound DNA duplexes; a series of filters can be checked for the stable duplex remaining at a given series of temperatures; or the dissociated single-stranded nucleic acid melted from the filter DNA duplex can be recovered at each step in the temperature elution program (Figure 7).

The procedure is as follows:

(1) At the end of the chosen reaction the series of filters are washed in the chosen manner. For example, after reaction in 2 × SSC at 65°C the filters are washed once in 15 ml of 2 × SSC and once in 15 ml of 1 × SSC at 65°C. The remaining buffer is carefully drained off and the filters dried. The extent of hybrid reaction and the proper controls are then assayed in a toluene-based liquid scintillation system.

(2) The filters are then removed from the counting fluid, dried, and washed in 10 ml of 1 × SSC at 50°C.

(3) For convenience the filters can then be mounted on nonreactive pins for actual thermal melting.

(4) The filters are then incubated for 10 min in 3 ml of 1 × SSC each at 5°C steps, commencing at 50°C.

(5) At the end of the 10 min interval at a given temperature the filter is removed, the remaining buffer carefully drained off, and the filter transferred to a new preequilibrated 3 ml 1 × SSC fraction. This routine is continued to 95°C.

(6) Each 3 ml fraction of 1 × SSC is subsequently made 5% with respect to TCA after the addition of 150 γ of carrier RNA or bovine albumin.

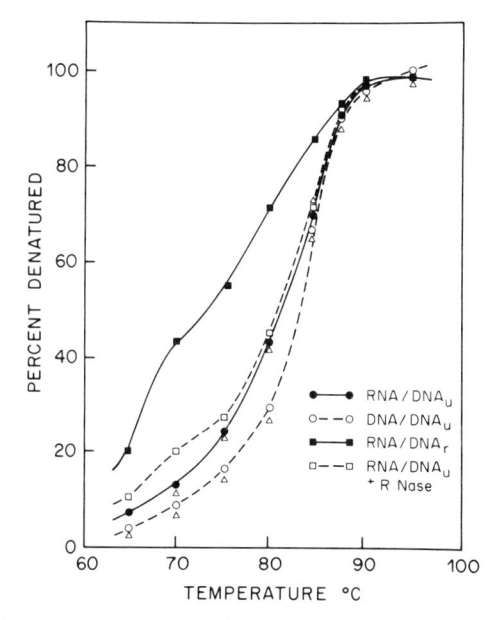

FIGURE 7. Thermal stability of RNA/unique DNA, RNA/reiterated DNA, and DNA/DNA duplexes. The thermal stability of single copy DNA (DNA_u) and reiterated DNA (DNA_r) isolated from mouse L-cells after reassociation with total mouse DNA; hybridization with total cellular brain RNA in 0.12 M PB at 60°C. The reiterated C_0t 220 DNA_r (10µg) was bound to a filter and the reaction carried out in 0.2 ml 0.12 M PB for 16 hr with 100 µg ^{32}P-mouse brain RNA. The reaction with unique DNA (C_0t 220) involved 2 µg/ml brain RNA, 0.5 µg/ml unique DNA hybridized for 14 days in 0.12 M PB at 60°C. Total DNA/^{3}H-unique DNA (1.5 mg/ml) reassociation was carried out to C_0t 5000 in 0.12 M PB at 60°C. Some duplicate thermal stabilities were monitored by optical density of the eluent (△), otherwise all profiles were assayed by elution from HA with 0.12 M PB at 5°C temperature increments. One sample of the RNA/^{3}H-unique DNA incubation mixture was treated with ribonuclease (15 µg/ml) for 30 min at 37°C after the hybridization reaction and before the thermal stability analysis. The resulting data was all normalized to a 0 equal to the cpm in the duplex at 60°C relative to the accumulated eluted cpm at 95°C.

(7) After cooling, the TCA precipitate is collected on Whatman GF/C glass filters or an HAWP Millipore membrane filters. Alternatively, the 3 ml aqueous fraction can be added to 10 ml of toluene-POP-POPOP scintillation cocktail containing 1/3 vol Bio-Solv BBS-3 Solubilizer (Beckman).

(8) Filters are dried and counted in a toluene-based liquid scintillation system.

The accumulated dissociated fractions can then be plotted against temperature to yield the normal melting profile.

Alternatively, a series of filters can be placed in the chosen buffer (that is, 1 × SSC at 50°C) after the normal post incubation washing but before counting.

(1) The temperature is increased by 3–5°C intervals and at the end of each 10 min equilibration period, duplicate filters are removed from the buffer wash fraction and the excess buffer carefully drained off and the filters dried and counted.
(2) The temperature is then raised by the chosen interval and after the chosen equilibrium period (that is, 10 min) two more filters are removed, drained, and dried as before.
(3) The process is continued until the temperature is above 95°C.

In this method the stable duplex is assayed. The dissociated molecule in the wash fraction can be precipitated or counted directly by the procedures outlined above to verify the melting profile. It is useful to consider monitoring of both double-stranded duplex and single-strand dissociate fractions since the DNA eluted from the filter can be readily assayed at the same time. The second procedure may be the method of choice when the RNA or DNA molecules are of low specific activity. This method maximizes the counts being assayed in the duplex. The DNA which is eluted from the filters with increasing temperature must be monitored since not only DNA but RNA/DNA will cause errors in the calculation of T_m. A different label in the filter-bound DNA is the easiest and most accurate way of checking DNA elution and filter DNA concentration.

Thermal Melting of RNA or DNA/DNA Duplexes from UV Gels or Agar

The basic procedure for the thermal elution of RNA/DNA or DNA/DNA duplexes from UV gels or agar is in principle similar to the previously described technique for filter-bound DNA. The immobilized DNA matrix is washed with 1/10 × SSC at successively higher temperatures commencing at 40°C. The labeled nucleic acid molecules which are melted from the duplex are precipitated from the buffer wash with TCA and collected or solubilized directly and counted.

Because of the serious DNA leaking problem at elevated temperatures these techniques are of more limited use for analysis of melting profiles than assays on HA or membrane filters. The technique has been used successfully for echinoderm RNA/DNA hybridization studies by Whiteley, McCarthy, and Whitely [1966].

Thermal Melting of RNA or DNA/DNA Duplexes from Hydroxyapatite

The thermal stability of duplexes formed in in-solution hybridization reactions can be assayed by chromatography on HA. Properly prepared HA recognizes structure in nucleic acid molecules [Bernardi, 1965,1971]. Therefore, double-stranded nucleic acids can be eluted from HA by increasing the salt concentration or melted by increasing the temperature with the concomittant elution of the single-stranded molecules thus dissociated at 0.12 M phosphate buffer.

The procedure is as follows:

(1) At a predetermined time the reassociation reaction is halted and the duplex may be subjected to nuclease action, dilution, etc. If the reassociation conditions include formamide it is necessary to dilute the formamide to below 1% with the appropriate buffer (usually 0.12 M PB) before adsorption of the double-stranded DNA to the HA [McConaughy et al., 1969].

(2) The reassociation mixture or nuclease-resistant duplex (as the case may be) is then loaded onto HA in 0.12 M PB at 60°C or other appropriate temperature (see section on HA analysis).

(3) The single-stranded molecules are eluted from the HA column with 3–5 bed vol of 0.12 M PB at 60°C.

(4) The temperature is then raised by 3 or 5°C intervals allowing sufficient time for the buffer washing the HA to reach equilibrium at each temperature step until the water bath has reached over 95°C.

(5) The dissociated nucleic acid will elute from the HA by 2–5 vol of 0.12 M PB. The flow rate will depend on the size of the column and the load of nucleic acid relative to HA capacity or ability to distinguish structure [Church and Brown, 1972].

(6) The dissociated single-stranded nucleic acid can be monitored optically at 260 mµ or labeled nucleic acid precipitated from each fraction, after addition of appropriate carrier, by making the solution 5% with respect to TCA or solubilized and counted directly. The precipitated nucleic acid is collected on membrane filters, dried, and counted as usual.

(7) If formamide is present, the optical density is monitored at 270 mµ. In some batches of HA, considerable elution of $CaPO_4$ may occur at high temperatures. A correction for this light scattering can be estimated from $A_{300\ m\mu}$. The concentration of nucleic acid being estimated from $A_{260} - A_{300}$.

(8) Necessary controls for the assay of DNA/DNA duplexes include the melt-

ing of native sheared DNA and the inclusion of an appropriate differentially labeled bacterial DNA to monitor C_0t during the incubation and influence of base composition. The ability to melt and elute all of the nucleic acids loaded onto the HA column can then be asaayed.

(9) Controls for the assay of RNA/DNA duplexes melted from HA include loading a HA column with a labeled bacterial DNA—a differentially labeled RNA mixture following reaction conditions similar to the RNA/DNA duplex incubation under study. The ribonuclease-resistant fragments will contribute to the column background (see HA reassociation analysis), and will be melted and eluted to contribute to the error in DNA excess reactions where the radiolabel is in the RNA. In RNA excess reactions, this is not a problem since the label monitored is in the DNA. However it is essential to include a control based on the melting of any homologous DNA/DNA duplex formation which may have occurred in the reassociation of a bacterial RNA/DNA reassociation reaction.

RNA secondary structure such as seen in tRNA, poly A sequences or other naturally occurring hairpin regions of mammalian RNA will be recognized as having structure by HA. Therefore, in labeled RNA/DNA in-solution reactions, particularly in vast DNA excess, the column should be washed with 0.24 M PB at 60°C. Under these conditions RNA/RNA and RNA with secondary structure will be eluted from HA. Recently, some very important observations concerning the parameters affecting nucleic acid hydroxylapatite interactions have been reported by Martinson [1973 a,b].

Other methods of eliminating RNA background on HA are considered elsewhere and utilize up to 2% sodium dodecyl sulfate (SDS) or 7 M urea.

The results of DNA filter, HA, and optical reassociation melting analysis are shown in Figure 7. The absorbance changes during the thermal denaturation of DNA/DNA and RNA/DNA can be plotted as the percent hyperchromicity at a given temperature on normal probability paper according to a method suggested by Knittel et al. [1968] for analysis of component elements.

Spectrophotometric Analysis of RNA/DNA and DNA/DNA Duplex-Melting Profiles

The absorbance change during thermal dissociation has been used for many years to ascertain the T_m and melting profiles of native DNA. In the same way it is possible to monitor the melting profiles of DNA/DNA and RNA/DNA reassociation duplexes. Britten and Kohne [1968] first observed the complete reassociation profile of complex DNA in a specially designed recording spectrophotometer. In most laboratories a Gilford 2400 or Beckman ACTA V recording spectrophotometer fitted with a temperature controlled cuvette housing are used to monitor reassociation and denaturation. Absorbance is measured at 260 mμ in the absence of formamide and 270 mμ in its presence. The temperature should be raised slowly enough so that 3–5 OD observations can be recorded per degree rise in temperature.

SECTION V

DNA Reassociation Analysis

Reassociation of DNA molecules isolated from higher organisms was pioneered by Britten and his coworkers, with the demonstration that the half-period for DNA reassociation is inversely proportional to the DNA concentration at a given criteria and proportional to the genome size of the organism [Britten and Kohne, 1968]. The definition of C_0t and parameters of the rate of reassociation were discussed in a previous section. For the C_0t concept to have meaning in the comparison of genome sizes, the term unit genome was introduced by Laird [1971]. Unit genome is defined as the chromosomal DNA of a cell such that the least frequent nucleotide sequences are present only once, and all nucleotide sequences are represented in the preparation in the proportions found in the cell. A homogeneous population of DNA fragments must be used in order to interpret reassociation experiments, therefore fragments of 200–500 nucleotides are used (that is, 400 nucleotides corresponds to a template for a polypeptide of about 130 amino acids). The estimate of the nuclear DNA content in the meiotic cells of a species is crucial to the interpretation of DNA reassociation results. In the mouse 1.8×10^{12} dalton or 3 pg of DNA are present in the sperm cell [von Gelder et al., 1971; Laird, 1971]. DNA reassociation experiments containing an internal standard are an essential part of any reassociation study [Britten and Kohne, 1968; Laird, 1971] since the significance of repeated sequences can only be extrapolated relative to an internal control of known genome size and complexity.

The data presented in Figure 1 for the reassociation of DNA from various sources included, an internal standard of ^{14}C-E. coli DNA, an excess of unlabeled total mouse DNA and small amounts of ^{3}H single copy mouse DNA incubated in one reassociation reaction. In the elegantly documented analysis of DNA reassociation presented by Laird [1971] it is shown that DNA's from widely related sources, such as E. coli and mouse, reassociate independently of each other. The C_0t of reassociation being calculated from the concentration of DNA present in vast excess.

The renaturation of DNA is a two-step process involving nucleation, a bimolecular reaction involving the collision and complementary pairing of a few base-pairs to form a short stable duplex. The homology of the nucleic acids will determine the stable minimum length which is required to permit further growth of the duplex. This initial reaction product has a reversible thermally unstable component [McCarthy and Church, 1970]. The second-order rate constant of the nucleation reaction depends upon the number of complementary nucleotides required to form the stable duplex, hence nucleation is a measure of base sequence homology over short sequences. The second step, "zippering," is a unimolecular reaction in which helical growth follows stable nucleation. The complexity of the total reassociation reaction kinetics depends on the heterogeneity of the paired sequences base-paired. Therefore the presence of reiterated sequences may have different apparent reassociation rates depending on the stringency of the incubation-reassociation conditions.

The expected or theoretical second order rate constant for all sequences present only once per genome can be calculated from the computer generated profile [Britten, 1970] or by the curve fitting method of Laird and McCarthy [1969]. They use the equation

$$C/C_0 = 1/(1 + k_2 C_0 t)$$

where C_0 represents the single-stranded DNA concentration at time zero and k_2 is the rate constant which would be obtained if all the sequences in a DNA were present only once.

The data in Figure 1 show that mouse DNA reassociates approximately 900 times more slowly than E. coli and 9000 times more slowly than DNA from T4. If the data is corrected for the effect of base composition [Wetmur and Davidson, 1968] the rate constant for the reassociation of mouse DNA is approximately 700 times less than for E. coli DNA. This is in very close agreement with the fact that mouse sperm contains about 700 times more DNA than E. coli. The data in Figure 1 also shows that $C_0 t_{1/2}$ for the second order rate curve for single copy mouse sequences is approximately 1850. Correlations between kinetic and analytical complexities of various DNAs have been presented by Britten and Kohne [1968] and Laird [1971]. The data presented in Table II is from Laird [1971] and Church and Schultz [1973].

DNA reassociation can be measured in a variety of ways, each depending on some easily monitored physical difference between single- and double-stranded DNA. Hence the optical assay of reassociation is based in the fact that dissociated or denatured DNA absorbs more UV radiation than native DNA does. The extent to which phosphate groups are exposed, and the entropy of

TABLE II. Kinetic and Analytical Complexity of DNA

Source	% G + C	% Single copy	$C_0 t_{1/2}$ Corrected for repeated sequences	$C_0 t_{1/2}$ relative to E. coli	Minimum daltons	Genome size base pairs
T4	34	100	0.19	0.056	1.3×10^8	2.0×10^5
E. coli	50	99	1.8	1.0	2.6×10^9	4.0×10^6
Mouse	41	63	1850	700	1.8×10^{12}	2.7×10^9

the structure of DNA, are the basis for differential binding to HA. Some exonucleases have a high substrate specificity for single-stranded DNA which allows the digestion of DNA tails in DNA/DNA reassociation and RNA excess hybridization. In the following pages each of the three methods of reassociation analysis are discussed.

It must be stressed that it is desirable to have two independent measures of the extent of reassociation in any experimental system. An accurate estimation of genome size is required for interpretation of the relative abundance of reiterated sequences since proportionality between $C_0 t_{1/2}$ and genome size is only true in the absence of reiterated DNA sequences.

A. Hydroxyapatite Reassociation Analysis. Reassociation of sheared, denatured DNA isolated from higher organisms can be analyzed by HA chromatography [Walker and McLaren, 1965; Britten and Kohne, 1968; Laird, 1971; Bernardi, 1971; Church and Brown, 1972].

(1) The mixture of DNA's to be analyzed is denatured in phosphate buffer at greater than 95°C for 15 min. A typical internal control reassociation mixture consists of 2 mg/ml sheared unlabeled total mouse DNA, 1 μg/ml ^{3}H-labeled unique mouse DNA ($C_0 t$ 220) and 10 μg/ml ^{14}C-E. coli sheared DNA set up in 0.5 ml of 0.12 M PB at 60°C in a tightly sealed glass vessel.

(2) Alternatively 50 μliter aliquots are sealed in capillary tubes (Corning, micropipets) before denaturation at 95°C for 15 min, and cooled to 60°C for incubation.

(3) Aliquots of 50 μliter or capillary tubes (containing 50 μliter) are removed at various times and analyzed immediately by stopping the reaction by addition of 2 ml of cold 0.12 M PB. The $C_0 t$ aliquots can also be frozen at −20°C and the experiment analyzed at one time.

(4) The aliquots are applied to 1 ml of HA equilibrated with 0.12 M PB at

60°C. Multiple samples are easily handled by using 2 1/2 cc syringes or pasteur pipets as columns mounted in a mouse cage connected to a water bath. Constant head volumes are not required for elution by known bed volumes by gravity flow.

(5) The HA column is washed with 5 bed vol of 0.12 M PB at 60°C to elute the single-stranded DNA, over 90% of the single-stranded DNA is eluted in the first bed volume. Capacity of HA is usually about 100 μg DNA/ml.

(6) The HA column is then washed with 0.4 M PB to elute the double-stranded DNA. Approximately 80% of the double-stranded DNA is eluted in the first bed volume.

(7) The fractions are analyzed at A_{260} to determine the concentration of unlabeled DNA which is reassociated (that is, total mouse DNA), and an aliquot precipitated with an equal volume of 10% TCA with carrier and counted to assay radioactive DNA reassociation (that is, ^{3}H-mouse unique DNA and ^{14}C-E. coli DNA). Water-jacketed columns 2 X 5 cm are convenient columns for pumping the buffer (LKB Variopex 2.5 X 10) through the column: OD can be monitored continually (LKB Uvicord) and fractions collected [Brown and Church, 1971].

(8) An aliquot taken at zero time is the denaturation blank while an acid-precipitable assay series is set up in a set of parallel incubations to estimate degradation during incubation.

(9) For thermal stability analysis the temperature is raised by 5°C steps from 60°C in 0.12 M PB. After temperature equilibration 2 bed vol of 0.12 M PB are used to elute the melted single-stranded DNA from the HA column before raising the temperature the next 5°C step.

(10) For reassociation of complex DNA's from species with a large proportion of unique sequences 0.1% SDS should be added to the phosphate buffer to prevent degradation. Lower temperatures and formamide may be of value (see earlier section) in these reassociation studies.

(11) Control experiments must ascertain the HA background binding of nucleic acids. A dilute DNA solution (^{3}H-DNA, 10 μg/ml) in 0.12 M PB is denatured and rapidly cooled to 4°C in an acetone dry ice bath. The sample is diluted 100-fold with 0.12 M PB, the temperature raised to 60°C and loaded onto HA at 60°C. The sample is immediately washed with 5 bed vol of 0.12 M PB followed by 5 bed vol of 0.4 M PB. The DNA bound after the 0.12 M PB washing and eluted in the 0.4 M PB wash is the nonspecifically retained background at C_0t 0. Normally about 0.5% of the total DNA is bound to the column, with 98% nucleic acid recovery from HA with 0.4 M PB elution.

(12) As pointed out in another section and shown in Figure 2 DNA fragment size greatly influences the apparent reassociation as estimated on HA. The OD and HA reassociation profiles come into closer agreement as DNA fragment size approaches 250 nucleotides [Laird, 1971; Bell, 1971; Grouse et al., 1972]. The disparity between the two values for longer DNA fragments is consistent with the existence of physical linkage between slowly reassociating single copy sequences and the more rapidly reassociating reiterated sequences in the same long fragment.

B. DNA/DNA Optical Reassociation. DNA melting profiles and DNA/DNA reassociation kinetics can be monitored on a continuous recording spectrophotometer with an automatic 0 to correct for drift and a programmable temperature controlled cuvette chamber (that is, Gilford 2400 or Beckman ACTA V). A cuvette containing a blank of known OD must be present at all times. The buffer concentration should be below 0.12 M PB or 1 X SSC and should be boiled to evaporate trapped gases before use.

(1) The spectrophotometer is set to continuously monitor optical density in an overlapping concentration series. A spectrophotometer which records temperature continuously is desirable but not essential. For melting profiles a temperature program rise of not more than 1°C/min is used in conjunction with a high capacity circulating bath.

(2) The cuvettes containing DNA samples for melting and reassociation studies are placed under partial vacuum to remove dissolved air. Each sample is then covered with silicone oil and the cuvette's glass stopper put in place.

(3) The OD is monitored at 260 mμ in water jacketed quartz cuvettes connected to two water baths in parallel. One bath is programmed to increase the temperature to 100°C, with glycol, for melting the DNA and the other bath is set at a constant 60°C for reassociation. It is then possible to melt the DNA sample with the first bath and quickly switch to the 60°C bath for DNA reassociation.

(4) The DNA samples are first melted by programmed temperature increase to greater than 95°C and held for 15 min at this temperature. The $OD_{260 \, m\mu}$ at this point represents complete denaturation and time zero.

(5) The cuvette is rapidly cooled to 60°C with the second circulating bath and the $OD_{260 \, m\mu}$ at the time the cuvette reaches 60°C called time 0. The apparent instant reassociation is due in part to base stacking effects (5% for mouse DNA, [Laird, 1971]), renaturation of sequences held in register by cross linkage [Alberts and Doty, 1968] and by very rapid reassociation of highly reiterated sequences [Britten and Smith, 1970]. The apparent instant reassociation can be minimized by homogenous populations

of DNA fragments 400–500 nucleotides long which have been passed over Chelex-100 or SE-Sephadex and extensively dialyzed.

(6) Reassociation in 0.12 M PB at 60°C is monitored continuously at 260 mμ for the first 24–48 hr and twice daily for 1/2 hr thereafter. Other conditions, as appropriate, can be used since the rate reaction can be increased by higher salt and the temperature lowered by addition of formamide.

(7) The fraction of DNA renatured at time $\underline{t}$ is plotted against the log of the equivalent $C_0 t$ of the DNA solution. The equivalent $C_0 t$ is the $C_0 t$ value multiplied by a salt correction factor to correct the rate of reassociation at any given Na^+ or formamide concentration to that of the standard condition of 0.12 M PB (0.18 M Na^+). The amount of DNA renatured at any particular time is calculated from the hyperchromicity of each sample after melting the sheared DNA at time zero. The reassociation profile based on hyperchromicity can be compared to that calculated from a computer analysis of the profile [Britten, 1970].

(8) A 1 cm path-length cuvette can usefully contain 0.2 OD_{260}/ml (approximately 10 μg/ml) and a 1 mm path-length cuvette 2.0 OD_{260}/ml for melting and reassociation. Two further cuvettes with 1 cm and 1 mm path-lengths, containing only buffer serve as blanks [Bell, 1971].

C. Exonuclease Assay of DNA Reassociation. Optical monitoring of DNA/DNA reassociation requires access to an accurate programmable spectrophotometer with a temperature controlled cuvette for extended periods of time, while the analysis of DNA duplexes on HA can be very tedious and time consuming. Alternatives exist, which utilize exonucleases specific for single-stranded DNA. The specificity of all nucleases presently in use for such studies is open to some question, however, very rapid analysis of DNA reassociation can be achieved by the use of the Sutton [1971] S_1 and Fraser, Rabin, and Allen [1970] single-stranded exonucleases.

The exonuclease (S_1) isolated from Aspergillus oryzae (Takadiastase, Sankyo Co.) has a high specificity for single-stranded DNA [Sutton, 1971] and is easily prepared. In contrast the exonuclease prepared from Neurospora crassa conidia is more fully characterized but tedious to prepare [Fraser et al., 1970]. In either case the exonuclease can be used to digest unmatched sequences and tails of DNA/DNA reassociation duplexes presumably leaving base-paired structures. The use of an exonuclease is analagous to the ribonuclease treatment of RNA/DNA duplexes after hybridization reactions.

Reassociation can be conveniently monitored by the use of the exonuclease as follows:

(1) The DNA/DNA reassociation reaction is set up in the normal manner and 1 μg aliquots of DNA removed at the desired $C_0 t$ values.
(2) The aliquots are frozen until the reassociation is complete and all enzyme digestions run at once.
(3) To each 1 μg DNA aliquot which contains single-stranded DNA, double-stranded DNA, and molecules with both single- and double-stranded region, is added 1 ml of the exonuclease solutions, (that is, for the S_1 exonuclease, the reaction includes 10 units S_1 nuclease in 0.03 M NA acetate, pH 4.5, 3×10^{-5} M $ZnSO_4$, 0.1 M NaCl and 50 μg/ml sonicated, denatured E. coli DNA at 50°C for 40 min or with 100 units of S_1 for 10 min.
(4) At the end of the enzymatic digestion the reaction is stopped by making the solution 5% TCA after addition of 50 μg rRNA carrier at 4°C.
(5) The precipitate (double-stranded DNA) is collected on nitrocellulose filters and washed with 3 vol of 5% TCA at 4°C; or, spun down in a centrifuge tube and the pellet recovered.
(6) The double-stranded DNA pellet is washed with 0.12 M PB several times and assayed for enzyme efficiency and thermal stability.
(7) The reassociation plot calculated by this quick and easy precipitate-filter method requires an adequate zero time point and an optical or HA assay of enzyme efficiency. An example of such a reassociation curve is shown in Figure 8.

Caution in interpretation of such results include the fact that at zero time 5% of the DNA appears double-stranded based on enzyme activity. This may be due to cross-linking, to base stacking effects, or some as yet poorly understood characteristic of the enzymes. In addition these enzymes seem to have ribonuclease and endonuclease activity under certain reaction conditions.

Preparation of Hydroxyapatite

Hydroxyapatite (HA) is a crystalline form of calcium phosphate first prepared for chromatography by Tiselius et al. [1956] to recognize structure in macromolecules. The HA used for the separation of single- and double-stranded nucleic acids can be prepared in the laboratory by the method of Bernardi [1969, 1971] or obtained commercially (BIO-GEL HTP, Biorad or Hydroxyapatite–clarkson). The fractionation of nucleic acids on HA is partly based on differences in the extent of phosphate groups exposed by molecules with secondary and tertiary structure and on the influence of cations on the physical

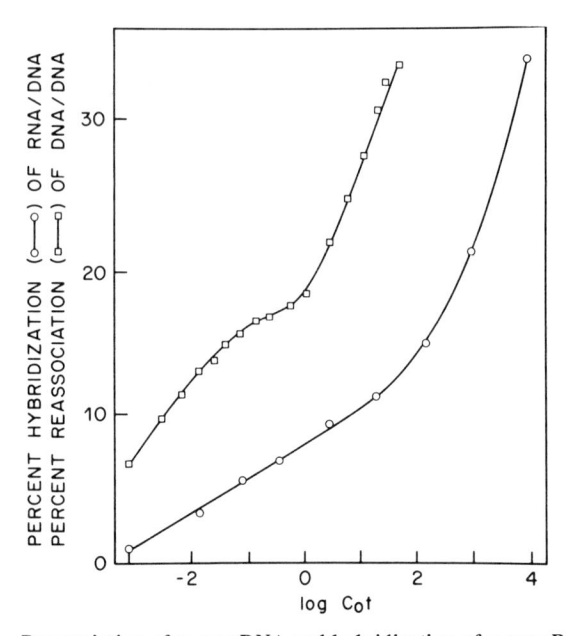

FIGURE 8. Reassociation of mouse DNA and hybridization of mouse RNA in vast DNA excess. The hybridization of equilibrium-labeled ^{3}H-mouse Taper ascites RNA with mouse DNA present in vast excess and the renaturation of mouse DNA plotted against log $C_o t$. The mouse DNA/DNA reassociation reaction was monitored optically at 260 mμ in 0.12 M PB, 60°C as described in the text. The RNA/DNA hybridization was also carried out in 0.12 M PB at 60°C with a RNA:DNA ratio of 1:80,000. The ^{3}H uniformly labeled mouse ascites (Taper) RNA had a specific activity of 107,000 cpm/μg. After appropriate incubation periods 50 μliter aliquots of the RNA/DNA mixture were removed, diluted to 10 ml with 0.12 M PB and treated for 30 min with 10 μg/ml ribonuclease. The ribonuclease-resistant duplex was precipitated with an equal volume of 10% TCA after addition of a carrier and collected on GF/C filters for analysis.

structure of the DNA molecule. Therefore single-stranded molecules with secondary structure will not be distinguished from double-stranded molecules.

Hydroxyapatite columns have high resolution with a relatively high flow rate. The capacity of each batch of HA to distinguish between different extents of structure, normally single- or double-stranded nucleic acids, must be checked. Capacity is usually about 100 μg DNA and 30 μg RNA/ml bed vol. The capacity depends on the HA crystal surface hence on the source and preparation of HA crystals. The larger the crystal size the higher the flow rate and lower the capacity. In our laboratory HA crystals (that is, HTP-BIO-GEL) are suspended in 100 vol of 0.01 M PB at pH 6.8. Any "fines" are gently decanted and the

HA fully equilibrated in the loading buffer, (that is, 24 hr at 4°C in 0.03 PB).

The column is prepared by pouring the slurry into a water-jacketed column or into multiple pasteur pipets stuck through the bottom of a plastic mouse cage. The mouse cage serves as a water bath when connected to a circulating bath after sealing the pipets and cage. If the column has a fine scintered glass bottom it will quickly clogg with HA particles unless a glass wool or cellulose layer is in place before the slurry is poured. After 1 cm of HA has settled into place, the outlet may be opened and the column filled as required. Before the sample is loaded, 2 bed vol of the eluting buffer are passed through at the required temperature, usually in 0.03, 0.12, or 0.14 M PB, pH 6.8 at 60°C. Slight pressure will increase the flow rate but increased pressure will pack the HA and severely diminish flow rate particularly at high temperatures during thermal elution.

Hydroxyapatite can be stored in small amounts in 0.03 or 0.12 M PB with chloroform as a preservative. When HA crystals are being resuspended, care should be exercised to avoid excessive agitation which damages the crystals and aggregates.

The elution of DNA from HA is accomplished by 0.12 M PB (single-stranded) and greater than 0.4 M PB (double-stranded) at 60°C or with increasing temperature. Elution of RNA and RNA/DNA hybrids is slightly more complex due to the increased secondary structure of the RNA. RNA elutes from HA in the PB range 0.12–0.28 M. Addition of 0.4% SDS or up to 7 M urea to the normal PB prevents the elution of RNA into the RNA/DNA fractions. Formamide must be diluted to less than 1% for the usual stepwise PB elution of nucleic acids. It is possible to elute nucleic acids from HA with very shallow PB gradients from 0.14 M to 0.55 M PB and obtain separation in 30% formamide. Care must be taken to choose elution conditions which have the proper "window" such that double stranded molecules are not eluted prematurely [Martinson, 1973b]. Phosphate buffer molarity in the column effluent can be checked by refractive index. We have reused HA several times by regenerating the column with 10 bed vol of the loading buffer over a 1–2 hr period after elution of all adsorbed material is complete (4 vol 0.5 M PB).

Preparation of Reassociation Fractions of DNA

The complexity of the genome of higher organisms is so large and the nonspecific reassociation of repeated sequences and hybridization so difficult to interpret that kinetically homogeneous populations of DNA sequences are often of great value to the investigator. Therefore, methods have been developed which allow isolation of DNA sequences of similar reiteration frequency [Schultz, 1969; Britten and Smith, 1970]. These methods may be coupled in the future with methods of isolation of high molecular weight single-stranded DNA containing specific "gene sequences." In these latter studies, DNA or RNA is attached to a solid matrix such that the macromolecule is free to form a complementary duplex followed by elution of the sequence enriched fraction [Gilham, 1971; Alberts and Herrick, 1971; Robberson and Davidson, 1972].

A complex genome can be separated into populations of DNA sequences with similar rates of reassociation by separating reassociated DNA from single-stranded DNA molecules at different C_0t values. The DNA fractions can then be used as templates for cRNA synthesis [Saunders et al., 1972]; for analysis of RNA transcriptional activity [Church, unpublished] and for visual localization of genetic loci by in situ hybridization [Pardue and Gall, 1969].

There are numerous experimental regimes which are applicable to the isolation of specific populations of DNA with similar reiteration frequencies. I would like to outline three such programs as examples of the technique: (1) isolation of mouse DNA free of the very rapidly reassociating fraction, including satellite DNA; (2) isolation of several reiterated DNA sequence families; and (3) the isolation of single copy DNA sequences.

(I) The isolation of mouse DNA free from the 10% very rapidly reassociating sequences can be accomplished as follows:
  (1) Purified mouse DNA which has been passed over Chelex 100 or SE-Sephadex is sheared to a fragment size of less than 500 nucleotides.
  (2) The DNA is then denatured at less than 500 μg/ml in 0.03 M PB by heating to more than 95°C for 15 min before being cooled rapidly in an acetone–dry ice bath to 60°C.
  (3) The phosphate buffer concentration is quickly brought to 0.05 M PB to initiate reassociation at a rate approximately 10-fold less than 0.12 M PB [Britten and Smith, 1970].
  (4) The reassociation is stopped at an equivalent C_0t of 10^{-2} by addition of an equal volume of 2% formaldehyde, 1 M NaCl, 0.05 M PB at 60°C [Schmeckpeper and Smith, 1972].
  (5) The DNA solution is then mixed with sufficient preequilibrated HA to approach 75% capacity. The HA is preequilibrated with 0.05 M or 0.14 M PB, 1% formaldehyde at 40°C for 4 hr.
  (6) After gentle mixing, the HA slurry in 0.05 M PB is poured into a water-jacketed column at 40°C and the single-stranded DNA free of the very rapidly reassociating sequences eluted from the HA column with 2 bed vol of 0.14 M PB. Or: the 0.14 M PB HA slurry is placed in centrifuge tubes and spun at 500 × g for 5 min. The HA pellet is gently washed with 2 bed vol of 0.14 M PB twice more and the combined supernatants,

dialyzed against 100 vol of 0.03 M PB for 10 hr at 4°C, lyophylized, and the very rapidly reassociating sequence free single-stranded DNA taken up in an appropriate buffer [Flamm, Walker and McCallum, 1969].

(7) The very rapidly reassociating DNA (double-stranded) is eluted from the HA column with 2 bed vol of 0.4 M PB, dialyzed against distilled H_2O for 10 hr, lyophylized, and taken up in an appropriate buffer.

Separation of single- and double-stranded DNA by this differential absorption to and elution from HA columns is fast and convenient. In place of 0.14 M PB, 1% formaldehyde we have successfully used 0.4% SDS, 0.14 M PB at 60°C for reassociation and HA chromatography. Under these conditions single-stranded DNA passes through the column at 60°C in 4 bed vol of the 0.14 M buffer. Less than 2% of the single-stranded control DNA was adsorbed to the HA in 0.14 M PB, 0.4% SDS while less than 1% of the double-stranded control DNA failed to be adsorbed in the same buffer. If the concentration of DNA is kept below 75% of HA capacity, recovery is routinely greater than 98%.

(II) The isolation of a number of reiterated DNA sequence families contained in a genome is similar in principle to the above described procedure since the very rapidly reassociating fraction eluted from HA in 0.4 M PB is by definition a family of highly reiterated sequences. Saunders et al. [1972] have separated the reiterated sequence families found in human DNA into two types of reiteration populations by the use of salt and temperature elution from HA columns. The procedure was first described by Britten and Smith [1970] for the fractionation of calf thymus DNA. Reassociation analysis of the DNA fragments is accomplished by allowing reassociation to procede to different $C_0 t$ values and assaying the extent of reassociation by fractionation on HA columns. The reassociation profile of the DNA under study must be completed so appropriate $C_0 t$ values can be selected corresponding to the size of the reiteration families present in the genome. The procedure involves:

(1) Purified sheared DNA which has been passed over Chelex-100 is denatured and reassociation allowed to proceed in the usual manner (that is, 0.12 M PB, 60°C).

(2) At the desired equivalent $C_0 t$ the reaction is stopped by loading the solution onto a HA column preequilibrated with 0.12 M PB at 60°C and the single-stranded DNA eluted with 5 bed vol of 0.12 M PB, and the double-stranded DNA with 0.4 M PB.

(3) Alternatively, the reassociation reaction is poured into a slurry of HA in 0.14 M PB at 60°C and the single-stranded DNA which remains

in solution recovered by centrifugation or by column elution as described previously.

(4) The single-stranded fragments are recovered from the 0.12 M or 0.14 M PB fractions by dialysis against 100 vol of 0.01 M PB for at 4°C 10 hr, and lyophylized.

(5) The DNA fragments are then dissolved in distilled H_2O and the residual salt concentration determined by equating the refractive index measurements to a standard reference plot for phosphate buffer.

(6) The DNA fragments are then denatured once again for 5 min at greater than 95°C to ensure a single-stranded configuration and rapidly cooled to 60°C.

(7) The reassociation reaction is initiated by adjusting the salt concentration to that used initially (0.12 M PB, 60°C) and the reaction allowed to proceed to the next desired $C_0 t$ fractionation point.

(8) The double-stranded DNA fragments which remain bound to the HA in 0.12 M PB and are eluted in 0.4 M PB are concentrated by dialysis against 100 vol of H_2O for 10 hr at 4°C, lyophylized, and taken up in distilled H_2O.

(9) To ensure homogeneity of reiteration preparations the double-stranded (0.4 M PB) fraction must be denatured, reassociated to the same $C_0 t$ value once again, and fractionated in the same manner on HA. The DNA eluted with 0.4 M PB the second time is considered the pure $C_0 t$ fraction.

(10) The sequence is repeated until only unique or single copy sequences remain in the DNA population.

Two principle sources of error are apparent in the analysis of reiterated DNA/DNA reassociation kinetics. The effect of mispaired base sequences affects the second order rate constant by a factor of about 2 while the low hyperchromicity per unit DNA of isolated repetitive duplexes makes optical measurements difficult. In mouse the hypochromicity of the repetitive duplexes is about one half of that seen for sheared native DNA. This may result from some linkage of repetitive sequences to single copy DNA sequences [Britten and Kohne, 1968] such that these are free tails which do not reassociate. The treatment of DNA/DNA duplexes with exonuclease should increase the potential hypochromicity of the repetitive duplexes.

The following flow chart is an outline for the fractionation of human DNA into reiteration families by Saunders et al. [1972].

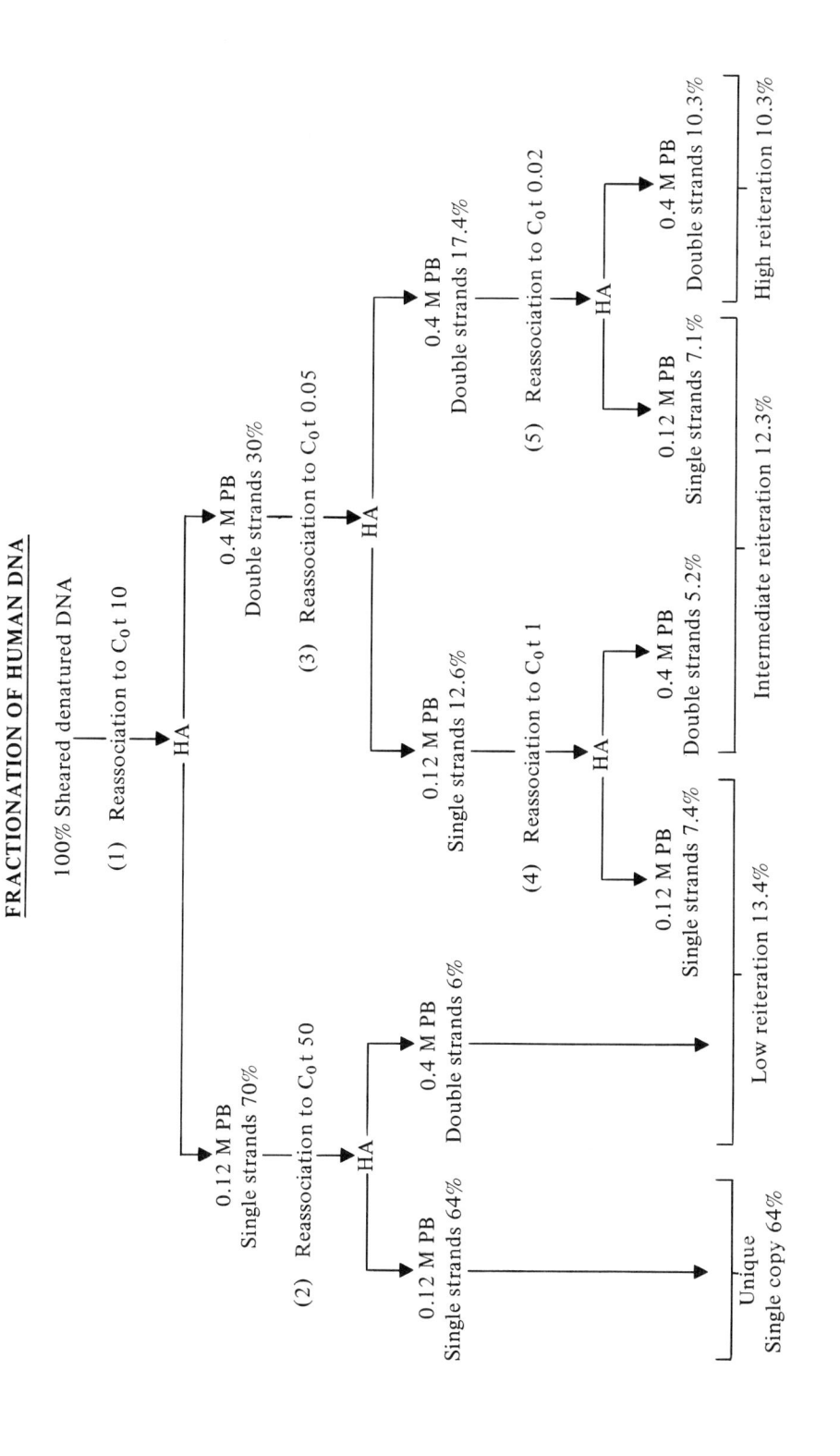

FRACTIONATION OF HUMAN DNA

100% Sheared denatured DNA

(1) Reassociation to C_0t 10
↓ HA

- 0.12 M PB Single strands 70%
  - (2) Reassociation to C_0t 50
    ↓ HA
    - 0.4 M PB Double strands 6% — **Low reiteration 13.4%**
    - 0.12 M PB Single strands 64% — **Unique Single copy 64%**

- 0.4 M PB Double strands 30%
  - (3) Reassociation to C_0t 0.05
    ↓ HA
    - 0.12 M PB Single strands 12.6%
      - (4) Reassociation to C_0t 1
        ↓ HA
        - 0.12 M PB Single strands 7.4% — **Low reiteration 13.4%**
        - 0.4 M PB Double strands 5.2% — **Intermediate reiteration 12.3%**
    - 0.4 M PB Double strands 17.4%
      - (5) Reassociation to C_0t 0.02
        ↓ HA
        - 0.12 M PB Single strands 7.1% — **Intermediate reiteration 12.3%**
        - 0.4 M PB Double strands 10.3% — **High reiteration 10.3%**

(III) The isolation of single copy or unique DNA sequences has enabled a number of studies of the complexity of RNA transcription to be carried out (see section V). After the complete reassociation profile of a particular DNA has been determined the proper $C_0 t$ value can be selected for the isolation of single copy or unique sequences. The $C_0 t$ reassociation value under given reaction conditions will correspond to the coincidence of the observed reassociation profile and the theoretical second order kinetics for a genome of that size. The mouse unique DNA sequences exhibit second order kinetics with a reaction rate about 1000 times slower than E. coli DNA, as would be expected from the differences in genome size. The reassociation profiles presented in Figure 1 illustrate both total mouse DNA and isolated unique sequences. It should be noted that the fragment size and reassociation conditions both affect the relative yield of unique and repeated sequences hence the division between each is arbitrary [Church and Brown, 1972]. The procedure is:

(1) Purified DNA fragments 400–500 nucleotides long are passed over Chelex-100 to remove heavy metals and heat denatured for 15 min at greater than 95°C followed by cooling.

(2) The reassociation reaction is initiated by raising the temperature to 60°C and adjusting the salt concentration (0.12 M PB).

(3) The reassociation is allowed to proceed to $C_0 t$ or $C_0 t$ equivalent of 220–250 before the reaction is stopped and the mixture separated on HA into single-stranded (0.12 M PB) and double-stranded (0.4 M PB) fractions at 60°C.

(4) The single-stranded material in 0.12 M PB is concentrated as described above or by vacuum dialysis [Brown and Church, 1972].

(5) The single-stranded fraction is heat-denatured (5 min, 95°C), rapidly cooled, and reassociated to the same $C_0 t$ once more.

(6) The single-stranded material is eluted in the 0.12 M PB fraction once more and concentrated as before. The 0.4 M PB usually contains about 5% of the DNA after the second reassociation. This DNA represents the double-stranded contamination in the first single-stranded 0.12 M PB fraction. The yield of single-stranded sequences is greatly reduced by increased fragment size which presumably contain unique and reiterated sequences. Fragment size must be less than 1.7×10^5 [Britten and Kohne, 1968].

(7) The unique sequences must be assayed for reiterated contamination by monitoring reassociation of 1 μg ^{3}H-unique DNA, 100 μg ^{14}C-E. coli DNA and 500 μg total sheared mouse DNA (2 mg/ml). Aliquots are collected at various $C_0 t$ values and assayed on HA. The $C_0 t$

values are calculated by using the concentration of unlabeled DNA [Hahn and Laird, 1971].

A representative flow pattern from Brown and Church [1972] for the isolation of unique sequences is presented below.

ISOLATION OF SINGLE COPY MOUSE DNA

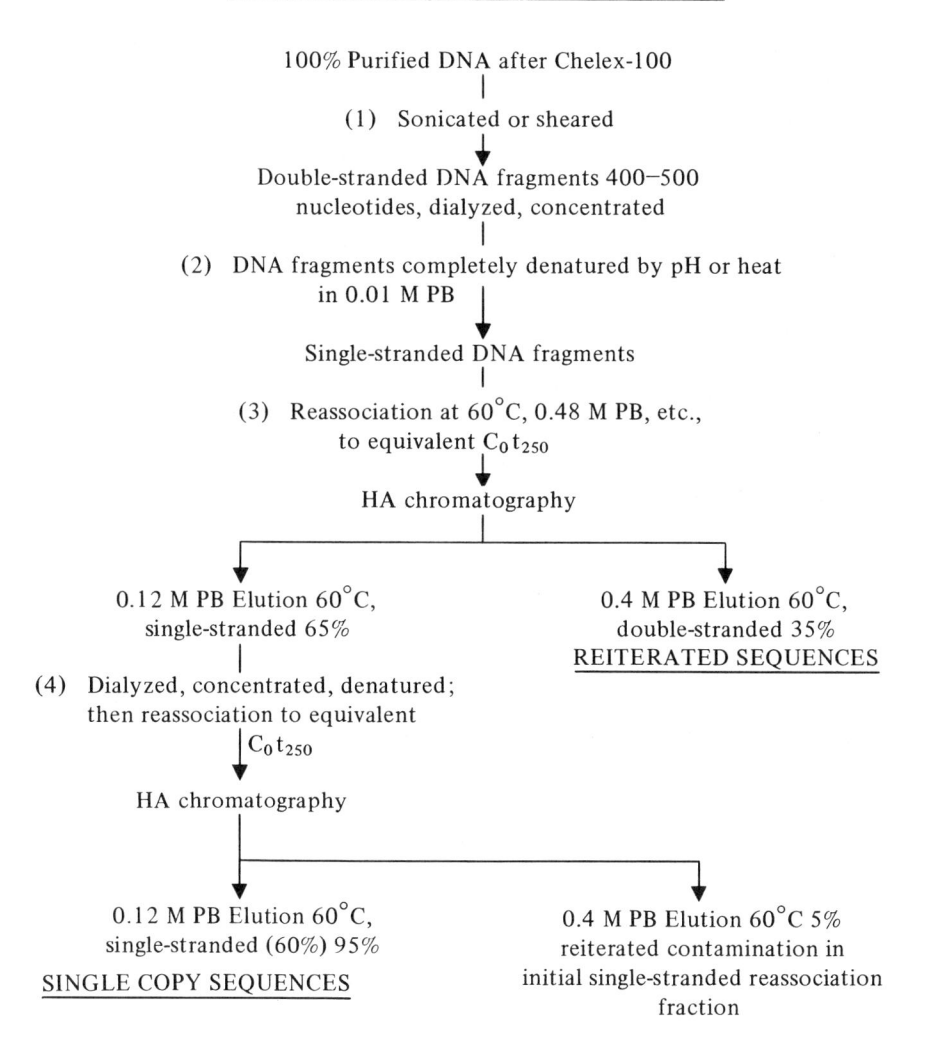

100% Purified DNA after Chelex-100
|
(1) Sonicated or sheared
↓
Double-stranded DNA fragments 400–500 nucleotides, dialyzed, concentrated
|
(2) DNA fragments completely denatured by pH or heat in 0.01 M PB
↓
Single-stranded DNA fragments
|
(3) Reassociation at 60°C, 0.48 M PB, etc., to equivalent C_0t_{250}
↓
HA chromatography
|
├──────────────────────────────┬──────────────────────────────┤

0.12 M PB Elution 60°C, single-stranded 65%
|
(4) Dialyzed, concentrated, denatured; then reassociation to equivalent C_0t_{250}
↓
HA chromatography
|
├──────────────────────────────┬──────────────────────────────┤

0.12 M PB Elution 60°C, single-stranded (60%) 95%
SINGLE COPY SEQUENCES

0.4 M PB Elution 60°C, double-stranded 35%
REITERATED SEQUENCES

0.4 M PB Elution 60°C 5% reiterated contamination in initial single-stranded reassociation fraction

The C_0t is in moles nucleotide per liter times the time of reassociation in seconds. The equivalent C_0t is a C_0t value corrected for the reassociation rate differences at salt concentrations other than 0.12 M PB [Britten and Smith, 1970].

SECTION VI

High C_0t RNA/DNA Hybridization with RNA in Vast Excess

The rate of hybridization or reassociation of nucleic acids depends on the effective concentration of complementary sequences, therefore, at low RNA concentrations and short reaction times only those transcripts complementary to repeated DNA sequences will have a chance to react. To analyze transcriptional activity of the nonrepeated DNA sequences contained in complex genomes of higher organisms, very high concentrations of nucleic acids or very long reaction times or both are required to permit the hybridization of RNA with complementary nonrepeated DNA (high C_0t hybrids [Kohne, 1968]). In-solution DNA/RNA reassociation reactions are preferred as the reaction rate is 20 times the filter reaction rate for the same system [McCarthy, 1967].

There are two methods presently in use for preparation of high C_0t hybrids. These involve the reaction of either a large excess of unlabeled RNA with a small amount of highly labeled DNA (RNA-driven reaction), first used by Kohne [1968], or a very large excess of DNA in reaction with a small amount of highly labeled RNA (DNA-driven reaction), first used by Britten [1969], and extended by Bishop, Pemberton and Baglioni [1972]. The RNA excess has been used to analyze the complexity of RNA transcription in the whole mouse embryo [Gelderman et al., 1968; Gelderman, Rake, and Britten, 1971], in the Xenopus oocyte [Davidson and Hough, 1969,1971; using <u>in vitro</u> labeled RNA], in various mouse tissues including brain [Smith, 1968; Hahn and Laird, 1971; Brown and Church, 1971,1972; Grouse, Chilton and McCarthy, 1972] and in slime mold development [Firtel, 1972]. The DNA excess procedure has been used for analysis of mouse embryo mRNA [Gelderman et al., 1968, 1971], histone mRNA transcription [Kedes and Birnstiel, 1971] and repetition of duck erythrocyte sequences [Melli et al., 1971]. This system, providing one can obtain very high specific activity RNA, makes it possible to measure the reiteration frequency of DNA sequences complementary to purified messenger RNA [Melli et al., 1971]. Wilt [1971] has recently discussed advances in high C_0t nucleic acid hybridization studies which involve the use of these methods for the analysis of differential gene activity.

The procedure involves the use of high specific activity DNA with excess (600- to 2000-fold) of RNA. Analysis of the DNA/RNA duplex is done on HA columns in 0.12 M PB at 60°C The labeled DNA may have "free" tails so the use of an exonuclease <u>may</u> be of advantage in the analysis. The extent or complexity of DNA molecules capable of forming complementary duplexes with each different RNA sequences is measured. The RNA should be in sufficient excess that the least frequent molecule has a chance to react with its transcriptional site. The thermal melting profiles of all such products examined so far suggest that the base-pair mismatching is minimal since RNA/DNA and DNA/DNA reassociation products show similar profiles and expected T_m's. The thermal stability of brain RNA/unique mouse DNA hybrids after reassociation to $C_0 t$ 8000 is 81°C [Brown and Church, 1972].

Although various salt concentrations can be used to change the rate of reaction, in combination with formamide, incubation temperatures can be lowered, and we prefer to use aqueous reaction mixtures at temperatures up to 70°C. The degradation of RNA at these high temperatures is proportionally low if the RNA is sheared to 6 S or less before the reaction. RNA passed over Chelex-100 and incubated at 70°C, in 0.12 M PB for 3 weeks is eluted in the void volume from G-75 Sephadex. It has an electrophoretic mobility, in 2.6% polyacylamide–SDS gels, similar to RNA molecules of molecular weights of greater than 60,000 [Brown and Church, 1972].

When DNA is present at low concentration, the RNA/DNA hybridization reaction driven by vast excesses of RNA appears to be a pseudo first-order reaction. Therefore, the rate of reaction is a function of the concentration of individual RNA sequences in the reaction. For very complex populations of RNA molecules, very high concentrations of RNA are required (60,000:1 for RNA:DNA) to enhance the hybridization reaction while holding the DNA $C_0 t$ constant. The saturation of complementary DNA sequences by increasing concentrations of RNA will only approach completion for RNA populations with low levels of complexity. This can be expressed as:

$$\frac{d[D]}{dt} = -K_2 [D]^2 - K_2^1 [D][R]$$

where [D] = concentration of single-stranded DNA at any time, t
[R] = concentration of RNA sequences complimentary to DNA
K_2 = the second-order rate constant for DNA reassociation
K_2^1 = the second-order rate constant for RNA/DNA hybridization

In reactions of vast [R] excess over [D], if one assumes $K_2 \doteq K_2^1$ then the integration of the above equation results in:

$$\frac{[D]}{[D_0]} = -K_2^1 R_0 t \quad \text{or} \quad \frac{[D]}{[D_0]} = e^{(-K_2 [R_0]t)}$$

where $[D_0]$ is the initial concentration of DNA complementary to RNA [Firtel,

1971]. Firtel [1971] has suggested the term R_0t for hybridization similar to C_0t for DNA reassociation. Therefore, sequences of RNA which are present in few copies will have little opportunity to hybridize unless very long (RNA/DNA R_0t or equivalent DNA C_0t of > 20,000) reaction times are used. In most cases the degradation of RNA will result in lower apparent RNA/DNA saturation at very long incubation periods (3 months). Therefore, in most cellular RNA populations, true saturation values cannot be easily attained in RNA-driven reactions. The estimates of saturation are a minimum of the extent of RNA sequences complementary to unique DNA sequences. Secondly, as pointed out by Brown and Church [1971] the RNA complexity in any given cellular preparation is the sum of all stable molecules synthesized up to that time by the tissue.

The usefulness of RNA hybridization reactions in the analysis of the complexity of gene activity has wide applications. However as Firtel [1972] has elegantly pointed out in his studies of RNA transcriptional complexity during slime mold development, the enormous complexity contained in mammalian genomes results in technical and interpretive difficulties. Not withstanding these considerations, the RNA-driven hybridization reaction is the most powerful tool presently available for analysis of RNA transcriptional complexity.

There are many variations to the in-solution RNA-driven hybridization reaction but all are based on the same principle. Since this technique assays total DNA in duplexes it is necessary to determine how much of the 0.4 M PB fraction is in DNA/DNA and how much in the RNA/DNA duplex. There are two control reactions to answer this question. First, if DNA is a contaminant in the RNA, it would increase the DNA C_0t and result in more DNA/DNA duplexes. A sample of RNA must therefore be treated with alkali (0.3 N NaOH pH 11.5 for 3 hr) or ribonuclease (20 μg/ml at 37°C for 30 min) prior to incubation with labeled unique DNA sequences. In such reactions with mouse unique ^{3}H-DNA less than 1% of the DNA is recognized as double-stranded by HA after incubation to C_0t 600. The effect of viscosity due to the high RNA concentrations has not been studied. The extent of HA 0.4 M PB background will be higher if the RNA preparation is contaminated with DNA. This control assay for DNA contamination must be included in any study using RNA-driven hybridization.

Secondly, the extent of DNA/DNA reassociation in the hybridization reaction must be assayed. The incubation mixture is loaded onto HA in 0.12 M PB and the duplexes are eluted in 0.4 M PB. The duplexes are then digested with preboiled pancreatic ribonuclease 50 μg/ml and 100 units/ml of T1 ribonuclease in 0.48 M PB for 10 hr at 37°C consistent with dialysis against 0.05 M PB. The RNA/DNA hybrid is sensitive to this combined ribonuclease attack while the DNA/DNA duplex is stable. The control reaction for DNA/DNA duplex stability contains know concentrations of the duplex DNA [Gelderman et al., 1971]. After the ribonuclease incubation the mixture is loaded onto HA in 0.12 M PB. The DNA which had been in the hybrid with complementary RNA will now elute in the 0.12 M PB fraction as single-stranded DNA while the DNA/DNA duplex will once again be eluted with 0.4 M PB. For unique mouse DNA incubated to an equivalent $C_0 t$ of 10,000 with 10 mg/ml brain RNA in 0.2 ml of 0.12 M PB approximately 0.2% of the DNA input is in DNA/DNA duplexes. Approximately, 8.0% of the DNA is in the form of RNA/DNA hybrids in this reaction. The technique of RNA excess hybridization may be outlined as follows:

(1) Sheared, denatured, unique-labeled DNA (i.e., $C_0 t_{250}$, specific activity $> 10^5$ cpm/µg) is mixed with unlabeled RNA in 0.03 M PB. The mixtures are set up in a ratio series of 60 to 10,000/1 (RNA:DNA) with 4–20 mg RNA/ml and 0.1–5 µg DNA/ml.

(2) The mixtures are heat-denatured for 5 min at $> 95°C$, quickly cooled to 60°C, and the hybridization reaction initiated by adjusting the salt to the desired concentration (0.12 M PB).

(3) 50 µliter aliquots are sealed in glass capillary tubes (Corning, micropipets) and incubated for the desired times at 60°C. The denaturation of both DNA and RNA can conveniently be done in the capillary tubes as well.

(4) At the selected time (equivalent $C_0 t$) intervals the tubes were removed and their contents quickly frozen at −20°C for analysis of all samples in a series at a later time. Alternatively, the tube is opened and the reaction stopped by dilution to 2 ml with 0.03 M PB at 4°C.

(5) The incubation mixture can be treated with Fraser et al. [1970] or Sutton [1971] S1 exonuclease at this stage to remove unpaired DNA tails (20 units/ml 0.2 M NaCl, 50°C for 1 hr) or if desired with 10 µg/ml pancreatic ribonuclease to remove excess RNA.

(6) The reaction mixture from (4) or (5) is loaded onto HA columns previously equilibrated with 0.03 M PB at 60°C. If large amounts of RNA are involved, the incubation and column buffer should contain 0.1% SDS or 4 M urea.

(7) The majority of RNA will pass through the HA column in the 0.12 M PB wash (5–10 bed vol) at 60°C if 0.1% SDS or 4 M urea is present. For low concentrations (6 mg/ml) of RNA, the SDS and urea are not required for separation of the RNA from the duplex.

(8) After exonuclease or ribonuclease treatment, the liberated nucleotides

will pass through the column in 0.03 M PB. Very limited amounts (5%) of ribonuclease-resistant cores will be eluted from 0.12 to 0.20 M PB.

(9) Degradation of nucleic acids can be minimized by careful attention to glassware cleaning and by passing all preparations over Chelex-100 to remove heavy metals and nucleases.

(10) The RNA/DNA hybrid can be eluted in 0.4 M PB at 60°C or melted from the HA in 0.12 M PB with increasing temperature steps to 95°C. Greater than 98% recovery should be obtained by either elution procedure.

(11) The unique labeled DNA eluted with 0.4 M PB or between 60 and 95°C in 0.12 M PB compared to the total precipitable DNA input in the control incubation (without RNA) at the end of the reaction is expressed as a percentage. Typical results are shown in Figure 7.

(12) Methods of analyzing the thermal stability of the RNA DNA hybrid are discussed in section III.

It is essential that the proper control experiments discussed in this chapter be included in the analysis of RNA transcriptional complexity by RNA-driven RNA/DNA hybridization. They include

(a) Assay of the extent of DNA/DNA reassociation
(b) Assay of RNA for contaminating DNA
(c) Incubation of RNA alone to detect degradation of acid-precipitable input
(d) Incubation of DNA alone to detect degradation and to calculate acid-precipitable input
(e) Incubation of control reactions which include a labeled bacterial DNA to act as an internal standard

Finally, as noted elsewhere in this chapter, formamide concentrations must either be below 1% or the duplex eluted with a very shallow PB gradient to prevent smearing of the RNA and single-stranded DNA into the double-stranded hybrid elution fractions.

SECTION VII RNA/DNA HYBRIDIZATION WITH A VAST DNA EXCESS

The size of the genome with its inherent base sequence complexity in higher species makes it impossible to isolate the complementary strands of DNA for analysis of RNA transcriptional complexity. Therefore, when DNA is hybridized with similar concentrations of RNA, the ensuing reaction is very complex since both the RNA and DNA sequences are competing for the same complementary DNA sequences. Hybridization experiments using some viral DNA can prevent DNA renaturation by strand separation while the immobilization of single-stranded DNA on various solid matrices is widely used to prevent self-renaturation of DNA in studies of higher species. There is a very strict limitation to the amount of DNA which is experimentally possible to obtain in these methods of limiting DNA self reassociation.

Britten [1970] found that, if DNA and RNA are allowed to reassociate in a reaction in which the DNA sequences, which are complementary to the RNA, are present in a very large excess, the kinetic properties of the hybridization reaction can be easily analyzed. Melli et al. [1971] developed the technique further and suggested that the method be termed "hybridization in vast DNA excess." Their experiments were designed to assay fractions of highly labeled cellular RNA to determine the reiteration frequency of their complementary DNA sequences. In further studies of the kinetics of hybridization Bishop [1972] has presented a detailed analysis of the vast DNA excess/RNA reaction which provided theoretical evidence that if the rate constants of the RNA/DNA and DNA/DNA reactions are the same, the proportion of RNA remaining single-stranded will be the same as the proportion of DNA remaining single-stranded. Therefore, the time and concentration dependence of the DNA/RNA hybridization reaction is related to that of the DNA reassociation reaction in the same reaction. The rate constant of DNA renaturation can be estimated from the hybridization of labeled complementary RNA sequences provided a sufficiently large excess of DNA is in the reaction, in the order of a 10^8-fold excess of DNA over RNA. The details of the definition of suitable conditions for DNA/RNA hybridization experiments in vast DNA excess and their interpretation for reactions utilizing nucleic acids from higher organisms have been elegantly outlined by Bishop [1972] with particular emphasis on temperature and salt concentration. Using suitable bacterial RNA, in vitro labeled complementary RNA and ribosomal RNA, calibration experiments have provided evidence for the theoretical estimation of the rate constant of the DNA/RNA hybridization reaction.

An example of the results of hybridization in vast DNA excess is shown in Figure 8. The figure shows an optical reassociation curve of rat spleen DNA monitored in 0.12 M PB at 260 mμ [Bell and Church, unpublished] and the hybridization of uniformly labeled nuclear RNA isolated from mouse ascites cells. The results suggest that the rapidly renaturing DNA sequences are poorly transcribed in vitro by the bacterial polymerase [Melli et al., 1971]. Significant amounts of ascites nuclear RNA seems to be transcribed from the rapidly renaturing DNA sequences. A component which corresponds to 35% of the nuclear RNA and to a DNA sequence reiteration of about 350 can be seen to reassociate with a $C_0 t_{1/2}$ of about 30.

To calculate reiteration frequency calibration, experiments are required in order to calculate the rate of hybridization. Bishop, Pemberton, and Baglioni [1972] has shown that in 2 × SSC at 70°C the $C_0 t_{1/2}$ of the hybridization transition was 8.1 for E. coli in vitro RNA and $C_0 t_{1/2}$ = 16 for rRNA from duck.

Therefore reiteration frequency (F) for duck rRNA can be calculated to be

$$F = \frac{C_0 t_{1/2}}{C_0 t_{1/2}} \times \frac{C(\text{duck})}{C(\text{E. coli})} \quad [\text{Bishop et al., 1972}].$$

From this equation and genome complexities of 0.8×10^{12} and 2.7×10^9 dalton for duck and E. coli, respectively, the duck DNA must contain approximately 150 copies of ribosomal DNA sequences. The rate constant of DNA renaturation derived from the DNA/RNA hybridization reaction utilizing a vast excess of DNA and in vitro synthesized complementary RNA and in vivo labeled duck haemoglobin mRNA has been determined [Bishop et al., 1972].

This DNA-driven reaction has some severe limitations in that it is seldom possible to obtain sufficiently high specific radioactivity in RNA labeled in vivo to be able to monitor the reaction. Therefore, in vitro synthesized complementary RNA from chromatin or specific DNA sequence templates may be the only source of sufficiently highly labeled RNA for the biological system under study.

Secondly, the excess of complementary DNA sequences over similar RNA sequences must be on the order of 10^8 for the reaction to even come close to completion. One should note that the vast excess of complementary DNA sequences will be greater than the gram weight of DNA for RNA sequences complementary to the reiterated DNA sequences present in higher organisms. The effect of RNA population sequence frequency in a cellular extract on the required ratio of single copy DNA:RNA to provide vast excess conditions depends on the least frequent sequence in the RNA molecule spectrum. If the RNA is not of sufficiently high specific activity, the very high concentrations of DNA required will be difficult to keep in solution.

As with the RNA-driven hybridization reaction the stability of RNA during the incubation is important since the molecular weight of the RNA will affect the rate of reaction. The size of the RNA has a direct effect on the nucleation rate of DNA/RNA hybridization. Differences in the rate of hybridization at the initial and later stages of the reaction have been noted [Bishop, 1972]. A high level of purity of nucleic acids would not seem to be required [Melli et al., 1971] since the proportion of labeled RNA forming a duplex is analyzed.

The heated and quenched samples never give a completely zero value of either hybridization or renaturation. In addition, the reaction never reaches completion even at the highest $C_0 t$ values studied in model bacterial systems [Bishop, 1972]. Bishop [1972] has reported an apparent renaturation of 0.13 and apparent DNA/RNA hybridization of 0.04 with both in vitro labeled complementary RNA and cellular mRNA. The apparent zero time DNA/RNA hybridization was defined as the ribonuclease resistance of the incubation mixture in the absence of DNA. The probable causes of the apparent zero time reassociation have been discussed in section II.

The vast DNA excess in the DNA/RNA hybridization reaction is a powerful technique in the analysis of reiteration frequency of DNA transcriptional sites or number of genes present in a genome, for a given protein analysis of RNA transcriptional complexity is possible when sufficiently high specific activities can be obtained for the various cellular RNA fractions to be analyzed in any given system.

Procedure: The basic procedure is based on the method developed by Bishop [1972]. The technique may be modified to suit the particular questions being asked either total or fractionated DNA in the reaction.

(1) Unlabeled DNA, isolated in large enough quantities to complete each set of experiments, should be free of detectable contamination by alkali-labile and cold TCA-soluble material.

(2) The DNA at 100–500 μg/ml in 1/10 SSC or 0.03 M PB is then sheared by sonication or by passage through a French Pressure Cell. The temperature of the solution during sonication or shearing should be maintained as close to 4°C as possible. A single-strand molecular weight of below 200,000 is required for the reaction, as measured by the method of Studier [1965].

(3) The DNA fragments are then dialyzed for 10 hr against 0.03 M PB, and 0.1 vol of 2 M sodium acetate, pH 5.6, added, and precipitated by volumes of ice cold ethanol at −20°C. After centrifugation, the pellet is dissolved in 30 ml of 0.3 M NaCl, 0.01 M sodium acetate, pH 5, and passed, in 10 ml aliquots, over a Sephadex SE-50 (2.5 × 50 cm) or Chelex-100 (2.5 × 15 cm) column which has previously been equilibrated with the same buffer. The DNA fragments eluted in the void volume are recipitated with 2 vol of ice cold ethanol and left overnight at −20°C. This final precipitate is then centrifuged, drained thoroughly, and dissolved in 1/10 × SSC or 0.03 M PB to a final concentration of 20 mg/ml. The final precipitate should be completely free of alkali-labile

and cold acid-soluble material. It may be necessary to heat this solution slightly to get the DNA into solution at the highest concentrations desired.

(4) DNA either alone at from 0.5 to 20 mg/ml or with the 1–100 μg/ml of labeled RNA present, dissolved in 1/10 × SSC or 0.03 M PB is heated to 97°C for at least 10 min in a water bath or alkali-denatured at pH 11.5 by the addition of 0.1 N KOH for 10 min fillowed by neutralization with 0.1 N HCl. Complete denaturation is <u>essential</u> and should be monitored by an analysis of hyperchromic shift or by the elution profile with a PB gradient from an HA column at 60°C. A measure of the instantaneous reassociation is obtained by removing an aliquot immediately and cooling by dilution with the appropriate ice cold buffer.

Bishop [1972] has suggested that 2 × SSC at 70°C is an optimal buffer concentration, and that 50% formamide, 3 × SSC at 50°C must retard thermal breakage of the labeled RNA by at least 4-fold to be of advantage over 2 × SSC at 75°C. In our laboratory we prefer 0.12–0.48 M PB at 70°C to any combination of formamide and SSC since, in our hands, less RNA degradation occurs during prolonged incubations. The salt concentration is, of course, a compromise between the greater precision of base-pairing required at high-criteria low-salt concentrations which result in low reaction rates, and the more rapid reaction rates and lower base-pairing precision of higher salt concentrations [McCarthy and Church, 1970].

(5) The main reaction mixture is then placed in a water or oil bath at the chosen incubation temperature, and after 30 sec, the salt concentration adjusted is the desired concentration. An aliquot is removed at this time and designated as 0 time. The sample containers are then sealed. Duplicate reaction mixtures are desirable with DNA concentrations of 0.5–20 mg/ml.

(6) At appropriate time intervals, aliquots are removed from the incubation reaction and diluted with ice cold H_2O to give a final concentration of 1/10 × SSC or 0.03 M PB as appropriate.

(7) In experiments which include formamide [McConaughy et al., 1969], all formamide should be added before the renaturation step. In reactions without formamide, up to 2% SDS can be added to the reaction to reduce degradation. The dilution after the reaction and before ribonuclease treatment must yield an SDS concentration of less than 0.01%. Salt concentrations are adjusted by using suitable dilution of 20 × SSC or 1 M PB at pH 5.5 and 6.7, respectively. The pH of the 10-fold diluted SSC solution is about 6.4.

(8) To determine the thermal stability and melting profile of the duplex formed at any given reaction time, the aliquots, removed from the incubation reaction in sectionVI, are diluted to the required buffer concentration at the incubation temperature. The thermal melting profile can be analyzed by the change in hyperchromicity monitored on a recording spectrophotometer equipped with a temperature controlled cuvette chamber and thermister probe, or by the quenched assay method described by Bishop [1972]. Alternatively, on aliquot can be diluted to 0.12 M PB, loaded onto a HA column, and the DNA/labeled RNA duplex melted from the column by increasing column temperature in 0.12 M PB (see RNA excess melting profile, p. 267) and the labeled RNA eluted at each temperature assayed. If formamide or SSC is present, the sample must be diluted at least 100-fold to obtain acceptable results from the HA column.

(9) Calculation of extent of DNA reassociation is the same for renaturation as for denaturation experiments [Bishop, 1972]. Aliquots of the incubation mixture described in section VI are diluted to 50 μg DNA/ml with 1/10 × SSC or 0.03 M PB. The extinction of the aliquot of the incubation mixture is recorded at 260 mμ if formamide is not present and at 270 mμ if formamide is used in the incubation reaction starting at 50°C in a recording spectrophotometer equipped with a temperature-controlled cuvette holder preferably with a thermister cuvette probe. The temperature is then raised by some previously calibrated temperature program to over 90°C. The increase in extinction observed from 50 to 90°C is due primarily to the denaturation of the reassociated DNA. Other considerations have been discussed in section II.

Bishop [1972] has developed the following equation for the estimation of the proportion of the total DNA in the form of a DNA/DNA duplex in a vast DNA excess reaction

$$d/C_0 = \frac{[(\text{extinction 260 m}\mu \text{ at 90°C}) - (\text{extinction 260 m}\mu \text{ at 50°C})]}{[H/(1 + H)] \text{ extinction 260 m}\mu \text{ at 90°C}}$$

where d is the concentration of DNA duplex and C_0 the initial DNA concentration both in moles of nucleotide/liter. In this equation H is the proportional increase in extinction of sheared native DNA from the same source. Therefore

$$(1 + H) = \frac{\text{extinction 260 m}\mu \text{ 90°C}}{\text{extinction 260 m}\mu \text{ 50°C}}$$

for native sheared DNA is handled in exactly the same manner. The H was found to be equal to 0.38 and 0.42, respectively, for E. coli DNA at 260 and 270 mμ [Bishop, 1972] and 0.40 for mouse DNA at 260 mμ. All estimations of reaction which include formamide in the incubation are calculated using the extinction recorded at 270 mμ (not 260 mμ) at 50 and 90°C.

(10) A method of calculating the amount of labeled RNA which has formed a stable duplex with complementary DNA sequences has been described by Melli et al. [1971].

Aliquots of the DNA excess/labeled RNA hybridization mixture are removed at appropriate $C_0 t$ values. The salt concentration is adjusted to 2 × SSC or 0.24 M PB and the sample divided into two equal parts. To one sample, 10–30 μg of ribonuclease/ml is added and both samples are incubated for 10–30 min at 37°C before stopping the ribonuclease reaction by cooling to 4°C. After addition of a carrier (Bovine serum albumin to a concentration of 150 μg/ml or E. coli rRNA to a concentration of 200 μg/ml), the sample is precipitated with an equal volume of ice cold 10% TCA. After 10 min with frequent shaking the precipitate is collected on Whatman GF/C glass filters or Millipore HAWP membrane filters, washed with 3 vol 5% TCA, once with ethanol, dried, and the radioactivity assayed in a toluene-based scintillation system.

The rate constants and the kinetics of DNA/RNA hybridization in vast DNA excess have been described by Bishop [1972] as

$$r/R_0 = 1 - [1/(K^d C_0 t + 1)^{K^h K^d}]$$

where r/R_0 is the proportion of labeled RNA forming a stable duplex at time t and K^h is the rate constant of the DNA excess/labeled RNA hybridization reaction. The results of this second order reaction generate a sigmoid curve similar to that discussed in section II for the Britten and Kohne [1966] analysis of DNA.

SECTION VIII CONCLUSIONS

Nucleic acid hybridization methods have now been in use for about one decade. Much of our knowledge of transcriptional activity has been derived from RNA/DNA hybridization. The specificity of reaction of bacterial and viral nucleic acids is widely accepted for both RNA/DNA hybridization and DNA/DNA reassociation homology studies. However, systematic studies of the RNA/DNA reaction with model bacterial systems are needed to understand the kinetics of reaction, the fate of the unstable RNA/DNA intermediate which contributes unduly to the initial rate of reaction and the reassociation parameters which affect the final hybrid in mammalian systems.

The tremendous complexity of the mammalian genome including the presence of reiterated sequences complicates the interpretation of RNA/DNA hybridization. However, with the preparation of reiterated DNA sequence populations, analysis of the function of these sequences in RNA metabolism is an experimental possibility. Reassociation fractionation also allows the preparation of single copy DNA sequences which can be used to estimate the complexity of transcription of the RNA molecules in a given preparation. On the basis of the results of RNA/DNA hybridization studies in many developing systems [see Hahn and Church, 1970; Schultz and Church, 1973] which show RNA spectrum changes, prompting Britten and Davidson [1969] to develop a model for gene regulation in higher organisms. Undoubtedly, the methods of reassociation and hybridization using mammalian nucleic acids will improve as refinements in the techniques are developed. Most of our understanding of differential gene activity in higher species will coincide with developments in and application of reassociation techniques for these systems.

ACKNOWLEDGEMENTS

I would like to thank Judy Crozier, Graeme Bell, and Anne Vipond for their assistance during development of the experimental methods presented in this paper. Appreciation is also extended to Grady Saunders and Gilbert Schultz for their comments on the manuscript. The work was supported by the National Research Council of Canada.

REFERENCES

[1] Alberts, B., and P. Doty. 1968. J. Mol. Biol. 32:379–386.
[2] Alberts, B., and G. Herrick. 1971. In Methods in enzymology. L. Grossman and K. Moldave (ed.). XXID:198–217.
[3] Arion, A., and G. P. Georgiev. 1967. Mol. Biol. Acad. Sci. U.S.S.R. 172:716–729.
[4] Bautz, E. K. F., and B. D. Hall. 1962. Proc. Nat. Acad. Sci. U.S.A. 48:400–412.
[5] Bell, G. 1971. M.Sc. thesis, University of Calgary.
[6] Bell, G., and R. B. Church. 1971. Unpublished, University of Calgary.
[7] Bellamy, A. R., and R. K. Ralph. 1968. In Methods in enzymology. L. Grossman and K. Moldave (ed.). XIIA:156–160.

[8] Bendich, A., and E. T. Bolton. 1968. In Methods in enzymology. L. Grossman and K. Moldave (ed.). XIIB:635–640.
[9] Bernardi, G. 1965. Nature 206:779–780.
[10] Bernardi, G. 1969. Biochim. Biophys. Acta 174:423–438.
[11] Bernardi, G. 1971. In Methods in enzymology. L. Grossman and K. Moldave (ed.). XXID:95–139.
[12] Birnstiel, M. L., B. H. Sells, and I. Purdon. 1972. J. Mol. Biol. 63:21–39.
[13] Bishop, J. O. 1969. Biochem. J. 113:805–819.
[14] Bishop, J. O. 1972. Biochem. J. 126:171–185.
[15] Bishop, J. O., R. Pemberton, and C. Baglioni. 1972. Nature New Biol. 235:231–234.
[16] Bolton, E. T., and B. J. McCarthy. 1962. Proc. Nat. Acad. Sci. U.S.A. 48:1390–1399.
[17] Bonner, J., G. Kung, and I. Bekhor. 1967. Biochemistry 6:3650–3656.
[18] Bostock, C. J. 1971. In Advances in cell biology. D. M. Prescott, L. Goldstien, and E. McConkey (ed.), pp. 116–174. Appleton Croft, New York.
[19] Britten, R. J. 1963. Science 142:963–964.
[20] Britten, R. J. 1969. Carnegie Instit. Wash. Yearbook. 68:300–307.
[21] Britten, R. J. 1970. In Problems in biology:RNA in development. W. E. Hanly (ed.), pp. 187–216. University of Utah Press.
[22] Britten, R. J., and E. H. Davidson. 1969. Science 165:349–358.
[23] Britten, R. J., and D. E. Kohne. 1966. Carnegie Instit. Wash. Yearbook 65:78–86.
[24] Britten, R. J., and D. E. Kohne. 1968. Science 161:529–540.
[25] Britten, R. J., and N. Smith. 1970. Carnegie Instit. Wash. Yearbook 69:167–175.
[26] Brown, I. R., and R. B. Church. 1971. Biochim. Biophys. Res. Comm. 42:850–856.
[27] Brown, I. R., and R. B. Church. 1972. Devel. Biol. 29:73–84.
[28] Brown, D. D., and C. S. Weber. 1968. J. Mol. Biol. 34:661–680.
[29] Chauveau, J., Y. Moule, and C. Rouiller. 1956. Exp. Cell Res. 11:317–331.
[30] Church, R. B. 1972. Unpublished. University of Calgary.
[31] Church, R. B., and B. J. McCarthy. 1967. J. Mol. Biol. 23:459–475.
[32] Church, R. B., and B. J. McCarthy. 1968. Biochem. Genetics 2:55–87.
[33] Church, R. B., and I. R. Brown. 1972. In Results and problems in cell differentiation. H. Ursprung (ed.), Vol. 3, pp. 11–24.
[34] Church, R. B., and G. A. Schultz. 1973. In Current topics in developmental biology. A. Moscona and A. Monroy (ed.), Vol. 8, in press.
[35] Commerford, S. L. 1971. Biochemistry 10:1993–2002.
[36] Crozier, J. 1970. Unpublished. University of Calgary.
[37] Davidson, E. H., and B. R. Hough. 1969. Proc. Nat. Acad. Sci. U.S.A. 63:342–349.
[38] Davidson, E. H., and B. R. Hough. 1971. J. Mol. Biol. 56:491–506.
[39] Denhardt, D. T. 1966. Biochim. Biophys. Res. Comm. 23:641–645.
[40] Firtel, R. 1972. J. Mol. Biol. 66:363–377.

[41] Flamm, W. G., P. M. B. Walker, and M. McCallum. 1969. J. Mol. Biol. 42:441–450.
[42] Flamm, W. G. 1972. Intern. Rev. Cytol. 10:1–51.
[43] Fraser, M. J., E. Z. Robin, and G. Allen. 1970. Can. J. Biochem. 48:501–509.
[44] Gelderman, A., A. Rake, and R. J. Britten. 1968. Carnegie Instit. Wash. Yearbook 67:320–325.
[45] Gelderman, A., A. Rake, and R. J. Britten. 1971. Proc. Nat. Acad. Sci. U.S.A. 68:172–176.
[46] Georgiev, G. P. 1967. Prog. Nucleic Acid Res. 6:259–352.
[47] Getz, M. J., L. C. Altenburg, and G. F. Saunders. 1972. Biochim. Biophys. Acta 287:485–494.
[48] Gilham, P. T. 1971. In Methods in enzymology. L. Grossman and K. Moldave (ed.). XXID:191–197.
[49] Gillespie, D. 1968. In Methods in enzymology. L. Grossman and K. Moldave (ed.). XIIB:641–668.
[50] Gillespie, D., and S. Spiegelman. 1965. J. Mol. Biol. 12:829–842.
[51] Grossman, L. 1968. In Methods in enzymology. L. Grossman and K. Moldave (ed.). XIIB:641–668.
[52] Grouse, L., M. D. Chilton, and B. J. McCarthy. 1972. Biochemistry 11:798–805.
[53] Hahn, W. E., and R. B. Church. 1970. In Cell differentiation. O. Schjeide and J. de Vellis (ed.), pp. 119–140. Van Nostrand-Reinhold Co., New York.
[54] Hahn, W. E., and C. D. Laird. 1971. Science 173:158–161.
[55] Hall, B. D., and S. Spiegelman. 1961. Proc. Nat. Acad. Sci. U.S.A. 48:1390–1396.
[56] Helmkamp, G. K., and P. O. P. Ts'o. 1961. J. Amer. Chem. Soc. 83:138–144.
[57] Kates, J. 1970. Cold Spring Harbor Symp. Quant. Biol. 35:743–752.
[58] Kedes, L. H., and M. L. Birnstiel. 1971. Nature 230:165–169.
[59] Kennel, D. E. 1971. Prog. Nucleic Acid Res. 11:273–324.
[60] Knittel, M. D., C. H. Black, W. E. Sandine, and D. K. Fraser. 1968. Can. J. Microbiol. 14:239–252.
[61] Kohne, D. E. 1968. Biophys. J. 8:1104–1112.
[62] Laird, C. L., B. L. McConaughy, and B. J. McCarthy. 1969. Nature 224:149–154.
[63] Laird, C. L. 1971. Chromosoma 32:378–406.
[64] Lawley, P. D., and P. Brookes. 1963. Biochem. J. 89:127–134.
[65] Lee, S. Y., J. Mendecki, and G. Brawerman. 1971. Proc. Nat. Acad. Sci. U.S.A. 68:1331–1336.
[66] Marmur, J., and P. Doty. 1959. Nature 183:1427–1429.
[67] Marmur, J., R. Rownd, and C. L. Schildkraut. 1963. Prog. Nucleic Acid Res. 1:231–274.
[68] Martinson, H. G. 1973a. Biochemistry 12:139–144.
[69] Martinson, H. G. 1973b. Biochemistry 12:145–150.

[70] McCarthy, B. J. 1967. Bact. Rev. 31:215-258.
[71] McCarthy, B. J., and B. H. Hoyer. 1964. Proc. Nat. Acad. Sci. U.S.A. 52:915-922.
[72] McCarthy, B. J., and R. B. Church. 1970. Annal. Rev. Biochem. 39:131-150.
[73] McCarthy, B. J., and B. McConaughy. 1968. Biochem. Genetics 2:37-53.
[74] McCarthy, B. J., R. W. Shearer, and R. B. Church. 1970. In Problems in biology:RNA in development. W. Hanly (ed.), pp. 285-314. University of Utah Press, Salt Lake City, Utah.
[75] McConaughy, B. L., C. L. Laird, and B. J. McCarthy. 1969. Biochemistry 8:3285-3294.
[76] McConaughy, B. L., and B. J. McCarthy. 1970a. Biochem. Genetics 4: 409-424.
[77] McConaughy, B. L., and B. J. McCarthy. 1970b. Biochem. Genetics 4: 425-446.
[78] Melli, M., and J. O. Bishop. 1970. Biochem. J. 120:225-237.
[79] Melli, M., C. Whitfield, K. V. Roa, M. Richardson, and J. O. Bishop. 1971. Nature New Biol. 231:8-12.
[80] Morrison, M. R., J. Paul, and R. Williamson. 1972. European J. Biochem. 27:1-9.
[81] Nass, M. M., and C. A. Buck. 1970. J. Mol. Biol. 54:187-195.
[82] Nyaard, A. P., and B. D. Hall. 1964. J. Mol. Biol. 9:125-142.
[83] Pardue, M. L., and J. G. Gall. 1969. Proc. Nat. Acad. Sci. U.S.A. 64: 600-606.
[84] Robberson, D. L., and N. Davidson. 1972. Biochemistry 11:533-537.
[85] Saunders, G. F., S. Shirakawa, P. Saunders, F. E. Arrighi, and T. C. Hsu. 1972. J. Mol. Biol. 63:323-334.
[86] Schildkraut, C. L., J. Marmur, and P. Doty. 1961. J. Mol. Biol. 3:595-617.
[87] Schmeckpeper, B. J., and K. D. Smith. 1972. Biochemistry 11:2344-2358.
[88] Schultz, G. A. 1969. Ph.D. thesis, University of Calgary.
[89] Schultz, G. A., and R. B. Church. 1972. J. Exp. Zool. 179:119-128.
[90] Schultz, G. A., and R. B. Church. 1973. In Biochemistry of animal development. R. Weber (ed.), Vol. 3. Academic Press, New York.
[91] Smith, K. D. 1968. Personal communication. Department of Biology, Johns Hopkins University, Baltimore, Md.
[92] Smith, K. D., J. L' Armstrong, and B. J. McCarthy. 1967. Biochim. Biophys. Acta 142:323-331.
[93] Soeiro, R., and J. E. Darnell. 1969. J. Mol. Biol. 44:551-562.
[94] Studier, F. 1965. J. Mol. Biol. 11:373-380.
[95] Sutton, W. D. 1971. Biochim. Biophys. Acta 240:522-531.
[96] Sutton, W. D., and M. McCallum. 1971. Nature 232:83-84.
[97] Thrower, K. D., and A. R. Peacock. 1968. Biochem. J. 109:543-547.
[98] Tiselius, A., S. Hjerten, and O. Levin. 1956. Arch. Biochem. Biophys. 65:132-144.

[99] von Gelder, I., R. Smith, and H. Tobler. 1971. Naturwissen 58:518–520.
[100] Walker, P. M. B., and A. McLaren. 1965. Nature 208:1175–1179.
[101] Waring, M., and R. J. Britten. 1966. Science 154:791–794.
[102] Wetmur, J. G., and N. Davidson. 1968. J. Mol. Biol. 31:349–370.
[103] Whiteley, A. H., B. J. McCarthy, and H. Whiteley. 1966. Proc. Nat. Acad. Sci. U.S.A. 55:519–527.
[104] Wilt, F. H. 1971. Devel. Biol. 26:357–359.

Index

Acid phosphatase, density labeling of, 85
  in subcellular organelles, 10
Actinomycin D, effect on RNA polymerase, 106
Aldolase, activity staining on gels, 36–37
  electrophoresis of, 34–36
  in rat organs, 29–37
  isozymes of, 29–37
  subunits of, 23
α-amanitin, effect on RNA polymerase, 106
Aminoacyl oligonucleotides, formation of, 214–218
Aminoacyl-t RNA, digestion with ribonuclease T_1, 213
  formation of, 207–209
Aminoacyl-tRNA synthetase, density labeling of, 89–90
  turnover of, 89–90
AMP, determination of label in, 147
  labeling of DNA with radioactive, 154
  labeling of RNA with radioactive, 144–145
  separation from other nucleotides, 147
ATP, luciferase assay of, 148
  quantitation of, 149
  specific activity of labeled, 152

Barley, acid phosphatase from, 85
  germination in H_2O and D_2O, 81
  peroxidase from, 87
Binding sites on proteins, determination of, 41–53
  for progesterone, 41

Chlamydomonas reinhardi, characterization of DNA, 131–137
Chloroplasts, isolation of, 122–123
  purification of DNA from, 128–130
  ribosomal RNA from, 204
  transfer RNA from, 217–219

Chromatography, by gel filtration with Sephadex gels, 55–73
  by reversed phase to separate tRNA's, 211
  with carboxymethyl cellulose, 218
  with DEAE cellulose, 100, 104, 218
  with hydroxypapatite, 137, 173, 250
  with phosphocellulose
  with thin layer gels (TLG), 77
  with thin layer plates (TLC), 135, 145
Competition hybridization, 264

de novo synthesis of protein, 79–92
Density labeling of protein, 79–92
Density shift, of acid phosphatase, 85
  of amino acyl-tRNA synthetase, 89
  of peroxidase, 86–87
Deoxynucleoside 5'-monophosphate, 136
Deoxynucleotides, separation of, 135
Deoxyribonucleic acid (DNA), analytic complexity of, 272
  base composition of, 134–137
  base sequence families, 281
  base stacking, 234, 275, 277
  denaturation, 234
  density of, 130–133
  deproteinization, 129
  enzymatic hydrolysis of, 135
  extraction from subcellular organelles, 128–130
  fractionation, 283, 285
  from different organisms, 99
  isolation of, 232–235
  kinetic complexity of, 272
  preparation of template, 97
  quantitation of, 124–126
  reassociation kinetics, 225, 282
  reiterated, repeated base sequences, 223, 224, 282, 285
  reiteration frequency, 251

Deoxyribonuleic acid (DNA) Continued:
  renaturation, 272
  second order reassociation kinetics, 224, 227, 258, 272
  separation of single and double stranded DNA, 137, 138
  single copy unique sequences, 227, 271, 285, 286
  size of genome, 223, 225, 255, 271
  snapback hairpins, 234
  template for RNA synthesis, 99
  ultrasonic fragmentation of, 235
Dictyostelium discoideum, RNA polymerase, 93
D_2O, density labeling with, 80
  germination of barley in, 81

Electrophoresis, with cellulose acetate strips, 31
  with polyacrylamide gels, 98
  with SDS-polyacrylamide gels, 204
  with starch gels, 87
Embryos, RNA synthesis in sea urchins, 141–163
Endoplasmic reticulum, electron microscopy, 11
  enzymatic activity of, 16
  isolation of, 10–16
  microsomal subfractions, 16
Equilibrium density gradients, 81–85, 131–133

Fingerprinting, 79
Formamide reassociation, 177, 234, 252–257, 279
Fractionation, of cytoplasmic organelles, 1–27, 119–123
  of proteins according to size, 55–75
French pressure cell, 235

Galactosyl transferase as a marker for cytoplasmic organelles, 10, 16, 21
Gel filtration, columns for, 63
  desalting by, 70
  elution volume, 60
  molecular weight determination by, 72
  principles of, 59
  protein fractionation by, 68, 71
  thin layer
  using Sephadex gels, 55–78

Gel filtration Continued :
  void volume, 59
Gene frequency calculation, 292
Glucose-6-phosphatase as a marker for cytoplasmic organelles, 10, 16, 21
Golgi apparatus, electron microscopy, 9
  isolation of, 3, 8
  marker enzymes, 10
Gradients, cesium chloride gradients, 81–85, 131–133, 225, 243, 263
  equilibrium density gradients, 81–85, 131–133, 225, 243, 263
  glycerol gradients, 105
  isopycnic gradients, 6, 13, 18, 26, 81–85, 131–133
  sucrose step gradients, 6, 13, 18, 26
  sucrose step gradients with cesium chloride, 16

Haploid genome, 224, 226
Hydroxyapatite, chromatography on, 173, 250
  column conditions, 257, 274, 278
  preparation of, 277, 279
  reactions with filter-bound DNA, 245–271
  reassociation analysis, 273
  separation of single and double stranded DNA, 137
  thermomelting, 269
Hybridization techniques, agar hybridization, 171, 239, 246, 247
  analytical RNA complexity, 260–262
  CsCl density fractionation, 172, 243
  CsCl gradients, 225, 243, 262
  Denhardt mixture, 245
  filter hybridization, 170, 172, 176, 177–178, 185–188, 248
  genome size, 223–225, 255
  hydroxyapatite columns, 173, 175, 178
  immobilization of single strand DNA 176–177, 185–189, 237–245
  membrane trapping efficiency, 193–195, 234
  methylated albumin (MAK) columns, 173
  molecular weight calculation, 235–237
  nitrocellulose filters, 170, 179–184, 237, 239
  optical reassociation, 275
  preincubation, 176–177, 245
  RNA transcriptional complexity, 260

INDEX

Hybridization techniques Continued:
  solution hybridization, 170, 175–176, 179–184, 257
  ultrasonic fragmentation of DNA, 235
  UV-gel hybridization, 240–247

Immobilization of single stranded DNA
  in agar, 239
  of density fractionated RNA, 243
  on membrane filters, 193–195, 241
  in UV gels, 240
Iodination with ^{125}I, 230–231
Isozymes, aldolase, 30
  catalase, 88
  density labeling of, 87–88
  peroxidase, 87
  separation of, 30–37, 87–88

Luciferin-luciferase assay, 148
Lysomes, isolation of, 21

Microsomes
  isolation of, 12, 119–121
  subfractions, 16
  see also, Endoplasmic reticulum
Molecular weight,
  of aldolase, 30
  of DNA fragments, 237–245
  of RNA-polymerase, 105
  relation to elution volume, 72
Monoamine oxidase, 10
Mouse satellite DNA, 225, 256

Nitrate reductase, turnover of, 91
Nitrocellulose filters, absorption of RNA-DNA hybrids, 172, 237–239
  immobilization of DNA, 170
Nucleation, 165, 224, 234, 258, 272
Nuclei, preparation of, 96, 119–123
Nucleotides, chromatography of, 145
  exchange of tritium label from, 151
  incorporation into RNA, 144–155
  radioactivity in, 147
  see also, AMP, ATP
Nucleoplasm, RNA polymerase from, 94
5′-nucleotidase, as marker of cytoplasmic organelles, 10, 16, 21

Organelles, integrity of, 118
  isolation of 1–28, 117–123

Organelles Continued:
  see also, Chloroplasts, Microsomes, Golgi

Peptide mapping, 79
Plasma membrane, electron microscopy of, 22
  enzymatic activities of, 21
  isolation of, 17–21
Progesterone binding proteins, 41
Proteins, cytoplasmic receptor, 40–41
  de novo synthesis of, 79–92
  density labeling of, 79–92
  fractionation by gel filtration, 68–71
  high affinity binding sites, 45–50
  progesterone binding to, 41–47
  steroid-binding, 31–41
  turnover of, 89

Rat, aldolase isozymes in different organs, 33
  fractionation of subcellular fractions from liver, 1–27
  steroid receptor proteins in the uterus, 39–53
Reassociation (of nucleic acids), see Hybridization
Reassociation kinetics, $C_0 t$, 74, 166, 224
  C_0, 166, 272
  low $C_0 t$, 245–277, 286–296
  high $C_0 t$, 271–277
Refractive index, determination of, 83–132
  monitor (automatic), 73
  of aqueous cesium chloride, 83–132
  relation to density, 132
Repeated or reiterated sequences, 226, 245
Ribonucleic acid (RNA), alkaline hydrolysis of, 146
  DNA-like, 94
  from sea urchins, 144
  hairpin structure of, 276
  hybridization with DNA, see RNA/DNA hybridization
  in vitro labeling of, 229–232
  in vivo labeling of, 142, 144
  isolation of, 227–229
  of subcellular fractions, 125
  precipitation of, 145
  quantitation of, 124
  synthesis of, 141
  t-RNA see transfer-RNA

RNA-polymerase, characterization of, 99
  effect of antibiotics on, 106
  in cytoplasmic organelles, 109
  purification of, 100–103
  solubilization of, 98
  stimulation by Mn^{++} and Mg^{++}, 109–110
  template specificity of, 99
RNA/DNA hybridization, agar hybridization, 171, 246
  base pair matching, mismatching, 167, 171, 226, 249, 250, 254, 257, 272
  competition hybridization, 166, 264–265
  control experiments membrane filter, 195–196, 249
  control experiments vast DNA excess, 167, 292
  control experiments vast RNA excess, 290
  exonuclease analysis, 276
  filter hybridization, 170, 179–188, 248
  first order reaction kinetics, 287
  gel hybridization, 247
  high $C_0 t$ reassociation, 286–290
  hybridization parameters, 168–169, 250
  low $C_0 t$ reassociation, 271–277
  nucleation, 165, 226
  presaturation competition, 264–265
  reaction conditions, 165, 225–227, 261–265, 270–275, 280
  reassociation criteria, 226
  reassociation reaction conditions, 227
  RNA complexity, 279
  RNA transcriptional complexity, 284
  saturation hybridization, 166, 257–263
  thermoelution, 262
  thermostability, melting profiles, 256, 265–270, 274
  vast DNA excess, 271, 278, 290–296
  vast excess RNA, 286
  zippering, 165, 224, 272

Satellite free DNA, 280
Scatchard plot, 44, 51
Sephadex gels, antimicrobial agents, 62
  available types of, 57
  column packing with, 64

Sephadex gels Continued:
  flow rates for, 66
  preparation of, 62
  properties of, 55–59
  to determine molecular weight, 72
Shearing of DNA, 235
Single copy, unique DNA, 227, 245, 271, 282, 284–285
Single stranded nuclease, 276
Sodium dodecyl sulfate (SDS), in gel electrophoresis, 203
  in solubilization of RNA, 202
  to separate subunits of RNA polymerase, 107
Spinach, isolation of chloroplasts from, 122–123
Steroid binding proteins, 39
Succinate-INT-reductase, 10, 16, 21
Sucrose gradients, isolation of subcellular organelles with, 5–21

Thermal stability of hybrids, from agar, 268
  from hydroxyapatite, 175, 269
  from membrane filters, 266
  from UV gels, 268
  melting profiles, 270
Transfer-RNA, changes during development, 201
  charging of, 206
  from cotton chloroplasts, 217–219
  from cotton cytoplasm, 217–219
  in cotton seed development, 215
  isoaccepting species of, 199
  loss of CCA-terminus of, 207
  on reversed phase columns, 211
  purification of, 202

Unit gernome, 271
Urchins, see embryos

Void volume of Sephadex gels, 59

Water regain value of Sephadex gels, 57

Zymogen, 80